T0133228

AMERICAN STUDIES – A MONOGRAPH SERIES
Volume 249

Edited on behalf
of the German Association
for American Studies by
REINHARD R. DOERRIES
GERHARD HOFFMANN
ALFRED HORNUNG

MARC PRIEWE

# Textualizing Illness

Medicine and Culture
in New England
1620–1730

Universitätsverlag
WINTER
Heidelberg

Bibliografische Information der Deutschen Nationalbibliothek

Die Deutsche Nationalbibliothek verzeichnet diese Publikation
in der Deutschen Nationalbibliografie;
detaillierte bibliografische Daten sind im Internet
über *http://dnb.d-nb.de* abrufbar.

Die vorliegende Studie wurde in einer früheren Version
im Oktober 2011 als Habilitationsschrift
an der Philosophischen Fakultät der Universität Potsdam
eingereicht.

UMSCHLAGBILD

John Winthrop, Jr. to Richard Odell, 27 November 1652, BMS C.56.1.
Mit freundlicher Genehmigung der Boston Medical Library
in der Francis A. Countway Library of Medicine, Harvard University.

ISBN 978-3-8253-6362-8

© 2014 Universitätsverlag Winter GmbH Heidelberg
Imprimé en Allemagne · Printed in Germany
Druck: Memminger MedienCentrum, 87700 Memmingen

Gedruckt auf umweltfreundlichem, chlorfrei gebleichtem
und alterungsbeständigem Papier

Den Verlag erreichen Sie im Internet unter:
www.winter-verlag.de

*Für Marla, Simon und Robin*

# Acknowledgements

I owe special gratitude to a number of people and institutions that have helped me during the research and writing process for this book. Rüdiger Kunow supported my project from its inception, providing valuable advice and direction at all junctures. Francis Bremer, Reiner Smolinski, Walter W. Woodward, Robert C. Anderson, David D. Hall, Udo Hebel, Dirk Wiemann, and Cristobal Silva offered useful suggestions on the intersections between medicine and culture in early New England.

In tracing primary sources I have received generous help from the following archivists and libraries: Diane Ducharme at the Beinecke Rare Book and Manuscript Library, Yale University, Caroline Sloat and Tom Knoles at the American Antiquarian Society, Jeremy Dibbell at the Massachusetts Historical Society, Arevig Caprielian at the New York Society Library, Jack Eckert at the Francis A. Countway Library of Medicine, Harvard University, and the staff at the Royal Society, the British Library.

Kevin Concannon, Jacqueline Grenz, Veronika Hofstätter, Stephanie Siewert, Dennis Mischke, and Sebastian Mühleis were faithful readers and helpful commentators. I am especially grateful to Dorothee Heinz, who read the first draft and helped to improve the book's accuracy and readability.

Special funding for this project came from St. Lawrence University, the German-American Fulbright Commission, and the German Research Foundation (DFG).

John Carlos Rowe and Julia Foulkes deserve a special shout-out for their intellectual and personal support during the past years. Dirk and Gisela Priewe have kept me sane and offered guidance and inspiration for as long as I can think. I could not have reached this point without Marianne Grenz, whose love and patience kept me going.

Berlin, June 2014

# Table of Contents

# Introduction

In 1640, after ten years of steady migration and settlement, English cultural norms and practices seemed to have been transplanted successfully to the North American colonies. Diseases, lack of provisions, internal frictions, and struggles with Native Americans constituted real and imagined obstacles to colonization and had, so far, mostly been averted. In looking back at the first decade of English colonialism in the "New World," the co-founder and governor of Massachusetts Bay, John Winthrop, recorded an observation about his son's attempt to uphold the values of a self-styled godly people in a hostile environment. Reflecting on the learnedness of his son, he wrote:

> Mr. Winthrop the younger, [...] having many books in a chamber where there was corn of divers sorts, had among them one wherein the Greek testament, the psalms and the common prayer were bound together. He found the common prayer eaten with mice, every leaf of it, and not any of the two other touched, nor any other of his books though there were above a thousand.[1]

The combination of books and corn in the younger Winthrop's room serves as an apt metaphor of the daily realities that learned men encountered at the periphery of the emerging British Empire, where intellectual and scientific activities had to be coupled with pragmatism and were undertaken in relative isolation. Regardless of whether the number of books recorded by his father is accurate or whether mice truly destroyed "every leaf" of the Anglican Common Book of Prayer, Winthrop's library was one of the largest and most encompassing book collections in early America. However, the impression conveyed by the Massachusetts Bay founder that his son's library consisted primarily of

---

[1] John Winthrop, *The History of New England from 1630 to 1649*, ed. James Savage, vol. 2 (Boston: Little, 1853) 24.

religious works and that, therefore, the preoccupation of its owner was geared solely toward theology, is misleading. Only a quarter of his book collection reflected his interest in religious topics, whereas more than half consisted of works on early science.[2] Next to some obligatory religious writings, the young colonist and physician owned books that tell us something about his immersion in contemporary European discussions about the occult tradition (astrology, magic, alchemy, and numerology) and the evolving science of medicine.[3] Aside from the symbolism of theology-hungry rodents, then, Winthrop's account indicates how New England colonists thought and wrote about three potentially contentious discourses and practices of healing bodies: Calvinist theology, the emerging medical sciences, and the remnants of European occultism. This is evident in many writings on illness from early New England and shall be investigated from a literary and cultural studies perspective in the present book.

## I.

When the elder John Winthrop penned his report, illnesses were a ubiquitous, life-shaping occurrence. In contrast to health conditions in Western societies of the late twentieth and early twenty-first centuries, diseases constituted life experiences throughout the early modern period. Especially at the fringes of the English sphere of influence, the confrontation with a new physical and cultural environment created a host of anxieties about the impacts of newfound lands on European bodies. Because most people (still) interpreted illnesses in supernatural terms, colonial physicians addressed both the spiritual and physical needs of their patients. When treating ill bodies, most practitioners, secular and clerical, combined the Galenic tradition based predominantly on herbs and bloodletting with remedies lately developed

---

[2] Herbert Greenberg, "The Authenticity of the Library of John Winthrop the Younger," *American Literature* 8 (1937): 449-452.

[3] Throughout this study, I employ a broad definition of the term "medicine." Except when used in conjunction with Native American cultures (see below), it refers to a substance, method, practice and/or science of treating human illnesses.

by proponents of the iatrochemical school (i.e., healing methods drawn from chemical innovations). During the second half of the seventeenth century, New England physicians, following their colleagues in Europe, also began to grapple with the religious and diagnostic implications of the iatromechanists (i.e., doctors devising disease treatment based on the laws of physics).[4] However, aside from a small group of colonial healers aware of these new approaches in the field of medicine, curative techniques more often than not rested on folk traditions, especially in New England frontier settlements. As one result, the colonial medical scene was marked by pluralistic approaches to illness and healing. Lacking a sufficient number of university-trained practitioners until well into the eighteenth century, colonists depended primarily on minister-physicians, folk healers, midwives, apothecaries, barber-surgeons, and "Indian doctors" for their health needs.[5]

---

[4] For useful discussions of seventeenth-century English medicine, see Doreen Evenden Nagy, *Popular Medicine in Seventeenth-Century England* (Bowling Green: Bowling Green State University Popular P, 1988); Andrew Wear, *Health and Healing in Early Modern England* (Aldershot: Ashgate, 1998); Andrew Wear, *Knowledge and Practice in English Medicine, 1550-1680* (Cambridge: Cambridge UP, 2000); Charles Webster, *The Great Instauration: Science, Medicine and Reform, 1626-1660* (1975; Frankfurt: Lang, 2002) 246-323; David Harley, "Spiritual Physic, Providence and English Medicine, 1560-1640," *Medicine and the Reformation*, ed. Ole Peter Grell and Andrew Cunningham (London: Routledge, 1993) 101-117; Roy Porter, "The Patient in England, c. 1660 - c. 1800," *Medicine in Society: Historical Essays*, ed. Andrew Wear (Cambridge: Cambridge UP, 1992) 91-118; Roger French and Andrew Wear, eds., *The Medical Revolution of the Seventeenth Century* (Cambridge: Cambridge UP, 1989); Lucinda McCray Beier, *Sufferers and Healers: The Experience of Illness in Seventeenth-Century England* (London: Routledge, 1987) 8-50.

[5] General overviews of the main medical concepts and practices during the first two centuries of New England settlement include: Oliver Wendell Holmes, *Medical Essays: The Writings of Oliver Wendell Holmes,* vol. 9 (Boston: Cambridge UP, 1891) 314-345; Henry R. Viets, *A Brief History of Medicine in Massachusetts* (Boston: Houghton, 1930); John B. Blake, *Public Health in the Town of Boston, 1630-1822* (Cambridge, MA: Harvard UP, 1959); Richard Harrison Shryock, *Medicine and Society in America, 1660-1860* (New York: New York UP, 1960); Philip Cash, J. Worth Estes, and Eric H. Christianson,

The presence of various healing providers in the early English colonies resulted in part from a lack of consensus over the boundaries of sound medical practice. The medical setting in colonial New England differed from that in Europe because the diversity of colonial health practitioners emerged under the watchful eyes of the clergy and the magistrates, who were by and large unsuccessful in regulating treatment methods and in monopolizing the meaning of illness. Most New England ministers followed the idea of divine pathogenesis and stressed the relationship between a person's thoughts and actions and his/her physical conditions on earth, arguing that a believer's corporeal state reflected his/her spiritual past, present, and future. Not only was sin seen as the main cause of afflictions; its presence as illness marked a manifestation and translation of the spiritual into human physicality. The patient's state of health (stagnating, improving, or declining) was often seen as an inscription of God's providence onto the "screen" of the body human and the body social (i.e., some illnesses were interpreted as a collective punishment, reminder, and/or test of faith). As such, illnesses became intricately linked to the omnipresent world of signs and wonders, an interpretation of the universe as suffused by portents, angels, demons, divine interventions, and strange occurrences. In order to facilitate recovery, religiously inclined medical practitioners urged patients to pray, confess, repent, and reform but also to make use of remedies drawn from nature. The various recourses to, and shuttling between, "spiritual" and "natural" approaches to medicine—God and Galen—form an important concern of this book. As I hope to show, at times, they correlated well, while at others they posed conflictual and irresolvable modes of healing.

When English religious dissidents immigrated to the "New World" in increasing numbers after 1630, European medical scientists, energized by the discovery of blood circulation by William Harvey, were developing new methods of analyzing and treating the human body. Historians have repeatedly claimed the seventeenth century as an era of transition from experience to science and, with regard to the explorative and explanatory dominance over the human body, from religion to medicine.[6] In England, the shift from a mystical occult epistemology to rationalism is often seen as coinciding with the Restoration and the founding of the Royal Society of London in 1661. The suggested rupture between epistemic systems is, however, misleading; the decline of Renaissance occultism has to be seen as a concomitant rather than a mere opposing force to the rise of the scientific revolution: both epistemic systems—the occult tradition and the new sciences—continued to coexist, often in the works of individual authors, for several decades. This coexistence was further complicated by the ambiguous positions and roles of the church, whose official reactions ranged from hostility to support with regard to both occultism and experimental science. Aside from its departure from occult traditions, the new sciences followed a mode of inquiry based on reason and empiricism, and, as a result, also began to discard assumptions about divine intention and intervention with regard to disease. Hence, with the emergence of medicine as a scientific field during the Renaissance, the efforts of healers to discover regularities, patterns, and functions of the body repeatedly collided with religious doctrines that saw the body as a fascinating manifestation of providence, whose proper workings were ultimately hidden from human knowledge.[7]

---

[6] For the slow and dynamic shift from occultism to science, see Charles Webster, *From Paracelsus to Newton: Magic and the Making of Modern Science* (Cambridge: Cambridge UP, 1982); Brian Vickers, ed., *Occult and Scientific Mentalities in the Renaissance* (Cambridge: Cambridge UP, 1984). For a focus on the medicine of early modern Europe, see Ole Peter Grell and Andrew Cunningham, eds., *Medicine and Religion in Enlightenment Europe* (Burlington: Ashgate, 2007) and, especially, Roger French and Andrew Wear, eds., *The Medical Revolution of the Seventeenth Century* (New York: Cambridge UP, 1989). Recent introductions to the history of medicine include: Lois N. Magner, *A History of Medicine*, 2nd ed. (Boca Raton: Taylor, 2005); Francisco Gonzalez-Crussi, *A Short History of Medicine* (New York: Modern Library, 2008).

[7] This is not to argue that medicine and religion were entirely at odds with each other during the early modern period. As Charles Webster reminds us,

In early New England, however, the competition and even hostility between religion and medical science was far less developed than in the mother country; in fact, both epistemologies and modes of practical healing at times complemented each other, not least because economic and demographic conditions produced the personal union of minister and physician as the primary healing figure in many colonial settlements. Only toward the end of the seventeenth century did New England attract a rising number of secular physicians, and colonists increasingly incorporated a practical openness toward scientific discoveries in the field of medicine. With the growing confidence in new medical inventions and achievements, the two knowledge systems slowly diverged, especially with regard to the hierarchy of authority over interpreting and treating the body adequately. The tensions between religious and scientific doctrines were generally based on contested principles that represented different medical approaches: if, for instance, certain bodily ailments constituted signs of divine punishment or tests of faith—as theologians repeatedly argued—then to what extent may or should human beings interfere in the course of illness and thus in God's will and omnipotence?

The field of tension between religion and science was further complicated by the persistence of folk healing techniques, particularly among the New England laity. As a cultural inheritance from Renaissance Europe, many colonists continued to trust occult medical practices that were drawn primarily from alchemy, astrology, and witchcraft. The application of amulets, charms, and performative rituals, for instance, had long been viewed with suspicion by Protestants, whose goals included the eradication of superstitious, idolatrous, and popish elements from religious practices. The extent to which occult healing methods were acceptable and even compatible with religious doctrines and why they were either tacitly tolerated or violently persecuted still

---

"throughout the Scientific Revolution, Christian eschatology provided an undiminishing incentive towards science, if not a primary motivating factor" (Webster, *Paracelsus to Newton* 48). The argument that Protestantism was generally conducive to the new sciences is further elaborated by proponents of the Merton thesis. See, I. Bernard Cohen, ed., *Puritanism and the Rise of Modern Sciences: The Merton Thesis* (New Brunswick: Rutgers UP, 1990).

needs to be accentuated and hence marks a main area of interest in this study.

## II.

At first sight, a focus on early New England culture may seem redundant, given the number of books and articles published since the nineteenth century.[8] Yet, a sustained investigation of how early Americans textualized body perceptions and illness experiences still remains to be undertaken.[9] Hence, this book explores how Puritanism served as a dominant cultural, ideological, and conceptual frame within which illness narratives operated. Since Calvinist doctrines increasingly lost their social and cultural influence during the second half of the seventeenth century and especially during the first decades of the eighteenth century, *Textualizing Illness* covers the period between 1620 and 1730.[10] By tracing how New England colonists conceptualized

---

[8] For a useful overview of the field, see John Coffey and Paul C. H. Lim, Introduction, *The Cambridge Companion to Puritanism*, ed. John Coffey and Paul C. H. Lim (New York: Cambridge UP, 2008) 1-15. The history of colonial New England has been the subject of numerous studies. See, for instance, Gloria L. Main, *Peoples of Spacious Land: Families and Cultures in Colonial New England* (Cambridge, MA: Harvard UP, 2001); David Archer, *Fissures in the Rock: New England in the Seventeenth Century* (Hanover: UP of New England, 2001); Joseph Conforti, *Saints and Strangers: New England in British North America* (Baltimore: Johns Hopkins UP, 2006).

[9] A notable exception is Cristobal Silva, *Miraculous Plagues: An Epidemiology of Early New England Narrative* (New York: Oxford UP, 2011), which investigates the intellectual treatment of epidemics in early New England. While my own work shares Silva's emphasis on medical topics, it deviates from *Miraculous Plagues* by studying a broader textual corpus and by placing questions of health, illness, and medicine in larger cultural and transnational contexts.

[10] With this time frame, I follow a common temporal limitation in Puritan New England studies. See, Francis J. Bremer, "The Puritan Experiment in New England, 1630-1660," and David D. Hall, "New England, 1660-1730," *The Cambridge Companion to Puritanism*, ed. John Coffey and Paul C. H. Lim (New York: Cambridge, 2008) 127-142; 143-158.

individual and collective illnesses in North America, I seek to explore further the discrepancies between the religious belief in predetermination and the perceived necessity of human self-determination that shaped the eighteenth century. Furthermore, a focus on textualized illness concepts and responses in early America promises to illustrate how medical and cultural trajectories unfolded and crossed in transnational force-fields energized by mobility, colonialism, religion, and the emerging sciences.

Against the background of a cultural history of disease, this study revolves around a set of guiding questions: How did the meaning-endowment of bodily conditions by men and women living in New England affect literary and other textual productions? To what extent did writing about medical issues change in the wake of the scientific revolution, increasing arrivals of non-Puritan settlers, and contacts with African slaves and Native Americans? In order to approach these and other related topics, I rely on a broad textual base, including letters, historical narratives, poetry, sermons and pamphlets, promotional tracts, confession of faith narratives, court records, medical handbooks, newspapers, diaries, and autobiographies. Colonial body perceptions and illness experiences are often hidden in these narratives and have to be unveiled—often across different texts and authors—to produce signification.

In colonial New England illness narratives did not constitute a genre of their own, nor were they linked to a particular genre.[11] While they may vary in scope anywhere between two sentences and a monograph, a decisive feature of colonial New England illness narratives is that they subjectively express cultural modes of communicating bodily changes,

---

[11] My conceptualization of illness narratives relies on arguments put forth by Shlomith Rimmon-Kenan, "The Story of 'I': Illness and Narrative Identity," *Narrative* 10.1 (2002): 9-27; Lars-Christer Hydén, "Illness and Narrative," *Sociology of Health and Illness* 19.1 (1997): 48-69; Harold Schweizer, "To Give Suffering a Language," *Literature and Medicine* 14.2 (1995): 210-221; John Wiltshire, "Biography, Pathography, and the Recovery of Meaning," *The Cambridge Quarterly* 29.4 (2000): 409-422; Barbara Duden, *The Woman beneath the Skin: A Doctor's Patients in Eighteenth-Century Germany*, trans. Thomas Dunlap (Cambridge, MA: Harvard UP, 1991) 1-37.

pain, and suffering. One of the aims of the present investigation is hence to identify and analyze the explanatory patterns and hermeneutic potentials of illnesses in colonial textual practices.[12] When thus approaching illness narratives, it is important to consider the co-presence of biological and cultural aspects in the experience, interpretation, and treatment of diseases. That is, while sickness constitutes a real experience of human pain and/or discomfort, its interpretation is consistently guided by how a given society attributes meanings to certain bodily conditions. In a similar vein, medicine as a discursive and practical field has constituted a biological as much as a social reality since its inception. Therefore, any investigation of illness and its narratives must take into consideration underlying social forces and cultural signification processes that affect individual and collective interpretations of disease over time and space. Although health matters are never distinct from cultural symbols and social imperatives, the latter are also never congruent with the corporal reality created by disease. As one consequence, the somatic and the semantic sides of illness and medicine, their biological and cultural facets, need to be considered in tandem rather than divorced from each other.

For such a biocultural perspective, *narratives* of illness play a central role.[13] Throughout cultural history, disease has not only been the object of verbal and written representations, it has often shaped the modalities of its narration(s). For instance, by the end of the seventeenth century, colonial medical practice had come to rely almost exclusively on

---

[12] In this sense, illness marks a temporary state of difference, a deviance from the normalcy of the healthy body that is both objective and subjective. Although there are significant semantic differences between "disease" and "illness," I will use both interchangeably, unless otherwise noted. The term "disease" normally refers to an objectifiable disorder of the body, triggered from the outside, whereas the term "illness" denotes subjective feelings of pain and/or malaise. Roy Porter, "What is Disease?" *The Cambridge Illustrated History of Medicine*, ed. Roy Porter (Cambridge: Cambridge UP, 1996) 82.

[13] The notion of bioculture (studies) constitutes a recent call for interdisciplinary approaches to, and mutual attentiveness between, practitioners from cultural studies and the biosciences. Lennart J. Davis, and David B. Morris, "Biocultures Manifesto," *New Literary History* 38.3 (2007): 411-418.

decoding illness signs on or in the body and on patients relating their histories of symptoms and conduct of life. The people of colonial New England expressed their illness experiences in various textual formats but consistently drew from a repository of signifiers that was part of talking and writing about illness. Whether serving as means of reflection in confession-of-faith narratives, muse and metaphor for poets, embedded in historical narratives, or expressed as cries for help in patient letters, reports on illnesses and treatment abound in early New England culture and necessitate further inquiry.

The symbolic encoding of illness in colonial texts often expressed a deep-rooted cultural linkage between morbidity and morality. According to this belief, some people deserved an illness due to their (sinful) behavior and for others it marked a necessary trial or corrective measure sanctioned by God. Illness was often perceived as compromising the patient's privacy, a space which modern societies generally attribute to bodily impairments. In colonial society, disease often sent the godly and the non-believers into the open, as it were, turning the individual over to the social. This process is vividly and retroactively illustrated in Nathaniel Hawthorne's representation of American Puritanism in *The Scarlet Letter* (1850), when the narrator—in the chapter entitled "The Leech"—comments on the troublesome relationship between the Reverend Arthur Dimmesdale and the medical expert Roger Chillingworth, stating that "[a] man burdened with a secret should especially avoid the intimacy of his physician."[14] This quote echoes religious convictions in colonial New England about a god-ordained connection between hidden or secret sin and illness, a connection that was potentially accessible to human knowledge. In addition, Hawthorne allegorizes the interaction between Chillingworth, the learned physician and alchemist, and Dimmesdale, the devout yet sin-prone minister, by letting them live in opposite rooms of a house in Boston. Carefully narrated through the nineteenth-century gaze on a seventeenth-century community, the physician is portrayed as a "diabolical agent" out to battle and destroy the not-so-innocent Puritan preacher and his spiritual approaches to healing. Among the things Hawthorne teaches is that

---

[14] Nathaniel Hawthorne, *The Scarlet Letter*, ed. Ross C. Murfin (1850; Boston: Bedford, 2006) 106.

illness constitutes a multiply encoded epiphenomenon that generates important physical implications, spiritual significances, and socio-political ramifications. *The Scarlet Letter* is also indicative of how outside the novel medical scientists in the course of the seventeenth and eighteenth centuries sought to draw interpretive authority over defining matters of health and illness away from theologians. As one result, the stigmatization of diseases and their carriers in colonial New England proved to be a highly complex cultural process, subject to change over time, and raised a number of problems for the religious, social, and political orders. While certain diseases (and their narratives) functioned to uphold and disseminate colonial power structures, others subtly undermined the subsumption of medical practices and theories under the auspices of the churches.

There was no linear movement from religion and folklore to reason and science, mind to body, or one medical theory or disease concept to another in early New England. It would thus be futile to suggest a shift from A to Z with regard to cultural representations of health and illness matters. Rather, a variety of traditions and new discoveries were coexisting, contesting, and intermingling to varying degrees. In order to begin to unravel the cultural vectors that informed New England illness narratives, the cultural history of medicine provides a heuristic window for identifying socio-cultural forces, responses, and structures underlying medical knowledge and treatments.[15] The present research and reading perspective is directed toward how social and cultural

---

[15] A useful and concise overview of various schools of thought in the historiography of medicine is offered by Mirko D. Grmek, Introduction, *Western Medical Thought from Antiquity to the Middle Ages*, ed. Mirko D. Grmek, trans. Antony Shugaar (1993; Cambridge, MA: Harvard UP, 1998) 1-21. For recent directions in the history of medicine, especially with regard to the subtle yet significant shift from social to cultural history, see Mary E. Fissell, "Making Meaning from the Margins: The New Cultural History of Medicine," *Locating Medical History: The Stories and Their Meanings*, ed. John Warner and Frank Huisman (Baltimore: Johns Hopkins P, 2004) 364-389. Another critical assessment of the contributions from anthropology and literary studies to the field of medical history is provided by Gert H. Brieger, "Bodies and Borders: A New Cultural History of Medicine," *Perspectives in Biology and Medicine* 47.3 (2004): 402-421.

factors, previously considered external to the field of medicine, resonated in sick persons or their acquaintances and were textualized as an "internal" positioning of an individual and of the community as a whole. Such an approach to medicine offers a better comprehension of how colonists in British America negotiated, contested, and appropriated existing interpretations of the body while, at the same time, adapting them to their particular cultural and physical experiences in the "New World."

A number of theoretical developments in literary and cultural studies inform this approach. Following the lead of Michel Foucault, medicine at large has been seen as a reflector and producer of social determinants, cultural values, and power relations before medical science and the emerging state apparatus coalesced to govern and monopolize the body in the eighteenth century.[16] Colonial illness narratives often employed medicine for the exercise or contestation of power. Medical theories and practices were unfolded in the interest of power and, in many cases, lay illness narratives subtly resisted the assimilation by power. Hence, a constructivist and new historicist reading of illness is particularly useful for texts that draw on the repertoire of the body, because the body's diseased state, aside from constituting a physical reality, is always culture- and power-bound.[17] An approach to medicine as both practice and narrative also traces changes in cultural processes and social structures, and illustrates, thereby, how disease and medicine have locked the universal and the particular into a perpetual dialectic.

One aspect of the medical transnationalism that undergirded early New England culture relates to the social and political framing of illness in colonial America—how class, race, gender, behavioral, and geographical differences were scripted in medical terms. As will

---

[16] Michel Foucault, *The Birth of the Clinic: An Archaeology of Medical Perception*, trans. A. M. Sheridan Smith (1963; London: Travistock, 1973) 111.

[17] For the recent scholarly interest in body issues pertaining to colonial America, see Martha L. Finch, *Dissenting Bodies: Corporealities in Early New England* (New York: Columbia UP, 2010); Janet Moore Lindman and Michele Lise Tarter, eds., *A Centre of Wonders: The Body in Early America* (Ithaca: Cornell UP, 2001); Kathleen M. Brown, *Foul Bodies: Cleanliness in Early America* (New Haven: Yale UP, 2008).

hopefully become clear, the differences of observed health disparities—between English and Natives, or among settler communities in and beyond the colonies—became medically encoded to denote differences of race, culture, and social status. Medicine thus served as a site of production of meaningful social categories and entailed both familiar and particularly English (and later, American) responses to disease that deserve sustained consideration.

## III.

An investigation of colonial illness narratives usefully begins by taking stock of salient theoretical concepts of, and practical approaches to, disease during the early modern period. It equally necessitates an analysis of culturally informed discursive practices that rendered illness meaningful and manageable for seventeenth-century Europeans, Africans, and Native Americans who met in New England. This marks a central cluster of interest in chapter one, which outlines how Calvinists approached human physicality with suspicion and aversion and, at the same time, how the body was considered as a plane of projection for God's will and sovereignty. For instance, with their responses to land-clearing Native American epidemics between 1616 and 1619 and again from 1633 to 1634 English colonists contributed to the emergence of a medicalization of alterity that played a crucial role in the settlement of New England. As evinced in William Bradford's *Of Plymouth Plantation* and in a number of reports and letters designed to advertise the advantages of life in early New England, by medicalizing physical differences that were ostensibly brought to light by "virgin-soil epidemics," English colonists were able to claim and justify ownership of land in North America.[18] This claim relied to a significant degree on the idea that an immunologically less prepared population was supplanted by divine providence and replaced by more "civilized" and healthy settlers. Medicine, in conjunction with zealous religiosity, hence became a tool of colonialism proper: with its help, Otherness could be

---

[18] Alfred W. Crosby, "Virgin Soil Epidemics as a Factor in the Aboriginal Depopulation in America," *The William and Mary Quarterly* 33.2 (1976): 289-299.

constructed along quasi-scientific lines and it could be employed to signify the cultural superiority of English settlers over their Native American neighbors.

The advances in medical knowledge since the time of the Renaissance required a reconciliation with diversifying religious tenets and teachings, especially within the emergent Protestant movement. New England theologians and intellectuals, living at the edge of the known world in the early 1600s and endowed with an aptitude for medicine, were faced with a variety of scientific, philosophical, and religious ideas, concepts, and approaches. Chapter two investigates how one particular colonist, John Winthrop Jr., positioned himself within the existing spectrum of ideas and traditions during an era of cultural transition, geographic expansion, and knowledge increase. Winthrop's approach to science, religion, and politics exemplifies a strain of Puritanism that eludes stereotypes of a narrow-minded social and cultural system.

Of special interest in the second chapter are medical request letters, most of them written during the 1650s, which members of the laity addressed to Winthrop Jr., who was widely revered and sought-after for his medical expertise. Rather than focusing exclusively on Winthrop's correspondence with other scientists and healers in Europe and the colonies—which is certainly useful for understanding health conditions and curative approaches at the time—I am particularly interested in the textual and cultural dimensions of illness letters written by common colonists, because they provide insight into conceptualizations and narrative representations of illness and healing "from below." What is perhaps most striking about these lay patient letters is that they present the sick human body in ways that deviate from official inscriptions of, and prescriptions for, disease by the clergy. Rather than focusing on the meaning of illness with regard to the patient's relation to God, lay illness letters often seek practical remedies and, in doing so, illustrate various aspects of the economic, religious, and social realities of colonial life in mid-seventeenth-century New England.

A similar focus on power issues underlies the next chapter, on gendered healing practices and pathologies. Because women (especially housewives, female servants, and midwives) provided most of the everyday medical services, they were at once respected members of colonial society and subject to incriminations that at times led to their banishment and even execution. The underlying argument presented in chapter three is that gendered medical reports appear with particular frequency and intensity during moments of social and cultural crisis in New England culture, among them the Antinomian controversy between 1636 and 1638 and witchcraft proceedings during the second half of the seventeenth century. These reports indicate how medical topics played a salient role in larger cultural struggles for interpretative authority over the female body. The argumentative arc of this chapter moves from elite women's healing networks, exemplified by the circle of medical experts surrounding New Haven minister's wife, Elizabeth Davenport, to the religious teachings of Anne Hutchinson, with a special focus on the official interpretation of her malformed birth, and ends with an investigation of documents that depict the role of physicians, midwives, and lay healers in various witch trials. Many of the narratives and documents surveyed for this chapter express an underlying cultural conviction that female medical practices were potentially contiguous to black magic. Witchcraft and medicine have indeed intersected in manifold ways throughout human history and especially since the Middle Ages, when Europeans widely believed in the ability of certain women (and only few men) to inflict and alleviate diseases through supernatural means. With regard to medicine in early New England, the witchcraft papers from Salem and other colonial towns are useful for the purpose of this study since they illustrate the interrelations and growing conflicts between spiritual and natural approaches to illness and healing.

Chapter four complements this study of textualized illnesses by comparing English and Native American conversion narratives. Confessions of faith in colonial meetinghouses and in Indian Praying Towns were partly constitutive of New England social formations: they marked norms and hierarchies of communal inclusion and exclusion and represented a culturally framed teleology of salvation bound by introspection and public declaration. In the recorded confessions of sins and professions of faith, illness and medicine play a recurring role, often by pointing the audience to the presence and sovereignty of God in earthly affairs. In most conversion narratives presented orally by colonists before a congregation and recorded in writing by the local minister, illness serves as a means for entering into a covenant with God and with the community.

The second section of chapter four centers on Native American conversion narratives, which by and large were published for a European audience and which played a significant political and cultural role in consolidating and legitimizing New English communities. This is one of the main points of interest as the focus shifts to John Eliot's *Indian Tracts* (1643-1671), with their staged contestation of Algonquian powwow practices. What Native American conversion narratives, viewed through a medical lens, demonstrate with particular force is that by implicitly and explicitly questioning the credibility of indigenous conversion, they threaten the validity of *all* narratives of assurance emanating from a self-examined and god-assured individual.

Chapter five concentrates on how illness-related passages in the Bible and concepts drawn from Galenic humoralism and Paracelsian iatrochemistry served as a repository of tropes and metaphors for seventeenth-century New England poets. One of the central questions underlying my reading of medical poems by Michael Wigglesworth, Anne Bradstreet, and Edward Taylor is the extent to which words were seen or used as healing devices; as bearing curative and redemptive powers both for the individual patient-poet and the collective readership. Michael Wigglesworth's illness poetics in "Meat Out of the Eater" (1670), for instance, draws exclusively on Scripture for solving in seeking riddles and for learning the lessons of illness. With regard to the collective, one of the central functions of the employment of body images in colonial poetry was to relieve a collective anxiety and siege mentality that resulted from contacts with the "wilderness," political changes in England after 1660, and an increasing migration of non-Puritan settlers to the colonies. The ensuing sense of declension is particularly evident in Michael Wigglesworth's poem "God's Controversy with New-England" (1661), in which the speaker employs many of the themes and rhetorical approaches common in sermonic jeremiads. Accordingly, the poem configures diseases as a just punishment for ungodliness and for the colonists' failure to align their society with the initial intent of building a heaven-directed society.

Such immediate references to the political, cultural, and religious state of New England are largely absent in the poetry of Anne Bradstreet. In her more personal reflections on illness collected in *The Tenth Muse Lately Sprung up in America* (1650) and the Andover Manuscript poems (c. 1678), the rebellious stance that can be detected in her love and grief poems (and which is often considered as the hallmark of Bradstreet's writing) remains largely unsupported. Rather than viewing her frequent poetic treatments of illness as a sign of her trembling faith or overwhelming doubt, the loss of health, similar to other losses experienced in the poet's life, functions as a religious catalyst that energizes devotional practice in poetic form.

This impetus for writing verse is also evident in Edward Taylor's *oeuvre*. His frequent recourse to the medical and alchemical practices of his time, especially in *Preparatory Meditations*, helps to understand more fully how religion, science, and the occult were not considered as divergent, mutually exclusive epistemologies but, rather, how they worked themselves palimpsestically into early New England literature.[19] In one of his final poems Taylor exemplifies how illness serves as a reminder of one's approaching death and of Christ's suffering at the cross for the benefit of the elect. However, in stressing the potentiality of words to transform suffering into edification, the poem conveys a lingering sense of uncertainty about language's ability to fully extract redemption out of the debilitating state of illness.

During the last decades of the seventeenth century, medical science increasingly contested the theological postulate of the supremacy of mind over matter, the immortal over the mortal. The discussion surrounding this development lies at the center of chapter six, in which Cotton Mather's attempts to reconcile religious and scientific explanations of diseases are investigated. The practical and theological difficulties of this negotiation became especially evident in 1721/1722, when Boston witnessed a severe smallpox epidemic and a concomitant

---

[19] For the context of colonial New England, scholars have often employed the term "literature" in a rather broad sense, denoting texts written for the purpose of relating information about the natural habitat (e.g., travel writings, promotional tracts) or to edify or teach the reader (e.g., sermons, captivity tales, historical narratives, poetry). In contrast to the term "text," which encompasses all forms of writing (including official records and documents, account books and wills), and deviating from a modern conceptualization of literature as a display of beauty and form that induces an emotional effect in the reader, I follow Michael Colacurcio, who claims that writings qualify as literature when they are "thoughtful and spirited." Michael J. Colacurcio, *Godly Letters: The Literature of the American Puritans* (Notre Dame: U of Notre Dame P, 2006) ix.

public debate about the ethics of artificial immunization. The controversy over inoculation brought to light an irreconcilable contradiction in the Puritan perception and understanding of illness. On the one hand, diseases were considered as a god-sent punishment or trial that believers needed to accept as actual signs of grace; on the other hand, colonists were to seek and employ preventive measures such as a healthy diet, exercise, continuous repentance, prayer, and inoculation. Having it both ways, inviting illness and preventing it, was deemed an irresolvable conflict by many settlers and hence presented Boston ministers, among them Cotton Mather, with intellectual challenges that were increasingly difficult to manage.

Mather's only medical book, *The Angel of Bethesda* (1724/1970), was informed by the belief that science should be divinely sanctioned. In responding to larger social and cultural changes, the posthumously published monograph can be seen as symptomatic of how colonists who wished to uphold and live God's covenant with New England struggled to reconcile the millennialist tradition and early Enlightenment ideas. What has so far been neglected in Mather studies is that the Boston minister—considered by some to be "the first significant figure in American medicine"— negotiated old and new medical concepts, as well as folk and scientific knowledge about the causes and cures of diseases.[20] In his book on medicine, the author extends the already transnational scope of medical discourse and knowledge in the Atlantic world of the early eighteenth century by including remedies offered by Native people and African slaves. As will be shown, this inclusion remained repressed by ideologies that demanded the disavowal of elements deemed unscientific and irreligious.

To place these developments in even larger cultural and historical contexts will be the task of the concluding chapter. By the early eighteenth century, New England, perhaps like no other geographic region in the early modern period, had functioned as an alembic for diverse medical practices and knowledge formations drawn from local and transnational sources: here, European medicine, in its early stages of

---

[20] Otho T. Beall, Jr., and Richard H. Shryock, "Cotton Mather: First Significant Figure in American Medicine," *Proceedings of the American Antiquarian Society* 63.1 (1953): 37.

emancipation from Greek humoral pathology and supplemented by new discoveries in chemistry, physics, anatomy, and physiology, had come into contact with healing knowledge derived from Native American and African sources. And in New England, a faction from the international Protestant movement had attempted to channel the perceptions and constructions of illness and healing in the wake of growing contacts and commerce with both the Atlantic world and the expanding *hinterland*. These observations do not necessarily play into the hands of American exceptionalism, but rather point to the transnational foundations of medicine and its representation in the British colonies.

In general, the illness narratives surveyed for this study drew from, and in part contributed to, social framings of corporeality and cultural constructions of the human body's biological (dys)functions. This relationship to the larger socio-cultural frame energized an illness rhetoric that often exceeded the borders of Puritan plain style. Overall, the textual renderings of illness experiences served as reminders and warnings, requests and reports, as cultural glue and boundary-setter, as expressions of hope and destitution, and perhaps even as a therapeutic means. The chapters that comprise this study demonstrate the plurivocal nature of illness narratives and the multidirectional flows of discursive power they both reflected and constituted.

# 1. Mobile Pathogens, Traveling Knowledge

When a small group of English religious dissenters reached the shores of New England in the winter of 1620, an eerie scene energized the travelers' fears and fervors about founding a new social order. After having spent almost a month searching for a suitable place to settle, the Puritan colonists entered a largely intact Native village, which was strangely devoid of inhabitants. Aside from a few untended fields and underground food storages, they encountered an empty and desolate wasteland, with "skulls and bones [...] in many places lying still above the ground," as William Bradford, *Mayflower* passenger and soon-to-be governor of Plymouth, reported retrospectively.[1] Even though leaders of the group knew before their departure that a mysterious epidemic had struck the area, they were unaware of the avalanche of disease that had killed approximately ninety percent of the indigenous population between 1616 and 1619. After the colonists set up shop at the abandoned coastal village, which the local Wampanoag called Patuxet, they not only swarmed the woods in search for food and building material, their bodies and livestock also swarmed with deadly pathogens. No sooner were their microbes unleashed (inadvertently, at first) than the indigenous population in the area further decreased, causing a foundational shift of demographics and power relations.[2]

---

[1] William Bradford, *Of Plymouth Plantation, 1620-1647*, ed. Samuel Eliot Morison (1856; New York: Knopf, 1952) 87.

[2] For studies treating early migrations of English settlers to North America, see David Cressy, *Coming Over: Migration and Communication Between England and New England in the Seventeenth Century* (New York: Cambridge UP, 1997); Virginia DeJohn Anderson, *New England's Generation: The Great Migration and the Formation of Society and Culture in the Seventeenth Century* (New York: Cambridge UP, 1991); Roger Thompson, *Mobility and Migration: East Anglian Founders of New England, 1629-1640* (Amherst: U of Massachusetts P, 1994).

Struck by the sight of dying and decaying Native bodies, the Anglican trader Thomas Morton noted that "the bones and skulls upon the severall places of their habitations made such a spectacle," that the coastal forest woods appeared as "a new found Golgotha," the hill of execution in Roman Jerusalem whither Jesus had carried his cross (cf. John 19:17).[3] Morton's apocalyptic scenario echoes Bradford's "skulls and bones" and, at the same time, contrasts John Winthrop's seminal metaphor of the Massachusetts Bay Colony as a glorious and promising "Citty upon a Hill" with a much gloomier image.[4] Morton's recasting of New England in biblical terms, on the one hand, complements Winthrop's *Ur*-narrative of American exceptionalism by consecrating the area in which English colonists erected their version of a godly society. On the other hand, Morton's use of Golgotha highlights the presence of violence and death, which is lacking in Winthrop's imagination of America. Morton thus acknowledges the contribution of the indigenous population to the present and future development of New England by establishing a parallel between Christ's redeeming sacrifice for humanity at the cross and Natives' disease-induced sacrifices for the salvation and advancement of Europeans in the "New World."

This chapter will lay the foundation for analyzing colonial illness narratives by outlining fundamental healing practices, disease concepts, and body perceptions in the seventeenth century. After carving out similarities and differences in the cultural framing of illness and healing

---

[3] Thomas Morton, *New English Canaan*, ed. Charles F. Adams, Jr. (1637; Boston: Prince Society, 1883) 132-133.

[4] Voiced in Winthrop's famous sermon onboard the *Arabella*, delivered at the eve of the Great Migration (1630-1640), the "city upon a hill" metaphor has since been adopted to denote the special position and mission of the United States in history and in the world. John Winthrop, "A Modell of Christian Charity (1630)," (Boston: Collections of the Massachusetts Historical Society, vol. 7, 1838) 47.

A textual note: In order to convey the historicity of the sources cited in this study, the original spelling and punctuation are replicated in accordance with the respective sources. In citing transcribed seventeenth-century documents, misspellings and omissions are retained, except that superscript letters are lowered and the thorn has been rendered as "th".

in indigenous and English communities, I will investigate salient responses and explanations to Native epidemics during the founding years of the Massachusetts Bay Colony. The dominant colonial rationalization of the demographic revolution stressed that health disparities were an intricate part of God's providential plan; however, some English observers attributed Indian epidemics to natural causes and cultural choices, while others pointed out the common humanity of both groups. By contrast, the majority of the remaining indigenous population in the area, paralyzed by physical and cultural annihilation, sought to understand their new reality by ascribing disease to English sorcery, Indian transgressions from cosmological principles, and/or the inadequacy of their deities.[5]

Native American Healing: Myths and Realities

Following the European imagination of America as an Edenic and inviting landscape, pre-colonial New England was initially seen as a health utopia. Giovanni da Verrazano, sailing the Atlantic coast of North America in 1524, described the indigenes of Narragansett Bay as "the most beautiful and have the most civil customs that we have found on this voyage. [...] They live a long time, and rarely fall sick; if they are wounded, they cure themselves with fire without medicine; their end comes with old age."[6] The myth of the lithe and healthy Native body

---

[5] For the encounter between Native people and Europeans in New England, see Francis Jennings, *The Invasion of America: Indians, Colonialism, and the Cant of Conquest* (Chapel Hill: U of North Carolina P, 1975); Alden T. Vaughan, ed., *New England Encounters: Indians and Euroamericans, ca. 1600-1850* (Boston: Northeastern UP, 1999). Native dispossession and English appropriation of land is investigated in, for instance, Jean M. O'Brien, *Dispossession by Degrees: Indian Land and Identity in Natick, Massachusetts, 1650-1790* (Cambridge: Cambridge UP, 1997); Stuart Banner, *How the Indians Lost their Land: Law and Power on the Frontier* (Cambridge, MA: Harvard UP, 2005); Gesa Mackenthun, *Metaphors of Dispossession: American Beginnings and the Translation of Empire, 1492-1637* (Norman: U of Oklahoma P, 1997).

[6] Giovanni da Verrazano, "The Written Record of the Voyage of 1524 of Giovanni da Verrazano as Recorded in a Letter to Francis I, King of France, July

was repeated time and again by accounts prepared by early seventeenth-century sailors, fishermen, and traders as well as by English settlers after 1620.[7] More often than not, European reports attempted to remedy a dominant sense of oddity about, and unintelligibility of, indigenous physique by linking it to preconceived conceptions of health and beauty drawn from ancient Greek and Roman images of corporeality. Such a conscious effort was often necessary as authors sought to modify "New World" conditions in order to legitimize their voyages and to acquire funding for further explorations and/or settlement.

The realities of Native health prior to contact are difficult to assess, however.[8] Although it is sketchy and inconclusive, skeletal evidence from many regions of North America indicates that, because of famines, wars, and illnesses, the average indigenous life expectancy ranged only between 21 and 37 years—similar to that of Europeans at the time.[9] Other archeological findings, as well as ethnographic research, suggest that Indian health in what was to become New England rested on a nutritious and balanced diet, small population numbers, and a way of life that included the isolation of the sick, which prevented the spread of

8th, 1524," trans. Susan Tarrow, *The Voyages of Giovanni da Verrazzano, 1524-1528*, ed. Lawrence C. Wroth (New Haven: Yale UP, 1970) 138-140.

[7] Howard S. Russell, *Indian New England Before the Mayflower* (Hanover: UP of New England, 1980) 35-39.

[8] For an overview of pre-contact Native health and disease in the Americas, see Martha Robinson, *"They Decrease in Numbers Daily": English and Colonial Perceptions of Indian Disease in Early America*. Diss., U of Southern California, 2005, 5-50. Given the dearth of first-hand knowledge about health practices and conditions in New England before cultural contact, scholars have to rely on reports by English observers supplemented by archaeological evidence. In many instances, the inventory of Native curative practices that emerges from these sources is full of inaccuracies, misconceptions, lacunae, and biases. For some of the methodological problems and difficulties involved in portraying Native New England cultures, see Kathleen J. Bragdon, *Native People of Southern New England, 1500-1650* (Norman: U of Oklahoma P, 1996) xix.

[9] Gerald N. Grob, *The Deadly Truth: A History of Disease in America* (Cambridge, MA: Harvard UP, 2002) 23.

communicable diseases.[10] Despite these health measures, pre-contact Native people in the Northeast often suffered from arthritis, rheumatism, and respiratory disorders due to a physically demanding way of life and cold winters. In addition, contacts with animals during hunting season most likely caused a variety of viral and bacterial infections, which, along with other environmental illnesses such as fungal infections, seem to have shaped health realities before the arrival of the Europeans.[11]

The assumption that Algonquians were more disease-prone than early reports indicate is further supported by English descriptions of Native healing knowledge and traditions.[12] According to a number of reports, local indigenes knew how to cauterize wounds, treat fractures and bone dislocations, used sweat baths for cleansing and as a panacea, applied animal oils for skin protection, and were experts in applying plants for medicinal purposes. Although medical practices differed among tribes, the aboriginal botanical repertoire, built during centuries of trial and error as well as through knowledge exchanges among tribes, included remedies for coughs, colds, fevers, digestive disorders, and syphilis; various plants, roots, and barks were used as antiseptics,

---

[10] John Duffy claims that before sustained contact, New England Natives "were exempt from malaria, typhoid, typhus, smallpox, measles, scarlet fever, diphtheria, venereal diseases and the host of other disorders besetting Europeans." *The Healers: A History of American Medicine* (Urbana: U of Illinois P, 1976) 2.

[11] Virgil J. Vogel, *American Indian Medicine* (1970; Norman: U of Oklahoma P, 1990) 161; Grob 21.

[12] In the following, I use the referent "Algonquian" to designate the New England indigenous population as a whole. Although the term encompasses Native people from the Northeastern region of the present-day United States and Canada, and even though it tends to obliterate cultural differences among New England tribes (including Wampanoag, Pawtucket, Massachusett, Nipmuck, Pocumtuck, Narragansett, Pokanoket, Niantic, Mohegan, Abenaki, Pequot, and others), it is useful when describing certain commonalities or when cultural specificities can no longer be traced. For more information on individual tribes and Native groups in New England, see *The Gale Encyclopedia of Native American Tribes. Vol. 1: Northeast, Southeast, Caribbean*, ed. Sharon Malinowski and Anna Sheets (Detroit: Gale, 1998).

emetics, cathartics, diaphoretics, narcotics, stimulants, and astringents.[13] This and other medical knowledge was mostly acquired, applied, and disseminated by elderly women, herbalists, and powwows (medicine person, shaman or priest-healer). During specific times of the year these tribal healers collected medicinal plants, boiled or pounded them into concoctions, and administered them orally, locally or rectally against common ailments. If a disease proved more serious, the patient or his/her family would ask the powwow to apply his special knowledge of, and connection to, the supernatural realm in order to facilitate recovery from illness.[14]

Native conceptualizations of health, illness, and medicine were, as with the Puritans, intimately tied to beliefs about humanity's role in, and relation to, the cosmos.[15] Its central components—the sky or upper realm, the middle or natural world, and the under(water) domain—were regarded as being intricately intertwined, as suffused by an impersonal force, often referred to as *manitou*, and described as non-human beings, guardian spirits, and mythical heroes. New England Natives believed in two main spirit beings that resided in the upper and the under(water) domains respectively and that significantly affected the course of health: Cautantouwit (or Keihtan) and Abbomocho (or Hobbomok). While the former was seen as the source of human existence, and the place to

---

[13] H. Russell 39; Barrie Kavasch, "Native Foods of New England," *Enduring Traditions: The Native Peoples of New England*, ed. Laurie Weinstein (Westport: Bergin & Garvey) 10-11, 16-19. For a supplementary perspective, see William N. Fenton, "Contacts between Iroquois Herbalism and Colonial Medicine," *Annual Report of the Smithsonian Institution for 1941* (Washington, DC, 1942) 503-526.

[14] For the traditional division of medical roles in Central and Western Algonquian societies, see Ake Hultkrantz, *Shamanic Healing and Ritual Drama: Health and Medicine in Native North American Religious Traditions* (New York: Crossroad, 1992) 23-42.

[15] Vogel points out the different meanings and uses of the word "medicine" in European and Native cultures. In addition to signifying the practice or property of curing illnesses, Native Americans generally ascribed magical and supernatural powers, something that remains inexplicable and unaccountable, to the term "medicine" (26).

which souls would return after death, the latter (Abbomocho), who often appeared as an eel, a snake or an other under(water)world dweller, was seen as having a more direct impact on matters of health. As Edward Winslow, one of the first English settlers to record the history of colonial New England, notes:

> Him [Abbomocho] they call upon to cure their wounds and diseases. When they are curable, he persuades them he sends the same for some conceived anger against them, but upon their calling upon him, can and doth help them; but when they are mortall and not curable in nature, then he persuades them *Kiehtan* is angry, and sends them, whom none can cure; insomuch as in that respect onely they somewhat doubt whether hee be simply god, and therefore in sicknesse never call upon him.[16]

Winslow's description of how indigenous people considered illness as a result of disrespect for spiritual forces illustrates primarily the cultural biases and lacunae in English depictions of indigenous medicine: colonial observers frequently recorded the actions of Native healers but generally failed to provide insight into their thought structure and cultural principles underlying their approaches to healing. For instance, in the above-cited passage the speaker suggests a correspondence between Cautantouwit and God as well as between Abbomocho and Satan.[17]

The Algonquian belief in disease etiology proved more complex than the divine anger suggested by Winslow and other observers. It drew on animism, the conviction that a greater power or supernatural spirits reside in all natural things on earth, a view which caused most Natives to proceed with caution when hunting animals or harvesting crops and

---

[16] Edward Winslow, *Good Newes from New England, or a True Relation of Things Very Remarkable at the Plantation of Plimoth in New-England* (1624; Early English Books Online, STC 25856) 53. For a similar description, see John Josselyn, *An Account of Two Voyages to New-England* (1674; Early English Books Online, J1091) 132-134.

[17] Bragdon points out, however, that instead of the good/evil dichotomy inherent in Western thought, the Natives described by Winslow regarded Cautantouwit as a benevolent deity with little influence in their daily lives, whereas Abbomocho combined forces of good and evil (190).

plants. Once offended, they believed, spirits might hide animals, destroy the harvest or intrude human bodies, causing illnesses. To be healthy thus meant to maintain the cosmological balance and to interact wisely with natural and supernatural beings.

New England Natives also ascribed illnesses to a person's dream soul, *Cowwéwonck*, which was thought to leave the body during sleep and illness, requiring powerful guardian spirits for protection and recovery. The help of denizens of the spirit world could be enlisted at certain natural places that were seen as points of fluid transition within the tripartite Native cosmos. Watery places such as the ocean, lakes, springs, or swamps, but also trees, which symbolically manifested the interrelation between sky world, surface world, and underworld, could serve as thresholds between different parts of Algonquian cosmography. These thresholds were frequently crossed by dream souls, shamans in non-human form, and various guardian spirits (often in animal shape). The spiritual power gained from travel and transformation in and by these places was considered essential for a person's health and well-being.[18]

In order to guide the dream soul toward recovery or to deploy friendly spirits for healing purposes, powwows—the intermediaries between the natural and the spiritual domains—had developed specific rituals. Captain Daniel Gookin, who served as English Superintendent of the Indians of Massachusetts Bay from 1661 to 1678, observed that

> [t]here are among them certain men and women, whom they call powows. These are partly wizards and witches, holding familiarity with Satan, that evil one; and partly are physicians, and make use, at least in show, of herbs and roots, for curing the sick and diseased. These are sent for by the sick and wounded; and by their diabolical spells, mutterings, exorcisms, they seem to do wonders. They use extraordinary strange motions of their bodies, insomuch that they will sweat until they foam; and thus continue for some hours together, stroking and hovering over the sick.[19]

[18] Bragdon 186, 192-193.

[19] Daniel Gookin, *Historical Collections of the Indians in New England. Of Their Several Nations, Numbers, Customs, Manners, Religion and Government, Before the English Planted There* (1674; Boston: Belknap & Hall, 1792) 14.

Gookin has been known for his unsympathetic view toward Native Americans but also for his relatively intimate knowledge of indigenous cultural practices. His commentary is typical of official New England discourse because it expresses a deep-rooted skepticism about shamanistic practices that is accompanied by a profound interest in them. Gookin's observation that "they seem to do wonders" indicates that some English commentators did not discard Native therapeutic practices as useless. In fact, one reason for the vociferous English rejection of Indian healing methods was precisely the recognition that there existed uncanny parallels between medical practices imported from Europe and those of the indigenous: both groups attached similar symbolic meaning to illness by placing it within a larger cosmos crowded with supernatural forces that intervened in the course of health.[20] Based on this belief, many colonists feared that the shaman's "diabolick skills" could afflict their own physical and/or spiritual well-being.[21] As one result, "the colonists could not rest easily until the Indian medicine men no longer had power to use against the English," as Karen Kupperman sums up a point that will be discussed in further detail in chapter four of this study.[22]

Largely due to their cultural prejudices, English commentators by and large condemned indigenous rituals as a heathen practice and thus fueled a more general process of satanizing the Native population. That

[20] William S. Simmons, *Spirit of the New England Tribes: Indian History and Folklore, 1620-1984* (Hanover: UP of New England, 1986) 37, 43.

[21] Cotton Mather, *Magnalia Christi Americana; or, The Ecclesiastical History of New England, Vol. II* (1702; Hartford: Andrus, 1853) 426. Even the most sympathetic English observers displayed their condemnation of what they considered witchcraft or devil worship. John Josselyn, for example, being both appalled and intrigued by shamanistic rituals, called New England shamans "Craftie Rogues, abusing the rest at their pleasure, having power over them by reason of their Diabolical Art in curing of Diseases, which is performed with rude Ceremonies" (*Two Voyages* 134).

[22] Karen Ordahl Kupperman, *Settling with the Indians: The Meeting of English and Indian Cultures in America, 1580-1640* (Totowa: Rowman and Littlefield, 1980) 118.

is, they recognized the healing abilities of certain powwows but discursively fixated their rituals as devil worship and thus sought to provide further evidence that the indigenous inhabitants of America were un-civilized and in dire need of proselytizing. This process at once positioned the Natives as Other and, at the same time, integrated them into the orbit of Puritanism: by attributing satanic qualities to Indian medical practices, English commentators could postulate the necessity for missionizing and acculturating New England's aboriginal inhabitants.[23]

Rather than "holding familiarity with Satan," as Gookin puts it, New England powwows claimed to deploy the support of Abbomocho and other spirit helpers through visions, trance or dreams, attempting to control the forces that were presumed to cause and cure illness. The diagnosis often began by consulting an animal oracle, designed to determine the chances of the patient's recovery. If certain death was predicted, no cure was administered; if healing was to be expected, the shaman collected a fee for his services and proceeded with the curing ceremony. Often equipped with charms, herbs, and medical tools, and his face smeared with black ashes to symbolize the liminal state of the afflicted between life and death, the powwow performed healing rituals that included drumming, chanting, singing, and dancing.[24] Once arrived in a state of trance, the powwow was believed to communicate with the spirit world and to gain access to metaphysical knowledge about the

---

[23] English colonists had inherited the notion that Native Americans were, individually and collectively, in cahoots with the devil from the writings of sixteenth-century Spanish explorers and conquerors. As David Lovejoy points out, the discursive relegation of Natives to the realm of Satan reached its peak with the arrival of Puritan settlers in New England and was prompted by the newcomers' self-righteousness about their exceptional position within human history. David S. Lovejoy, "Satanizing the American Indian," *New England Quarterly* 67.4 (1994): 603-621.

[24] "Letters of Samuel Lee and Samuel Sewall Relating to New England and the Indians," ed. George L. Kittredge, *Publications of the Colonial Society of Massachusetts* 14 (1912): 151; C. Keith Wilbur, *The New England Indians* (Chester: Globe Pequot, 1978) 71; William Wood, *New England's Prospect: A True, Lively, and Experimentall Description of that Part of America, Commonly Called New England* (1634; Early English Books Online, STC 25957) 83.

offended spirit and thus the cause of illness. If the shaman had previously diagnosed that a person's dream soul was lost, s/he could attempt to retrieve it by changing into non-human form and participating in the spirit world. While the soul of the powwow was in flight, it either became sensitive to supernatural beings or transformed into one and could thereby direct the spirit of illness away from a person.[25] Aside from treating soul-loss illnesses by intervening in a person's dream state, Native priest healers frequently attempted to suck the illness out of the body, as William Wood noted: "hee wrapt a piece of cloth about the foote of the lame man; upon that wrapping a Beaver skinne, through which hee laying his mouth to the Beaver skinne, by his sucking charmes he brought out the stumpe, which he spat into a tray of water, returning the foote as whole as its fellow in a short time."[26] This and other similar rituals were quite rational within a belief system according to which illnesses were caused by spirit intrusions.

It appears also that the efficacy of Native healing rituals often relied on diverting the mind of the afflicted from their state of suffering by suggesting that the ailment in question could be alleviated by the powwow's supernatural abilities. Aside from their mental effects, healing ceremonies also served an important social function because they often (re)connected the individual with the community and sanctified this connection cosmically. In addition, while some afflicted members were isolated from the rest of the tribe, Native therapeutics rested on a communal care system in which healthy members would attend the sick person, offering comfort and assisting the shaman's rituals. This communal practice proved detrimental when Algonquian communities were faced with highly communicable diseases which English explorers and settlers carried to North America after 1600.[27]

According to indigenous beliefs, health and wealth were intimately connected and hence, medicinal rituals often involved a sacrifice of material goods. Some of the shaman's payment for his efforts, especially

---

[25] Bragdon 203-204. A shaman was also believed to direct malevolent spirits toward a person, causing a corporeal affliction. This, many English colonists readily ascribed to while disavowing the healing power of powwow practices.

[26] Wood 83.

[27] H. Russell 40; Vogel 34.

sacred or symbolic objects, was often burned or buried in order to please Abbomocho and/or certain guardian spirits. Such giving-away ceremonies were central to the conceptualization and treatment of illness in a culture which placed a high value on reciprocity (exchanging gifts, sharing resources). Many Natives believed that property destruction and parting from possessions caused bodily and spiritual cleansing—that wealth could be exchanged for health. Since reciprocity was considered central to personal interactions as well as to the relationship between humanity and the spirit realm, Native people were convinced that ritual offerings, particularly during and after illness, would reaffirm the contract and connection with the divine. Burning personal belongings during times of sickness further echoed the cultural notion that renewal follows destruction, a notion which also played an important role in burial rites and agricultural practices.[28]

Based on the available archeological and ethnographic evidence, it is safe to say that the pre-contact Algonquian system of health was sufficient for curing or at least mitigating diseases common to the Native way of life. Undoubtedly, indigenous plant knowledge met the demands for healing the majority of ailments. Whereas the efficacy of some Algonquian medical applications appears questionable from the perspective of modern Western medicine, the Natives' belief in curative rituals seems to have facilitated recovery or at least ease from some diseases. As will be shown later in this chapter, indigenous therapeutics were severely strained after the arrival of English settlers and the pathogens they and their livestock carried across the Atlantic. As European germs infected a population that was immunologically unprepared for the new arrivals, they caused the virtual extinction of the indigenous population along the New England coast and the substitution of Native cultural practices and medicinal knowledge with those introduced by the newcomers.

---

[28] Josselyn, *Two Voyages* 134; Bragdon 43-44; Neal Salisbury, *Manitou and Providence: Indians, Europeans, and the Making of New England, 1500-1643* (New York: Oxford UP, 1982) 10-11, 42-45.

Bleed and Pray: Colonial Medicine in Early New England

When Puritans and other English settlers began to colonize North America during the first half of the seventeenth century, European medical science was still in its infancy, its healing methods almost exclusively drawn from ancient sources. The co-presence and interplays between scientific advances, therapeutic practices based largely on folk and Greco-Roman remedies, and the belief in illness and healing as divine interventions characterized European and Anglo-American medicine until well into the nineteenth century. Since the Greek beginnings of Western medicine, few systematic discoveries had produced a direct payoff for medical practice; however, since Antiquity, medicine had also been "defined as something over and beyond mere healing, as the possession of a specific body of learning, theoretical and practical, that might be used to treat the sick," and hence early modern Europeans eagerly sought to systematize ancient medical expertise into a scientific field comparable to physics or mathematics.[29]

After Renaissance Europe had awoken from its intellectual slumber, Christian theologians assimilated and de-secularized the Greek humoral system, consisting of four bodily fluids (phlegm, blood, yellow bile, black bile).[30] Until then, churches had been the most advanced and dominant institutions in the field of medicine, serving both as keepers of medical learning at a time when most Greek, Roman, and Arabic medical texts were forgotten in Europe and as spear headers of the hospital movement, which epitomized biblical calls for charity toward, and conversion of, humanity. Since the foundation of Christianity, the

---

[29] Vivian Nutton, "The Rise of Medicine," *The Cambridge Illustrated History of Medicine*, ed. Roy Porter (Cambridge: Cambridge UP, 1996) 53. Since it is an impossible task to provide an exhaustive overview of medical history, the following account will be limited to those ideas, concepts, and innovations that were particularly relevant to the objects of this study. For a more general and recent introduction to the history of medicine see, among many others, Lois N. Magner, *A History of Medicine*, 2nd ed. (Boca Raton: Taylor, 2005).

[30] For disease concepts in ancient Greece, see Mirko D. Grmek, "The Concept of Disease," *Western Medical Thought from Antiquity to the Middle Ages*, ed. Mirko D. Grmek, trans. Antony Shugaar (1993; Cambridge, MA: Harvard UP, 1998) 246-255. See also chapter five of the present study.

correlation between healing and holy (German: *heilen* and *heilig*) had been a salient, yet ambiguous doctrinal feature. This was largely due to Christendom's inherently ambivalent and complex attitudes toward the human body, which originated in Bible passages that depict body and soul as separate and conflictual but also as relational and complementary entities.[31] In Galatians 5:17, for instance, the Apostle Paul posits the body as the enemy of the soul: "For the flesh lusteth against the Spirit, and the Spirit against the flesh: and these are contrary one to another"; however, he also glorifies the body as "the temple of the holy Ghost" worthy of special care and maintenance (1 Corinthians 6:19). Early Christianity considered flesh (a person's physical being) as the prison-house of the soul, corrupt and in need of disciplining. That is, flesh was not considered as evil *per se* but represented humanity's sinful nature through various infirmities. This scripture-based conviction translated into a general abhorrence of the body in Western civilization, as Roy Porter explains:

> To a degree that is hard to imagine nowadays, visible, tangible flesh was all too often experienced as ugly, nasty and decaying, bitten by bugs and beset by sores; it was rank, foul and dysfunctional; for all of medicine's best efforts, it was frequently racked with pain, disability and disease; and death might well be nigh.[32]

Calvinism, in particular, stressed the depravity of human flesh and its subordination to the soul. In his treatise *Of the Combat of the Flesh and Spirit*, for instance, the Elizabethan theologian William Perkins explained the dichotomous relation between the soul and the body by describing the former as the "created quality of holiness" and the latter as "the naturall corruption or inclination of the mind, will, and affections to that which is against the law."[33] Although this notion of the inherent

---

[31] Nutton 64-69. Throughout this study, citations from scripture are taken from the Geneva Bible (1589 edition), which most New England Puritans studied and used until the 1680s when the King James Bible became standard.

[32] Roy Porter, *Flesh in the Age of Reason* (New York: Norton, 2003) 25.

[33] William Perkins, *Two Treatises: I. Of the Nature and Practise of Repentance. II. Of the Combat of the Flesh and Spirit* (1593; Early English Books Online,

immorality and wickedness of the flesh dominated theological doctrines and practices throughout the early modern period, the incarnation, bodily agony, and resurrection of Christ signaled a corporeal emphasis that was equally endemic to Christianity. The religious importance of bodily existence was further evinced by the belief that God created humanity in His image, by the transubstantiation of bread and wine into Christ's body and blood in Roman Catholicism, or by the promise that the soul of the believer, once it has ascended to heaven, would reunite with its physical body after the Last Judgment.

Against this background, Christian authorities conceived of bodily conditions as products and functions of divine omnipotence. Regardless of whether illnesses were inflicted by God directly or through natural or demonic mediators (Satan, evil spirits, witches), the etiology of disease lay almost exclusively in the metaphysical realm.[34] According to theological doctrine, sickness had entered the world and history as a punishment for Adam and Eve's original sin—the defiance of God's laws in order to gain knowledge that would elevate humanity to the level of divinity. Additional conceptualizations of illness and healing were primarily drawn from Exodus, Job, the Gospels, and the prophetic writings in the Bible. For instance, in Exodus 15:26 one reads that God grants immunity from disease if humans follows His laws, "for I am the Lord that healeth thee." Aside from His healing power, God's punitive

STC 1426:02) 73. This conviction was echoed time and again in English Puritan writings, for instance, in William Prynne's poem "The Soules Complaint against the Bodies Encroachment on Her" (1642): "What is the body, but *a loathsome Masse / Of dust and ashes, brittle as a glasse*" (Prynne quoted in Porter, *Flesh* 39; emphasis original).

[34] Satan played a relatively minor role in Protestant conceptualizations of illness. Since most Reformed Churches followed Luther's notion that the devil is God's devil, based on the depiction of Satan as belonging to the court of God in the Book of Job, demons were considered as intermediate agents of illness. Despite the cosmic dualism of good and evil forces within Christian theology, the devil could not appear on equal terms with God because if he did, the monotheistic character of Christendom would have been in danger. Furthermore, most Protestants held that while Satan might cause demonic possession that can either constitute or transform into an illness, his main role was luring human being to sin, for which God's punishment included disease.

measures were seen as consisting of various calamities and tribulations, including specific illnesses designed to make believers consider their actions carefully (cf. Deuteronomy 28:22; Leviticus 26:14-16).

Such a rather grim conceptualization of illness caused by an angry and vengeful deity is in part countered by the redemptive power of Christ. The New Testament's mutual implications of religion and health/illness is aptly illustrated by Christ's more than thirty healing miracles, which served as revelations of divine will, sovereignty, and compassion and established Christianity as a healing faith (cf. Mark 3:1-11). The Gospel generally describes disease as a potentially positive experience rather than as mere divine punishment, during which the afflicted learns to reform his behavior, strengthens his faith, and renews his/her devotion to God. As Steven Muir points out, the word "save" in the New Testament often refers to deliverance in both a theological, spiritual sense and in a medical, physical one. Similarly, healing combines the recovery of the body and the redemption of the soul through Christ. When, for example, the blind beggar Bartimaeus pleads for healing, Jesus replies that "thy fayth hath saved thee" (Mark 10:52), emphasizing not only the conjunctions between soul and body, as well as faith and saving for maintaining one's well-being but, equally important, the active role humans have to take in order to achieve deliverance from sin and sickness.[35]

Christendom's complex attitudes toward the body translated into ambivalent relations with medicine's evolution into a science since the late Renaissance. Because a person's physical body (flesh) and his/her spirit were regarded as God's property, Christians were held to glorify and care for both; a conviction which helped to legitimize the work of doctors and physicians.[36] At the same time, the ostensible separation

---

[35] Steven C. Muir, "Faith, Healing, and Deliverance in Mark's Gospel," *Healing in Religion and Society, From Hippocrates to the Puritans*, ed. J. Kevin Coyle and Steven C. Muir (Lewiston: Mellen, 1999) 85-104.

[36] Gary B. Ferngren and Darrel W. Amundsen, "Healing and Medicine: Healing and Medicine in Christianity," *Encyclopedia of Religion, Vol. 6*, ed. Lindsay Jones, 2nd ed. (Detroit: Macmillan Reference, 2005) 3846. Even though the Bible includes references to ancient physicians, midwives, and medical

between ennobled soul and depraved body precluded a valuation of medicine and practitioners on equal terms with the churches, for whom illness remained primarily a sign of divine anger at human indifference and carelessness, and healing an indication of His grace (cf. Psalm 107:17-20). Throughout Western history, Christian teachings often conflicted with natural medical approaches because mortal, sin-prone flesh was deemed inferior to the immortal and divine soul and thus deserved less attention. Many theologians hence considered the emerging medical sciences as countervailing the Christian distrust in the flesh because medicine approached disease from a somatic perspective that increasingly discarded the role and influence of spiritual and metaphysical aspects. Some early Christians had condemned medicine in principle, regarding its methods as futile, impious, and blasphemous interferences in God's sovereignty and this stance was to continue well into the early modern period.[37] Any secular attempt to discover regularities, patterns, and functions of the human body, some theologians argued, was in essence spurred by the desire to alter the necessary unfolding of God's will through illness, and to prevent divine punishment and correction. In addition, aside from religious misgivings about the aspirations of scientific medicine, scholars rightly pointed out the practical inadequacy, uncertainty, and even danger of many medical techniques. As one result, after physicians and scientists had begun to shift disease etiology from God to natural causes, institutions and organizations with pretensions to authority over illness and healing matters frequently quarreled over the effectiveness of medical procedures—from anatomical studies to the suitability of secular healing methods—and, particularly, over the role of God in matters of health and illness.[38]

Christianity and Western medical science were, however, not necessarily and exclusively engaged in a hostile and competitive relation

---

treatments, natural causes or remedies make only rare appearances, as healing and illness are placed almost exclusively in supernatural terms.

[37] Plinio Prioreschi, *A History of Medicine. Vol. 1: Primitive and Ancient Medicine* (Lewiston: Mellen, 1991) 526.

[38] Bertrand Russell, *Religion and Science* (1935; New York: Oxford UP, 1968) 7-18.

with each other; the two often co-existed without much interaction, or even complemented each other. The coexistence of medical and theological approaches to healing during the sixteenth and seventeenth centuries can be seen as the outcome of an attitude developed already during the Middle Ages, when "health, healing, and disease were no longer viewed solely as direct results of divine intervention, or only as the direct expression of the vicissitudes of the soul but were seen as phenomena that depended on natural and regular events, which the physician might and *must* investigate."[39] The increasing church-sanctioned interest in medicine marked a partial shift of emphasis within Christian theology from Exodus 15:26 ("for I am the Lord that healeth thee") to Ecclesiastes (Sirach) 38:4: "The Lord hathe created medicines of the earth, and he that is wise, will not abhorre it." As a result, the heightening repute of physicians paved the way for increasing inquiries into the structure and functions of the human body and culminated in significant discoveries that were to change Western medical practices. In brief, between the advent of the Renaissance and the initial colonization of New England, physicians increasingly differentiated diseases rather than viewing them as minor variations of a general body state; new inventions facilitated knowledge production and the improvement of treatment methods; universities across Europe gathered, evaluated, and disseminated past and present medical theories, discoveries, and practices; astrology, alchemy, and folk knowledge remained strong pillars of the healing arts.

In spite of these changes and continuities, medical practice remained relatively consistent throughout the seventeenth century. Inspired by Greek teachings, medical practitioners believed that diseases could transmute (e.g., a cold might turn into pneumonia and then into tuberculosis), and were caused either by miasma (putrid gases rising out of the ground) or by contagion (person-to-person transmission, usually by touch). As a result, almost all physical remedies during the early modern period were geared toward re-establishing the body's humoral

---

[39] Jole Agrimi and Chiara Crisciani, "Charity and Aid in Medieval Christian Civilization," *Western Medical Thought from Antiquity to the Middle Ages*, ed. Mirko D. Grmek, trans. Antony Shugaar (1993; Cambridge, MA: Harvard UP, 1998) 179 (emphasis added).

balance by emitting putrid or toxic elements. Since most available pharmaceuticals were comparatively ineffective—except for cinchona against malaria and opium against pain—a number of treatments took recourse to the occult sciences (magic, astrology, alchemy). For instance, Europeans based most of their botanical therapeutics on the doctrine of signatures, a central principle in ancient, folk, and Paracelsian medicine, which held that certain plants signal their application by their shape (resembling a certain part of the human body) and their color (e.g., red plants were thought to be useful in treating illnesses attributed to the blood). The doctrine of signatures was based on the notion of correspondences or analogies according to which all objects in the cosmos exert sympathetic influences on each other and can be manipulated to cure diseases. Most healers believed that by generating correspondences throughout the universe, the macrocosm "signed" every plant, animal, herb or stone and that the medico-alchemical adept could decipher its shape, color, taste or smell and correlate it to a specific therapeutic application.[40]

Before any treatment could be prescribed the patient had to be examined. Physical examinations of the entire body were not only considered morally questionable but were, moreover, impossible given the lack of diagnostic instruments and techniques. It had been common medical practice since Antiquity to detect illnesses by inspecting certain parts of the body, especially the tongue, smelling odors, listening to coughs, feeling the pulse, and tasting the patient's urine. In addition, the physician had to rely on conduct-of-life narratives that the patient offered. The interpretation of illness and life (hi)stories required an implicit agreement on a specific cultural code system that rendered certain symptoms and causes of illness intelligible to both health seeker and giver.[41]

---

[40] Miles Weatherall, "Drug Treatment and the Rise of Pharmacology," *The Cambridge Illustrated History of Medicine*, ed. Roy Porter (Cambridge: Cambridge UP, 1996) 274; Magner 21; Walter Pagel, *Paracelsus: An Introduction to Philosophical Medicine in the Era of the Renaissance* (Basel: Karger, 1958) 37-38, 69-70.

[41] Roy Porter, "What is Disease?" *The Cambridge Illustrated History of Medicine*, ed. Roy Porter (Cambridge: Cambridge UP, 1996) 96.

In the course of the seventeenth century, English Protestants brought European conceptualizations of disease and medical practices to their new habitats in North America. The impetus from Galenic humoralism guided New England medical practice in a number of ways, as the Reverend Thomas Palmer of Middleborough, Massachusetts explained: "it was necessary for the healer to follow basic Galenic principles when called to the sickbed of a parishioner: the first thing he should do is 'consider whether it [the illness] be a humoural Distemper & what Humours are most afflictive, & what parts of the body are most distempered, & where the seat of the disease lyes.'"[42] Although early colonists made some adaptations to contemporary Western medicine, for instance by including Native plant knowledge, "the institutional and intellectual environment of the New World was not sufficiently different from that of the Old World to produce more than variations in degree" during the first decades of settlement.[43] Due to the inadequacies of medical procedures at the time, and because of their intense religious convictions, most colonists approached the burden of disease, the actual health problems that affected them, theologically. Along with the conception of the body as depraved, they inherited the scholastic view that suffering and illness were primarily the result of sin. Conceptually, this notion challenged the traditional Christian body-soul dichotomy because illness was seen as connecting the two: it rendered malevolent thoughts and actions tangible in and on the body and, in doing so, caused painful repercussions and ramifications.

John Cotton, one of the most influential New England ministers of the first generation, illustrates the inextricable implications between body and soul as well as medicine and theology as follows:

[42] Thomas Palmer, *The Admirable Secrets of Physick and Chyrurgery*, ed. Thomas R. Forbes (1691; New Haven: Yale UP, 1984) 36.

[43] Eric H. Christianson, "Medicine in New England," *Medicine in the New World: New Spain, New France, and New England,* ed. Ronald L. Numbers (Knoxville: U of Tennessee P, 1987) 101-153. Rpt. in *Sickness and Health in America: Readings in the History of Medicine and Public Health*, ed. Judith W. Leavitt and Ronald L. Numbers, 3rd ed. (Madison: U of Wisconsin P, 1997) 66.

Physitians tell us there is no better medicine to purge out the most
gloomy and clammy obstructions of the stomach, and to dry up such
superfluous humours, then taking some bitter thing, as Aloes, and
Centaury, or the like: That is the true nature of this gracious look upon
Christ, it will cleanse the foule from what ever keeps us off from
fellowship with God, it purges out al clammy and cholerick distempers,
it preserves the frame of the spirit sweet and savoury, bitternesse is not
the wisdome which is from above [...] when once it hath wrought the
heart to this heavenly wisdome, then it makes a man gentle and meek
without partiality, &c.[44]

Cotton's linkage between "physick" and religion is more than
metaphorical. He considers sin as an ensemble of corruptions that
constantly affect the human condition. Just as the body evacuates
polluted matter to maintain its health, the soul has to be cleansed from
sin. This view ties in with the religious conviction that rotten matter in
nature (miasma) and society (corruption) are equally hazardous to health
and are, as a result, in need of constant disclosure, regulation, and
removal. This mutual interaction and intertwinement between the
spiritual and bodily constitution of the individual, on the one hand, and
putrid materials, thoughts, and actions that surround the faithful, on the
other, is central for understanding Puritan conceptualizations of health
and illness on both sides of the Atlantic and especially in the "New
World." By associating sickness with sin, the application of medical
treatments could be conceived as an assault on wickedness and thus
functioned to advance one of the central goals of the New England
experiment. When medicine was successful, sin and sickness were
momentarily banned from the world, marking a victory of the godly
over the devil. The failure of medicine, however, could imply that God
had something else in store for the afflicted and/or signified a reminder
that the assault on wickedness would always be limited by the
persistence of sin in the world.

Such an intimate linkage between sin and illness was far from
arbitrary. It served to promote the religious and political agendas of the

---

[44] John Cotton, *The Way of Life, or, Gods Way and Course* (1641; Early English
Books Online, C6470) 63.

power elite in colonial New England by allowing authorities to claim that a moral failure haunted those that had contracted an illness. In doing so, the sin/illness connection cemented the church's role in human affairs by providing a gateway to the body and the soul. Health and disease, accordingly, were seen as aggregate and complex outcomes of morality; however, these outcomes were as dynamic and hidden from view as the proper diagnosis of most diseases at the time. Most Puritans believed that God intended illness as a punishment; as such it potentially served as a means toward spiritual maturity and redemption. Deliverance from spiritual and physical adversities could only be gained through silent suffering, akin to Job and Christ, and by the constant awareness that illness marked a divine visitation whose end result was uncertain. Hence, instead of fearing disease as a "messenger of death,"[45] many colonists considered illness as a source of strength needed to fight the adversities of life in the "New World," an occasion to increase their ministerial efforts after healing, or as a sign that reunion with God in heaven was imminent.

Given the ubiquity of pain and suffering from sickness and injuries during the early modern period, religious faith often provided the only efficacious comfort and played an important role in making individual and collective afflictions of the body bearable. For instance, the men and women who settled Massachusetts interpreted an epidemic illness at Charlestown in 1630 (shortly after its founding) as an indication of divine wrath that could only be remedied by a communal gathering during which members asked God "to withdraw His hand of correction from them, so as also to establish and direct them in His ways."[46] This

---

[45] Cotton Mather, *Magnalia Christi Americana; or, The Ecclesiastical History of New England, Vol. I* (1702; Hartford: Andrus, 1855) 500.

[46] Bradford 235. The notion that God sends epidemics as a collective punishment was echoed time and again in sermons, promotional tracts, and historical writings during the seventeenth century and played a central role in official lamentations about the loss of the original vision and purpose for settling New England. See, for instance, Increase Mather, *A Brief History of the Warr with the Indians in New England* (1676; Early American Imprints, Series 1, no. 220) 32.

"ritual enclosing of sickness"[47] in prayer and fasting illustrates that colonists believed that illness could be as much a sign of individual sins as of collective guilt and transgression and that, thus, recovery was incumbent upon personal and communal acts of repentance.

Since the Middle Ages, disease had no longer been exclusively viewed as the result of individual or communal sins but also as a test of faith, patience, and obedience, especially in old age. Most New England colonists built their ideal approach to illness around the Book of Job, in which God inflicts an illness as a trial during which the afflicted must prove his/her allegiance. As part of the purification of church practices, English Protestants argued that miracle healings had ended with the apostles and hence rejected Catholicism's reliance on pilgrimages, exorcism, relics, unction, and saint worship as a feasible means of recovery from disease.[48] Instead, the Puritan patient was asked to engage in prayer, introspection, and repentance. Such a strategy would be beneficial regardless of whether the afflicted survived the illness or not: if the person recovered, s/he would be able to continue a reformed life in Christ; if not, s/he had at least done all that one could in preparation for death.

Because of the immensity of human suffering before the rise of medical science in the late nineteenth century, some ministers coded illness as a cause for ultimate celebration rather than despair. Given the

[47] David D. Hall, *Worlds of Wonder, Days of Judgment: Popular Religious Belief in Early New England* (New York: Knopf, 1989) 3, 192-200. Cf. James H. Cassedy, *Medicine in America: A Short History* (Baltimore: Johns Hopkins UP, 1991) 13.

[48] Andrew Wear, "Religious Beliefs and Medicine in Early Modern England," *The Task of Healing: Medicine, Religion and Gender in England and the Netherlands, 1450-1800*, ed. Hilary Marland and Margaret Pelling (Rotterdam: Erasmus, 1996) 145-169, points out the structural similarities in health conceptions among Protestants and Catholics in early modern England. He claims that differences with regard to medical theory and practice between Calvinism and Catholicism were primarily concerned with the issue of miracle healing. Cf. Calvin's critique of anointing the sick as a sacrament, based on James 5:14-15 and Mark 6:12-14, in John Calvin, *Institutes of the Christian Religion*, book IV, chapter 19, trans. Henry Beveridge (1536; Grand Rapids: Christian Classics Ethereal Library, 2002) 1023-1025.

ubiquity of disease and the scarcity of efficacious healing techniques, such a cultural construction of disease was vital in ensuring a mentality geared towards spiritual and material progress. Calvinist theology integrated illnesses into its belief system by postulating suffering as an occasion for reform, thus (at times literally) urging true believers to beg for more and regret not being afflicted more often. The faithful were expected to consider illness and recovery as an ultimate cause for rejoicing because they were seen as indicators of spiritual growth and "proof that they are the children of God."[49] Such a perspective on illness in terms of possible reassurance marked a central pillar of Puritan religious culture because it entailed a self-perception of the individual and the collective as both outcast and chosen. Any corporeal affliction represented sinful behavior that needed to be extracted from the body (social) and, at the same time, constituted God's incarnated presence, interest, and power. Illness thus allowed the individual and the community to display its own faith through suffering, perseverance, and acceptance. In addition, a sick person became an important collective tool of religious pedagogy and charity, offering healthy individuals and the community a chance to heal, minister, and coalesce.

Such an empowering encoding of illness was only possible, however, when the positive significance of an illness was present. In many instances this was hardly the case. What if, for example, an illness became chronic after the afflicted testified in public that s/he had returned to Christ? Or what to make of illnesses that visited respected and seemingly elect members of the community? Was a particular disease associated with certain sins or did it rather mark a general test of faith? The ambiguities contained in religious interpretations of disease (punishment of the wicked; trial for the righteous) and healing (as a possible manifestation of grace) forced colonists into an impossible task of deciphering the meanings of their bodily conditions: in order to receive glimpses into their individual and collective prospects for salvation, they engaged in almost incessant interpretation of what

[49] Darrel W. Amundsen and Gary B. Ferngren, "Medicine and Religion: Early Christianity through the Middle Ages," *Health/Medicine and the Faith Traditions*, ed. Martin E. Marty and Kenneth L. Vaux (Philadelphia: Fortress, 1982) 94-95.

appeared as signs all around them and even those who considered
themselves among the elect often expressed doubt and confusion about
the implication of divine wonders and portents such as diseases (and
storms, comets, the death of a loved one, or other providential signs).
Hence, when illness broke out, devoted colonists sought meaning and
recovery by engaging in intensive prayer, fasting, self-examination,
confession, and writing.

One typical example of how Puritans considered illness as an
occasion for introspection and its publication is found in Thomas
Hooker's letter to John Cotton, written in Holland while suffering from
a fever:

> I have looked over my heart, and life, according to my measure; aimed
> and guessed as well as I could: and entreated his Majesty to make known
> his mind, wherein I missed; and yet methinks I cannot spell out readily
> the purpose of his proceedings; which I confess have been wonderful in
> miseries, and more than wonderful in mercies to me and mine.[50]

First and foremost, sickness marks a sign sent by God calling on the
faithful to examine meticulously his/her thoughts and actions. The
divine message of this sign is, however, not self-revealing as Hooker
finds it difficult to decipher "the purpose of his proceedings." This is no
cause for doubt or even anger towards God; rather, even the most severe
affliction posits an occasion for rejoicing for the devout believer, who is
convinced that "miseries" and "mercies" are two sides of the same
divine coin. Hooker, as well as most people in New England, recognized
that the theological interpretation of disease appeared to be necessarily
shrouded in ambiguity. Since the enigma of illness remained insoluble,
it potentially strengthened the belief in, and devotion to, God's
providence as the wise, sovereign, and mysterious force that guided the
universe.

While God was perceived to intervene constantly in the affairs of the
world, He does not, however, govern all details on earth directly. Rather,
He establishes His power through a double mechanism: a general
providence comprised of transcendent laws that function as first causes,

---

[50] Thomas Hooker, quoted in Mather, *Magnalia* I:340.

and a special providence which God has entrusted to secondary causes. This dual structure of ordering and executing God's will was conceived as being constantly present, marking the necessary core of divine government of the world. Until approximately the end of the seventeenth century, Protestants and other Christians believed that certain illnesses, especially epidemic diseases, reached a person through direct intervention from God, while others, for instance colds, upset stomachs or other common illnesses were delivered through secondary causes. Regardless of its exact path—divine or natural—which eluded complete understanding, the cause and course of the illness was thought to rest with God's providence.[51]

Yet, as indicated above, Puritans did not consider religious and naturalistic etiologies and remedies to be contradictory as long as medical theory and practice were authorized by, and subservient to, theology. It is hence misleading to assume that even the most devout Puritan relied on providence exclusively. Placing illness in divine hands did not absolve the faithful of the desire and the necessity to seek and apply natural or human-made cures; however, God remained the essential and ultimate healer, as Cotton Mather's report on Theophilus Eaton, co-founder of New Haven Colony, exemplifies:

> But by the difficulties attending these journies, Mr. Eaton brought himself into an extream sickness; from which he recovered not without a fistula in his breast, whereby he underwent much affliction. When the *chirurgeon* came to inspect the sore, he told him, "Sir, I know not how to go about what is necessary for your cure;" but Mr. Eaton answered him, "God calls you to do, and me to suffer!" And God accordingly strengthened him to bear miserable cuttings and launcings of his flesh

---

[51] For the role and functions of providence in English Protestantism, see Alexandra Walsham, *Providence in Early Modern England*, (Oxford: Oxford UP, 1999); Keith Thomas, *Religion and the Decline of Magic: Studies in Popular Beliefs in Sixteenth and Seventeenth-Century England* (1971; New York: Penguin, 1982) 91-132. New England perspectives are investigated in Michael P. Winship, *Seers of God: Puritan Providentialism in the Restoration and Early Enlightenment* (Baltimore: Johns Hopkins UP, 2000); Hall 77-94; Perry Miller, *The New England Mind: The Seventeenth Century* (New York: Macmillan, 1939) 15-18.

with a most invincible patience. The *chirurgeon* indeed *made* so many wounds, that he was not able to *cure* what he had made; another, and a better, hand was necessarily imployed for it; but in the mean while great were the *trials* with which the God of heaven exercised the faith of this his holy servant.[52]

In light of the realities of surgical interventions in the seventeenth century, Mather's report functioned as an advertisement for placing human fate in God's hands. Before the introduction of anesthesia and aseptic techniques in the mid-nineteenth century, surgery was a gruesome undertaking that had to be limited to minor interventions and medical emergencies, e.g., phlebotomy, lancing, amputation, lithotomy, teeth extraction, bone setting, and wound treatment. These operations caused a rise in morbidity and mortality rates and necessitated a culture of indifference to suffering among those who practiced surgery at the time. Hence, Mather's invocation to trust "another, and a better, hand" is more than a mere compensation for bodily pain; it highlights the inadequacy of medical procedures without the help of God and dichotomizes the surgical culture of *indifference to* pain with a religious culture of *redemption through* pain.[53]

As Mather's *Magnalia Christi Americana* (1702) continues to report, one of the most prominent surgeons in early New England was Samuel Fuller, passenger onboard the *Mayflower* and among the region's best-trained medical practitioners for almost one hundred years. Equipped with a Bible, a few handbooks, and a medicine cabinet, Fuller treated the array of illnesses afflicting Plymouth settlers as well as neighboring colonists and Natives. In 1628 and 1630, John Endecott (Salem) and John Winthrop (Charlestown/Boston) sent for Fuller's medical

---

[52] Mather, *Magnalia* I:152 (emphasis original).

[53] Pain, as a human experience that proved highly influential for illness narratives, will be discussed in more detail at various points in the following sections and chapters. For a useful introduction to the significance and ubiquity of pain in colonial times, see E. F. Crane, "'I have suffer'd much today': The Defining Force of Pain in Early America," *Through a Glass Darkly: Reflections on Personal Identity in Early America*, ed. Ronald Hoffman, Mechal Sobel, and Fredrika J. Teute (Williamsburg: Omohundro Institute of Early American History and Culture, 1997) 370-403.

assistance of newly arrived settlers. In answering the governors' requests, Fuller helped to unite the emerging colonies; the experience of sharing and applying medical knowledge, as part of a broader array of cultural practices brought from England, strengthened the colonial body (politic).[54]

One may assume that Fuller's greatest medical challenge occurred immediately after the arrival of the *Mayflower* when the Pilgrims, having relied mostly on dried and salted foods and having traveled on an overcrowded ship for almost three months, suffered from nutritional disorders (scurvy and beriberi) and communicable diseases (influenza and typhus).[55] After reaching Plymouth in December 1620, many had died and the majority of the remaining passengers were weak, branded by sickness, fearful of the challenges ahead, and hence in no condition to embark on an "errand into the wilderness." Significantly, the first dwelling which the Pilgrims built during their first grim New England winter was a communal sickroom, used for treating *Mayflower* passengers. William Bradford, relating the scene of sickness and death ensuing arrival, noted:

> So as there died some times two or three of a day in the foresaid time, that of 100 and odd persons, scarce fifty remained. And of these, in the time of most distress, there was but six or seven sound persons who [...] with abundance of toil and hazard of their own health, fetched them

---

[54] Fuller had spent eleven years in Leyden before settling in Plymouth. Even though no records exist, it seems more than likely that he attended at least some of the (public) medical lectures at Leyden University, which housed one of the most prestigious medical programs in Europe at the time. Henry R. Viets, *A Brief History of Medicine in Massachusetts* (Boston: Houghton, 1930) 9-17. For an additional overview of Fuller's life and work, see Thomas F. Harrington, "Dr. Samuel Fuller, of the Mayflower (1620), the Pioneer Physician," *The Johns Hopkins Hospital Bulletin* 14 (October 1903): 263-270; Norman Gevitz, "Samuel Fuller of Plymouth Plantation: A 'Skillful Physician' or 'Quacksalver,'" *Journal of the History of Medicine* 47 (1992): 29-48.

[55] The story of the *Mayflower's* journey and arrival, as well as the ensuing fate and endeavors of its passengers has been told and retold numerous times. For a recent account, see Nathaniel Philbrick, *Mayflower: A Story of Courage, Community, and War* (New York: Penguin, 2006) 3-120.

wood, made them fires, dressed them meat, made their beds, washed their loathsome clothes, clothed and unclothed them.[56]

The Plymouth chronicler retroactively signs the heroic beginning of English settlement, and thus colonialism proper, by a language of hardship and suffering. Suspended in a state between life and death, the arrival scene described by Bradford conveys the uncanniness and insecurity at the outset of sustained English colonialism in North America. Illness thus obstructs a religious reading of arrival in terms of deliverance and induces a lingering sense of doubt and vulnerability. At the same time, Bradford's after-the-fact report about nursing and caring for the sick reveals a pragmatic optimism that is energized by a firm belief in the providential mission of the *Mayflower* passengers.[57]

Many early colonists encountered an environment that proved unfavorable to their health. Until approximately 1640, English newcomers and settlers frequently suffered from diseases caused by dietetic deficiencies, a harsh environment, and/or contact among each other: stomach aches, fluxes, smallpox, malaria, respiratory disorders, and pestilential fevers were among the most common afflictions in the colonies.[58] And even though babies born in New England later on had a higher chance of reaching adulthood than babies in Europe, during the first decades of colonization, morbidity and mortality rates, especially among children, were particularly high, partly because the basic

---

[56] Bradford 77.

[57] For an insightful reading of Bradford's rendition of the Pilgrims' arrival, see Kathleen Donegan, "'As Dying, Yet Behold We Live': Catastrophe and Interiority in Bradford's *Of Plymouth Plantation*," *Early American Literature* 37.1 (2002): 9-37. For a reading of the initial landfall, see, among many others, David Laurence, "William Bradford's American Sublime," *PMLA* 102.1 (1987): 55-65; Ursula Brumm, "Transfer and Arrival in the Narratives of the First Immigrants to New England," *The Transit of Civilization from Europe to America: Essays in Honor of Hans Galinsky*, ed. Winfried Herget and Karl Ortseifen (Tübingen: Narr, 1986) 29-36; Ulrike Brunotte, *Puritanismus und Pioniergeist. Zur Faszination der Wildnis im frühen Neu-England* (Berlin: De Gruyter, 2000).

[58] Duffy, *Healers* 9-12.

infrastructure of settlement (housing, roads, fields, wells) and public health measures (legislation, educated physicians) were still developing.[59]

Some early observers explained the general health difficulties among settlers during the founding decades of New England by invoking body concepts embedded in humoral theory and natural philosophy. According to the Galenic/Hippocratic tradition, health rested on a precarious connection between the four humors, human behavior, and the environment. Hence, the notion that there existed a powerful relationship between place and disease caused profound anxieties about English bodies moving to another location.[60] William Bradford, for example, reported how Protestants, in considering the advantages and disadvantages of permanent removal to the "New World," feared that that the climate in North America would disturb the precarious equilibrium of humors, moisture, and temperature in the English body, thus rendering it more susceptible to illnesses.[61] The idea that the translocation to America and the particularities of the New England environment had mental effects (producing fears and anxieties about leaving home and beginning a new life in an unknown land) as well as corporeal repercussions (the body adapting to a different surrounding) for the colonists was common among early commentators. Many believed that English bodies needed up to two years to adjust to "the rigors of untried climate" as well as to the new physical and socio-cultural environment, a process that was often referred to as "seasoning."[62]

---

[59] Ernest Caulfield, "Some Common Diseases of Colonial Children," *Publications of the Colonial Society of Massachusetts* 25 (1942): 4-65.

[60] For a more extensive discussion, see Andrew Wear, "Place, Health, and Disease: The Airs, Waters, Places Tradition in Early Modern England and North America," *Journal of Medieval & Early Modern Studies* 38.3 (2008): 443-465.

[61] Bradford 26.

[62] John Endecott, quoted in Harrington 268. For a more sustained analysis of how the English conceptualized the North American environment in relation to their bodies, see Karen Ordahl Kupperman, "Fear of Hot Climates in the Anglo-American Colonial Experience," *The William and Mary Quarterly* 41.2 (1984):

Other English writers discarded these and other anxieties about translocation and, instead, advertised America as beneficial to English health, especially when compared to urban areas in Europe. Francis Higginson's 1629 description of the New England environment marks a typical example of geographic boosterism, an attempt to encourage settlement by highlighting the region's conduciveness to health:

> there is hardly a more healthfull place to be found in the World that agreeth better with our English Bodyes. Many that have beene weake and sickly in old England, by comming hither have beene thoroughly healed and growne healthfull and strong. For here is an extraordinarie cleere and dry Aire that is of a most healing nature to all such as are of a Cold, Melancholy, Flegmatick, Reumaticke temper of body.[63]

Indeed, beginning in the second half of the seventeenth century, colonial New England witnessed a temporary increase in fertility, immigration, and life expectancy, which led to a significant rise in

---

213-240 & "The Puzzle of the American Climate in the Early Colonial Period," *American Historical Review* 87 (1982): 1262-1289.

[63] Francis Higginson, *New-England's Plantation. Or, A Short and True Description of the Commodities and Discommodities of that Countrey* (1630; Early English Books Online, STC 1352:04) 9. In a similar vein, William Wood regarded the "medicineable Climate" of New England (9) as one of many reasons for migrating to New England. In 1630, John Winthrop wrote to his son in England: "these Afflictions we have mett with need discourage none, for the Country is exceeding good, and the climate verye like our owne." John Winthrop to John Winthrop, Jr., 23 July 1630, *Winthrop Papers* II, 306. For a more elaborate celebratory account of the New England climate, see John White, *The Planters Plea, Or The Grounds of Plantations Examined, and Usuall Objections Answered* (1630; Early English Books Online, 25399). However, as with all early reports one has to be aware of the reality of news doctoring, in which colonial officials such as John Winthrop and others ensured that certain information about unfavorable conditions and developments of life in New England were omitted from correspondences with benefactors and potential emigrants in England. Cf. Robert C. Black, *The Younger John Winthrop* (New York: Columbia UP, 1966) 49.

population numbers.[64] But although the overall health of the colonists improved around 1650, disparities among villages remained. As Cotton Mather noted, "[p]estilential sicknesses have made fearful havock in divers places, where the *sound* perhaps have not been enough to tend the *sick*; while others have not had one touch from that *angel of death*."[65] Mather does not offer an explanation for these health disparities but vaguely argues that illness is caused by divine anger about human "carelessness" and "wickedness."[66] In doing so, he chooses to leave the mysteries of divine providence hidden from human understanding, refusing, as he does on several occasions in his history of New England, to disclose whether prayer or medicine protected colonists from certain death. Such a stance not only insinuates that providence works in mysterious and arbitrary ways but, moreover, aims to ensure that colonists continue to seek solace in Christ and thereby to uphold the power of congregational churches.

Preachers such as Cotton Mather played an important role in medicine throughout the history of Christianity. Because the division of labor between priests and physicians that was emerging in post-Renaissance Europe was not feasible in early New England—a region that failed to attract professional physicians from the mother country until the early eighteenth century—many colonial ministers attended to both the spiritual and the corporeal needs of their congregations. In her seminal study on the cultural phenomenon of the preacher-physician in early New England, Patricia Watson explains that "[t]he clergy, as the authorized interpreters of the exclusive faith, felt it their sacred duty to familiarize themselves with the epidemics, as well as the individual

---

[64] Grob (61) points out that the initial mortality rate in the first sustained Puritan settlements, Salem (est. 1628-1629) and Charlestown (est. 1630) ranged between approximately 21 percent and 30 percent, respectively. By 1660, however, the health conditions in established Puritan settlements had improved significantly. Infant and child mortality ranged around 25 percent and was thus lower than in Europe at the time. In addition, life expectancy rose substantially: a male adult, having reached 21 years, could expect to celebrate his 69th birthday (Grob 50-55).

[65] Mather, *Magnalia* I:88 (emphasis original).

[66] Mather, *Magnalia* I:92.

ailments, of their parishioners so that they could interpret and justify God's will to the community."[67] This "angelical conjunction," the combination of religious and secular duties of the New England preacher-physician, was not only a result of the intertwinement of faith and healing rooted in Christian theology; the reasons for striving for the double occupation were also quite worldly because medical practice often constituted a means of improving meager clerical salaries.[68] Since New England preachers expected periods of low or no income and because medical knowledge could be a criterion for ordination especially in communities lacking healing experts, many chose to supplement their studies of divinity by reading medicine. With their combination of theological doctrines and proto-scientific knowledge, some preacher-physicians had to struggle with congregations whose members resisted the prescribed remedies and adhered to folk healing, a tradition that the clergy viewed with suspicion because of its perceived grounding in superstition.

At the same time, visits to individual members of a community allowed many preacher-physicians to disseminate their specific medicinal knowledge among the laity and, in doing so, to cement the hegemony of the church in body matters.[69] As part of his clerical duties, the local minister was also responsible for relating information on

[67] Patricia Ann Watson, *The Angelical Conjunction: The Preacher-Physicians of Colonial New England* (Knoxville: U of Tennessee P, 1991) 9. For short biographical sketches of noted medical practitioners in seventeenth-century New England, among them a number of minister-physicians, see James Thacher, *American Medical Biography: Or Memoirs of Eminent Physicians Who Have Flourished in America* (Boston: Richardson & Lord, 1828) 17-19.

[68] Mather, *Magnalia* I:493. For reasons of practicability, New England pastor-physicians avoided a public debate about whether their double calling (i.e., ministry and medicine) was compatible with scripture. John Cotta, *A Short Discouerie of the Vnobserued Dangers of Seuerall Sorts of Ignorant and Vnconsiderate Practisers of Physicke in England* (1612; Early English Books Online, STC 5833) 89. For the tradition of priest-physicians in rural England, see Charles Webster, "English Medical Reformers of the Puritan Revolution: A Background to the 'Society of Chymical Physitians,'" *Ambix* 14.1 (1967): 21-22.

[69] Ola Elizabeth Winslow, *A Destroying Angel: The Conquest of Smallpox in Colonial Boston* (Boston: Houghton, 1974) 15; Watson 42.

diseases and epidemics to his parishioners during church services. This information, as well as knowledge about new treatment methods, were often obtained through a communicational exchange network with colleagues in other towns.[70] Minister-physicians could, however, also function as agents of contagion during their visits to the sick and their frequent contacts with other members of the local and regional community. In outlining the duties of ministers "to 'Visit the Sick,' in times of Epidemical and Contagious Distempers," Cotton Mather attempts to balance the physical and, more importantly, spiritual needs of a congregation with the health of its minister. Aware that visitations of those afflicted with a contagious disease could potentially cause an infection of the minister, he alleviates men of the cloth of their duty to visit the sick in certain cases and advises modes of long-distance healing (i.e., prayer). If, however, a parishioner asks to relieve his/her conscience before dying, then the minister must attend the sick, resting assured that God would protect him in this endeavor. The minister, once he enters the sickroom of his parishioner, lays aside his primary public function (ministering to the congregation) and henceforth engages in "private services." These, however, become imminently public in cases of epidemic diseases, when a minister is called to visit several if not most households of his congregation.[71]

One of the most prominent seventeenth-century minister-physicians was Thomas Thacher, who arrived in Boston in 1635 at the age of 15, became minister at Weymouth in 1645 and of Boston's Third Church in 1669. Revered by Cotton Mather for his exceptional ability "to make *natural* and *spiritual* health accompany each other," Thacher's claim to historical fame rested primarily on having written the first medical publication in colonial New England after a smallpox epidemic had

---

[70] Watson 81-82, 95-96. Although Watson provides some useful insights into the practices and thoughts of New England preacher-physicians, she explains Puritan medicine exclusively within the confines of New England culture, as if all cures were derived from Europe and not from other sources of knowledge, e.g., Native Americans or Africans.

[71] Mather, *Magnalia* II:250.

reached Boston with particular severity in July 1677.[72] In his broadside on smallpox and measles, posted for all to read, the suggested treatments draw significantly on the English physician Thomas Sydenham (*Methodus curandi febres*, 1668), who was well known on both sides of the Atlantic for his unobtrusive medical prescriptions. Thacher's recommendation to apply rest, cordials, and a light diet and to avoid early bloodletting, purging, and sweating are strikingly commonsensical and almost devoid of religious overtones. Although it ends with a formulaic reference to the guiding hand of God, the publication illustrates a pragmatic rather than an exclusively religious approach to illness.

Despite the lack of religious instruction as a means of treating disease, however, Thacher's identification and depiction of smallpox bears significant social and theological allusions. Much as God employs disease as a natural means to sever "the impure from the pure [blood particles]," so He has set in motion a socio-religious process of separating pure Christians from corrupt Anglicans and Roman Catholics, establishing the former as the true body of God's Church and the latter as its pathologized Other.[73] Yet, this separation, achieved by migrating to New England, does not ensure infinite earthly bliss for the settlers. Hence, Thacher's publication instructs its audience how to read disease symptoms as signs indicating the chances of recovery, implying that if they are low, patients should consider their afflictions in providential terms and prepare for imminent death.

Despite the virtual absence of secular, university-trained physicians in seventeenth-century New England, colonists living in larger settlements were often able to choose from a variety of medical practitioners, ranging from ministers, barber-surgeons, and midwives to apothecaries, bloodletters, and "cunning folk." American medicine lacked public hospitals, education, and professionalization until the

---

[72] Mather, *Magnalia* I:494 (emphasis original). Other prominent minister-physicians treated in Mather's *Magnalia Christi Americana* include John Fisk (I:476-480) and John Ward (I:521-524).

[73] Thomas Thacher, *A Brief Rule to Guide the Common-People of New-England How to Order Themselves and Their in the Small Pocks, or Measles* (1677/78; Baltimore: Johns Hopkins P, 1937).

eighteenth century. Therefore, anyone who read a few books or served a seasoned medical expert as an apprentice could call himself "doctor" and practice "physick" in colonial New England.[74] Such a non-regulated system of healers was prone to abuse. As early as 1631, Massachusetts Bay officials attempted to control deviant medical practices, when they fined Nicholas Knopp (or Knapp) five pounds "for takeing upon him to cure the scurvey by a water of noe worth nor value, which hee sold att a very deare rate."[75] And in 1647 the General Court followed a suggestion by Reverend John Eliot to regulate the craft and practice of medicine by recommending future physicians and surgeons "to reade anatomy, and to anatomize once in foure yeares some malefactor" and two years later ordered that

> no person or persons whatsoever that are implied about the bodies of men, weomen, or children, for preservation of life or health, (as phisitians, chirurgions, midwifes, or others,) presume to exercise or put forth any act contrary to the knowne rules of art, nor exercise any force, violence, or cruelty upon or towards the body of any, whether yong or ould, (no, not in the most difficult or desperate cases), without the advice and consent of such as are skilfull in the same art, if such may be had, or at least of the wisest and gravest then present, and consent of the patient

---

[74] Next to Sydenham, the most popular medical authority for seventeenth-century New England practitioners was the astrological physician Nicholas Culpeper, especially his *Pharamacopoeia Londinensis; or the London Dispensatory* (1653), *The English Physician* (1652), and *Medicaments for the Poor, or Physick for the Common People* (1656). For a typical example of other popular medical handbooks printed in England and available in the colonies, see Owen Wood, *An Alphabetical Book of Physicall Secrets* (1639; Early English Books Online, STC 25955). Many colonists, especially in rural areas, also relied on almanacs (the first one was issued in 1647), whose medical sections often included information on herbs, treatment methods, and astrology. For the cultural significance of almanacs, see Hall 58-61; Francisco Guerra, *American Medical Bibliography, 1639-1783* (New York: Harper, 1962) 14-15; F. N. L. Poynter, "Nicholas Culpeper and the Paracelsians," *Science, Medicine and Society in the Renaissance: Essays to Honor Walter Pagel*, vol. 1, ed. Allen G. Debus (London: Heinemann, 1972) 201-220.

[75] Quoted in Edmund S. Morgan, *The Puritan Dilemma: The Story of John Winthrop*, 3rd ed. (New York: Pearson Longman, 2007) 89.

or patients, if they be mentis compotes, much lesse contrary to such advice and consent upon such punishment as the nature of the fact may deserve; [...].[76]

By issuing a colonial variation of the Hippocratic oath, leaders sought to institutionalize a medical code of conduct as well as distinct medical fields. In recognizing the presence of an unspecified group of medical Others (including quacks and Indian doctors), the decree exerted authority over unregulated, un-orthodox medicine that appealed especially to poor and rural segments of the population. While this instance of biopolitical control was relatively successful in Boston, its enforcement proved more difficult in frontier regions of New England. There especially, the urban European distinction between physicians, who entertained medical theories and treated internal illnesses, surgeons, who did the blood work and thus ranked below physicians in the medical pecking order, and apothecaries, who prepared medicines prescribed by doctors, was virtually non-existent. The realities of medical practice in fact varied considerably across New England. Whereas the colonial center, Boston, housed a relatively broad and diversified medical scene by 1700, rural settlements frequently had to rely on preachers, itinerant healers, and midwives to treat common illnesses.[77]

---

[76] *Records of the Governor and Company of the Massachusetts Bay in New England, Vol. 2, 1642-1649*, ed. Nathaniel B. Shurtleff (Boston: White, 1853) 201, 278-279. For similarly sporadic legislative measures to maintain or restore the public health in early New England (e.g., sanitary laws, quarantine regulations, food laws, and days of fasting) see John Duffy, *The Sanitarians: A History of American Public Health* (Urbana: U of Illinois P, 1990) 9-19; John B. Blake, *Public Health in the Town of Boston, 1630-1822* (Cambridge, MA: Harvard UP, 1959) 1-22. For the (minor) role of anatomy in early New England medicine, see Watson 134-139.

[77] This is not to say that health services *per se* were less available in rural than in urban sections of New England. As Eric Christianson points out, due to a lower population density and a comparatively large number of doctors traveling the country-side, many rural New Englanders actually had better access to health care than their compatriots in larger settlements (56). For the origins of the medical profession in Old and New England, see Richard Harrison Shryock,

In light of the relative scarcity of trained physicians in the early modern period, non-expert healers often administered medical care on both sides of the Atlantic domestically. As James H. Cassedy explains, "English people at home, particularly in rural areas, had always doctored themselves according to traditional practices, old family recipes, and local herbal lore," before resorting to more professional help.[78] This pattern persisted in colonial America, especially in frontier settings, where the necessity for self-reliance suffused daily lives and where lay medicine was disseminated through almanacs, popular handbooks, and by way of mouth. As will be shown in more detail in chapter three, women were often the main distributors of this medical knowledge and practice: they planted medical herbs, prepared poultices and concoctions, nurtured the ill, attended childbirths, and functioned as links between patients and doctors, when domestic treatment of illness proved insufficient.[79]

Lay medical practices rested to large degrees on European folk traditions, which, once transplanted to the "New World," proved quite compatible with, and susceptible to, indigenous applications of herbs and charms. Whether folk and/or Native healing methods, both of which relied on practices that a devout Protestant would consider as superstition, were tolerated in a given English settlement often depended on the presence of a minister and his acceptance by the congregation. As David Hall has shown, the common men and women of New England, especially those living close to the frontier, developed a rather pragmatic approach to healing, one that often entailed an eclectic fusion of orthodox rituals and methods drawn from accepted medicine and from folk traditions.[80]

*Medicine and Society in America, 1660-1860* (New York: New York UP, 1960) 1-18.

[78] Cassedy 11.

[79] Rebecca J. Tannenbaum, "The Housewife as Healer: Medicine as Women's Work in Colonial New England," *Women's Work in New England, 1620-1920. Annual Proceedings of the Dublin Seminar for New England Folklife* (Boston: Boston UP, 2003) 160-169.

[80] Hall 202. Morton (152-153) indicates that colonists also sought the help of Native healers. See also David Dary, *Frontier Medicine: From the Atlantic to*

While it is impossible to trace conclusively the exchanges between and betwixt colonial medicine and indigenous healing techniques, it is evident that the increasing contacts after 1600 changed medical practices on both sides of the cultural divide. In many instances, Native expertise about the curative and nutritional properties of plants exceeded that of their English neighbors, who, almost immediately after making landfall, explored the woods in search for raw materials, food, and soil, but also for medicinal plants. Because their own medical practices by and large rested on botanical therapeutics, many colonists considered indigenous acquaintance with plants as potentially valuable knowledge. For example, in 1603, the English explorer Martin Pring built a small fort near modern-day Truro (Cape Cod) to harvest sassafras, which Europeans found useful for treating syphilis and for cleansing the body. In the ensuing decades, some Native medicinal plants were appropriated by the emerging capitalist order of Europe, where angelica, guaiacum, tobacco, sarsaparilla, and many other herbs, roots, and barks became sought-after health commodities.

Whereas most New Englanders viewed Algonquian cultural practices with disdain, some realized the potential of indigenous knowledge and turned to Native healers for help and advice. One of the most striking depictions of indigenous medicinal knowledge is provided in John Josselyn's *New-England's Rarities Discovered* (1672) and *Two Voyages* (1674), based on his travels in 1638 and 1663. Rather than a mere inventory of New England plants and animals, Josselyn's observations describe a world of cross-cultural medical exchange: Algonquians acquired European medical knowledge and adopted imported plants such as dandelion, mullein, shepherd's purse, tansy or plantain to treat various afflictions. Conversely, some English settlers adopted indigenous plant applications, especially if they lived at the periphery of the colony, where the influence of colonial officials and European medical science was less pronounced.[81] English attempts to

---

*the Pacific, 1492-1941* (New York: Knopf, 2008) 37. For the spatial circumference and limitation of clerical power and influence in New England, see Hall 16-17.

[81] John Josselyn, *New-England's Rarities Discovered in Birds, Beasts, Fishes, Serpents, and Plants of that Country* (1672; Early English Books Online, J1093)

appropriate curative knowledge from Native people were grounded in the European conviction that every region of the world housed site-specific maladies that could (only) be cured by remedies found there.[82]

Despite the compatibility of indigenous botanical knowledge with English and early American medicine, certain aspects of Native healing approaches were either inassimilable or only tacitly integrated into Anglo-American medicine in the course of the seventeenth and eighteenth centuries. As pointed out earlier, English physicians, whose healing methods were embedded in Christian theology, vilified Native Americans for their reliance on rituals and supernatural healing. In

41-91; Josselyn, *Two Voyages* 59-82. Other references evincing the integration of Native New England remedies can be found in Palmer, *passim*; John Lederer, *The Discoveries of John Lederer*, ed. William P. Cumming (Charlottesville: U of Virginia P, 1958) 36-37. Vogel cites over 170 drugs which Anglo-Americans had adapted from North American tribes by 1890 (267-414). By 1920, about 30 Native New England natural curatives were (still) part of the official pharmacology of the United States. For specific examples of indigenous medicinal plants adopted by English settlers, see Josselyn, *Two Voyages* 69-76 and *New-England's Rarities* 52-66. An often-cited instance of a Native New England healer, who helped English settlers, is Joe Pye, who administered a cure for typhus fever (Vogel 119). See also, Josselyn, *New-England's Rarities* 61-62. For the "infection" of heterodoxy in New England fringe settlements, see Carla Gardina Pestana, *Quakers and Baptists in Colonial Massachusetts* (Cambridge: Cambridge UP, 1991) 8.

[82] Martha Robinson, "New Worlds, New Medicines: Indian Remedies and English Medicine in Early America," *Early American Studies* 3.1 (2005): 98-100. Unaccustomed to the abundance of snakes in colonial New England and other parts of North America, English settlers were especially interested in the Indians' application of snakeroot. Almost all English medical practitioners used a native plant known as puke weed or Indian tobacco (*lobelia inflate*) for treating food poisoning and asthma (Christianson 65). In contrast, Vogel claims that early New Englanders did not pay much attention to Native healing methods, pointing out that "[p]erhaps the gulf separating the Pilgrim and Puritan saints from the 'Salvage Hounds' who inhabited the forests was too wide to permit interest in any aspect of their culture" (39-40). This assumption is contradicted by, among others, Bradford, Williams, Winslow, Wood, and Josselyn, who repeatedly record early colonists' interest in indigenous cultural knowledge, especially when its practicability was evident.

addition, indigenous approaches to health lacked medical theories comparable to the ones that emerged in the "Old World" at the time of contact.[83] Although still steeped in religious premises, Galenic humoralism, and folk tradition, Western medicine was beginning to shift from spiritualism to rationalism and by the late eighteenth century, it had "defined itself in opposition to the presumed irrationality and superstition of indigenous medicine," as David Arnold observes.[84] In British America, the continuing colonial disavowal and misrecognition of Native healing methods is exemplified by Benjamin Rush, co-signer of the Declaration of Independence and prominent Philadelphia physician, who proclaimed: "We have no discoveries in the *material medica* to hope for from North American Natives. It would be a reproach to our school of physic, if modern physicians were not more successful than the Indians, even in the treatment of their own disease."[85] Despite his intellectual curiosity that led him to study American Indian medicine in the first place, Rush's statement is typical of how Anglo-American cultural bias and the overestimation of Western medicine had precluded systematic investigations of indigenous approaches to healing. It also illustrates how by the end of the colonial period, indigenous knowledge and bodies had been relegated to the fringes of an emerging American society and culture. The foundational narrative of this society and culture rested in part on the seemingly apparent health disparities and on the medicalization of perceived cultural differences between Natives and newcomers, a tradition of thought that had accompanied English colonization of North America from its beginnings.

[83] For a recent study of early Anglo-Native exchanges of medical theories, see Kelly Wisecup, *Communicating Disease: Medical Knowledge and Literary Forms in Colonial British America*. Diss. U of Maryland, 2009, esp. 36-88.

[84] David Arnold, "Introduction: Disease, Medicine and Empire," *Imperial Medicine and Indigenous Societies*, ed. David Arnold (Manchester: Manchester UP, 1988) 18.

[85] Benjamin Rush, *An Oration, Delivered February 4, 1774, before the American Philosophical Society, Held at Philadelphia: Containing, an Enquiry into the Natural History of Medicine among the Indians in North-America* (1774; Early American Imprints, Series 1, no. 13592) 60.

Exceptional Bodies: Responses to a Demographic Revolution

In 1605, when the French explorer Samuel de Champlain reached the coast of soon-to-be New England, he prepared a map depicting a healthy and thriving village, which its Native inhabitants called Patuxet.[86] Fifteen years later English separatists and adventurers reached the same village, rejoiced in the absence of dark-skinned and "uncivilized" pagans, unpacked their scarce belongings, and began to build a settlement. It seems unlikely that the Pilgrims would have succeeded in their colonial endeavor if the aboriginal villages in the area had remained as intact as Champlain's map indicates. The settlers' "fortune" rested primarily on a crossfire of disease which had reduced the indigenous population of New England from approximately 90,000 to 9,000 shortly before the *Mayflower* arrived.[87] No written Native accounts of the land-clearing epidemics are available. Yet, drawing on reports by French and English sailors who explored the Eastern seaboard of North America and/or fished in the area during the early decades of the seventeenth century, recent scholarship has been able to assemble many pieces of an historical disease puzzle. The sailors' reports that reached England after 1616 present a contact scenario characterized by illness and death, and thereby illustrate the overlaps between disease transmission and flows of people, commerce, and culture from Europe to the Americas during the early modern period.[88]

---

[86] William L. Grant, *Voyages of Samuel de Champlain 1604-1618* (New York: Scribner's Sons, 1907) 71-73.

[87] Bragdon 25. These figures have to be viewed with caution because they represent estimates rather than solid data. The pre-contact number is based on seventeenth-century calculations undertaken by Daniel Gookin and has generally been accepted by modern experts. In the recent past, however, the degree of Native depopulation in the wake of European colonialism has been subject to heated debates, which are often undergirded by political and ideological motives. See, Charles C. Mann, *1491: New Revelations of the Americas Before Columbus* (New York: Vintage, 2005) 102-118.

[88] The gauntlet of disease had fostered European colonization of the "New World" since Columbus and, especially, since Cortes' conquest of Mexico in 1519-1521. The fate of the indigenous population was similar throughout the

The discrepancy between early descriptions of idyllic Native habitations and later accounts of dying villages is striking, especially when one considers how little time had passed between these two kinds of reports. In 1614 John Smith echoed Champlain's account by noting prospering Algonquian settlements along the Atlantic coast. Exploring the islands in the Massachusetts Bay, he marveled at a region "planted with Gardens and Corne fields, and so well inhabited with a goodly, strong and well proportioned people [...] who can but approove this a most excellent place, both for health & fertility?"[89] Only two years later, Ferdinando Gorges, an English colonial entrepreneur sailing the coast of Maine offered a radically different report. He testified that the local Algonquians "were sore afflicted with the Plague, for that the Country was in a manner left void of Inhabitants."[90] In 1619, the Englishman Thomas Dermer wrote in a similar vein: "I passed alongst the Coast where I found some antient Plantations, not long since populous now utterly void; in other places a remnant remains, but not free of sicknesse. Their disease was the Plague, for wee might perceive the sore of some that had escaped, who described the spots of such as usually die."[91]

Western Hemisphere: imported diseases decimated and paralyzed the Native population; after a short epidemiological respite, new diseases attacked, making concerted military resistance against colonization virtually impossible. See, for instance, Tzvetan Todorov, *The Conquest of America: The Question of the Other*, trans. Richard Howard (New York: Harper, 1984) 133-138; Mann 68-102.

[89] John Smith, *A Description of New England; or, Observations and Discoveries in the North of America in the Year of our Lord 1614* (Boston: William Veazie, 1865) 28.

[90] Ferdinando Gorges, "A Briefe Narration of the Originall Undertakings of the Advancement of Plantations into the Parts of America (1658)," *Sir Ferdinando Gorges and his Province of Maine, Vol. II*, ed. James Phinney Baxter (Boston: Prince Society, 1890) 19.

[91] Thomas Dermer, "To His Worshipfull Friend M. Samuel Purchas, Preacher of the Word, at the Church a Little within Ludgate, London (1619)," *Sailors Narratives of Voyages along the New England Coast, 1524-1624*, ed. George Winship Parker (Boston: Houghton, 1905) 247. Salisbury states that the Pilgrims carried a copy of Dermer's report, which suggested the recently depopulated village of Patuxet/Plymouth as a suitable place to start colonizing the area (109).

Gorges's and Dermer's reports imagine America as an empty land ("void"), a trope which prospective English settlers recognized and echoed in order to justify and explain their colonizing efforts as being in sync with their conceptualizations of natural and civil law as well as with their religious expectations. In 1620, English dissenters were convinced that God had sent what seemed an obvious sign that their destiny was on the other side of the Atlantic Ocean. Ensured that He had answered their prayers by sending a "wonderfull Plague," Puritans and adventurers could finally flee from religious persecution, social marginalization, and economic hardships in their homeland and start anew.[92]

Most scholars agree that the contacts and interactions between Native Americans and English explorers, traders, and settlers initiated an "ecological imperialism" in which disease played a central role.[93] Possibly due to their relative isolation from "Old World" pestilences or to a less heterogeneous gene pool, indigenous people were biologically unprepared for the arrival of members from the immunological "elite" of Europe. According to the dominant explanatory model in American historiography, this "elite" had earned a sufficient degree of resistance to a number of diseases (especially smallpox, measles, typhus, and influenza) after centuries of contact with other peoples from Europe, Africa, and Asia. Other reasons often cited by scholars include

---

[92] Granting a patent to Gorges and the Plymouth (Northern Virginia) Company on 3 November 1620, King James I expressed the official English view on the recent epidemic: "within these late Yeares there hath by God's Visitation raigned a wonderfull Plague, [...] in a Manner to the utter Destruction, Devastacion, and Depopulacion of that whole Territorye, [...] whereby We in our Judgment are persuaded and satisfied that the appointed Time is come in which Almighty God [...] hath thought fitt and determined, that those large and goodly Territoryes, deserted as it were by their naturall Inhabitants, should be possessed and enjoyed by such of our Subjects and People [...]." "Patent of the Council for New England, Nov. 3/13, 1620," *Select Charters and Other Documents Illustrative of American History, 1606-1775*, ed. William MacDonald (New York: Macmillan, 1904) 25. For the relationship between providentialism and pestilences in early modern England, see Walsham 156-166.

[93] Alfred W. Crosby, *Ecological Imperialism: The Biological Expansion of Europe, 900-1900*. 2nd ed. (Cambridge: Cambridge UP, 2004) 195-216.

Europeans' frequent intermarriages outside their immediate group, their comparatively close interaction with livestock, and poor sanitary conditions, particularly in cities.[94]

When English Protestants and their farm animals crossed the Atlantic, especially during the Great Migration (1620-1640), they were, in essence, a teeming infectious multitude that was acutely dangerous to their less immunologically protected neighbors. In New England, at least two major "virgin-soil epidemics" (i.e., communicable diseases which are introduced into a region hitherto unaffected) preceded and accompanied European settlers. The first recorded pandemic induced by colonial exchange occurred from 1616 to 1619 and killed between seventy-five and ninety percent of the coastal population, while sparing most Native settlements in the interior and west of Narragansett Bay (present-day Rhode Island and Connecticut). The exact nature and scope of the calamitous disease(s) is impossible to determine retrospectively; some early reports call it the "plague," others "a sore consumption," while still others claim that Native people turned yellow before dying. Based on these observations and archaeological evidence, historians have speculated that the first lethal epidemic may have been jaundice, influenza, typhoid, yellow fever, chicken pox, viral hepatitis, and/or smallpox.[95]

---

[94] William Cronon explains: "What the Indians lacked was not so much *genetic* protection from Eurasian disease [...] as the historical experience as a population to maintain *acquired* immunities from generation to generation [...]." *Changes in the Land: Indians, Colonists, and the Ecology of New England* (New York: Hill, 1983) 85 (emphasis original). Cf. Mann 112-118.

[95] Alfred W. Crosby, "'God ... Would Destroy Them, and Give Their Country to Another People,'" *American Heritage* 29 (1978): 38-43, speculates that either typhus or the plague caused Native depopulation before the arrival of the Pilgrims; Arthur E. Spiess and Bruce D. Spiess, "New England Pandemic of 1616-1622: Cause and Archaeological Implication," *Man in the Northeast* 34 (1987): 71-83, argue in favor of hepatitis; Dean R. Snow and Kim M. Lanphear, "European Contact and Indian Depopulation in the Northeast: The Timing of the First Epidemics," *Ethnohistory* 35.1 (1988): 15-33 and Timothy L. Bratton, "The Identity of the New England Indian Epidemic of 1616-19," *Bulletin of the History of Medicine* 62 (1988): 351-383, consider smallpox as the most likely candidate. It seems probable that the indigenous population was decimated by an

In 1633, Algonquians living near Windsor, Connecticut were among the first group of Indians faced with a second wave of epidemics. This time, Native Americans were afflicted by smallpox, which had been introduced in the Western Hemisphere by Spanish conquistadors in 1518 and continued to spread in seventeenth-century New England due to growing commercial contacts with Europe, Africa, and the Caribbean.[96] Transmitted from one individual to another by droplets of moisture expelled from the upper respiratory tract, by contact with pustules on the skin or by exposure to contaminated cloth, smallpox proved the most detrimental disease for Algonquian communities, reaching epidemic proportion in 1633-1634. Forced to witness helplessly how their villages succumbed to a particularly malignant strain of *variola major*, many Natives, most likely in panic, escaped to other settlements and thereby unwittingly fueled the disease, which soon ravaged indigenous communities from New England to the Great Lakes region and the St. Lawrence River valley. Because smallpox was frequently exacerbated by respiratory infections and gastrointestinal disorders, the epidemic had an estimated mortality rate of ninety percent among the already

unspecified combination of several European diseases hitherto unknown in the Americas. Cf. Sherburne F. Cook, "The Significance of Disease in the Extinction of the New England Indians," *Human Biology* 45 (1973): 458-508.

[96] The exact origins of epidemic illnesses and routes of transmission cannot be conclusively traced. Due to the relatively long voyage to America during the seventeenth century, the Atlantic Ocean functioned as a filter for a number of diseases which had already run their course before a ship reached soil. While endemic illnesses (e.g., respiratory ailments, digestive disorders, or venereal diseases) remained nonvirulent on ships from Europe and were often transferred to Native Americans after arrival, epidemic diseases such as smallpox and measles were most likely first introduced via northern fur-trading regions and the Caribbean (Cronon 86). A useful historical overview of smallpox outbreaks in colonial America is provided by John Duffy, "Smallpox and the Indians in the American Colonies," *Bulletin of the History of Medicine* 25 (1951): 324-341; Elizabeth A. Fenn, *Pox Americana: The Great Smallpox Epidemic of 1775-82* (New York: Hill, 2001) 13-43.

decimated Native New England population, with only a few English casualties.[97]

Seventeenth-century Algonquians, as well as many other American Indians previously and afterwards, were unprepared to cope with the imported epidemics—many of which had been childhood diseases in Europe—both physically and culturally: their medical repositories lacked sufficient treatment methods, their system of caring for the sick, which included familial gatherings at the bedside of the afflicted, fostered contamination and collapsed as the disease took its toll, and survivors were paralyzed and traumatized by the horrors they had to face. As a consequence, fields were left untended, hunts canceled, kinship networks destroyed, causing many hungry survivors to seek food, shelter, and companionship in neighboring Algonquian villages, which were often equally struck by epidemics. In short, the introduction of European diseases destroyed the foundations of a subsistence economy, leading to a growing dependence on trade with Europeans (especially fur), which in turn increased the transfer of pathogens, created new political alliances and causes for violence, and further destroyed the traditional socio-cultural fabric of indigenous communities.[98]

Aside from setting in motion a vicious circle of socio-political disorganization, cultural declension, and economic realignment, the two major epidemical waves elicited complex responses and explanations on both sides of the New England cultural divide. In Native and English communities, the meanings of disease relied significantly on social determinants and cultural trajectories that were similar in certain respects while incompatible in others. Because Algonquians and

---

[97] Bragdon 26-28. Grob asserts that the relative genetic homogeneity of Native Americans contributed to the high mortality rate because once a virus has adapted to the immune response of one person, it becomes more virulent in other persons who are genetically similar. In addition, the lack of knowledge about methods of contagion and the fact that Native dwellings often housed up to twenty people, often genetically related, increased the speed and severity with which viral infections spread (44-45).

[98] For the changes in the social infrastructure of New England tribes in the wake of disease, see Salisbury 103-105.

European colonists generally understood disease in supernatural terms, their interpretations revolved primarily around the question whose deity was more powerful. This spiritual reading of illness had far-reaching repercussions for both Native and New English societies as well as for their patterns of interaction.

In the wake of disease-induced social disorganization indigenous communities, the powwow's elevated status within many villages, which depended on his medical success, was inevitably questioned and caused a number of cultural reconfigurations. Some surviving priest-healers attributed the Narragansett's exemption from the first wave of epidemic diseases (1616-1619) to periodic sacrifices and, as a result, transformed and intensified their own healing rituals accordingly. Recent archaeological expeditions in New England indicate that both the quantity and the quality of critical rites (performed during famines, droughts, wars, and collective illnesses) changed after European arrival. Scholars believe that due to a shifting disease ecology, many Native people felt compelled to acquire more goods for sacrificial purposes. Seventeenth-century burial sites exhibit an increase in Indian and European artifacts, suggesting that healing rituals, too, sought to address the new realities.[99]

While some Native Americans modified their healing traditions to meet the new realities, others sought direct medical help from English settlers. Demoralized and traumatized by pandemics, many indigenes were convinced that the Protestant God was more powerful than their own celestial forces and hence asked their English neighbors to invoke

---

[99] Bragdon 239-241. Based on earlier archaeological evidence, Salisbury argues that the number of burial goods actually declined in the course of the seventeenth century, indicating that the epidemics caused an alienation of Native traditional rituals (106). For changes in burial practices after the arrival of Europeans, see Kevin A. McBride, "Bundles, Bears, and Bibles: Interpreting Seventeenth-Century Native 'Texts,'" *Early Native Literacies in New England: A Documentary and Critical Anthology*, ed. Kristina Bross and Hilary E. Wyss (Amherst: U of Massachusetts P, 2008) 132-141. Cf. Brenda J. Baker, "Pilgrim's Progress and Praying Indians: The Biocultural Consequences of Contact in Southern New England," *In the Wake of Contact: Biological Reponses to Conquest*, ed. Clark S. Larsen and George R. Milner (New York: Wiley, 1994) 37-39.

the help of their God to halt the epidemic. Others decided to convert to Christianity in order to avoid future illnesses. In 1633, John Sagamore, a Pawtucket leader, told John Winthrop before succumbing to smallpox: "diverse of them in their sicknesse, confessed that the Englishe mens God was a good God, & that, if they recovered they would serve him."[100] The severe challenges that epidemics posed to indigenous spirituality and medicine did not result in a complete demise of Algonquian cultural practices. For example, certain healing methods persisted by shifting and adapting over time and others survived as (suppressed) medical knowledge in colonial and later American culture and society. It is difficult, if not impossible to determine, however, why some belief structures and curative techniques crumbled under the impact of "Old World" pathogens while others persisted.

Most Natives recognized a causal, yet unspecified, link between the arrival of the English and the appearance and dissemination of hitherto unknown diseases. Matthew Mayhew, minister at Martha's Vineyard, reported how one shaman attempted to cure a woman whose affliction could not be remedied by other local priest-healers. The powwow determined that the illness was caused by "the *Spirit* an *Englishman* drowned in the Adjacent Sound," and after curing the woman advised that "*unless she removed to* Martha's Vineyard, *she would again be Sick, for being an English Spirit he could not long confine it.*"[101] Powwows often clung to their power and position within their communities by blaming illness on their European neighbors and particularly on English sorcery. In a similar vein, a number of New England texts relate how Squanto, the Native who reportedly taught the Pilgrims how to survive the first New England winter, warned other Algonquians that the English might have stored epidemics, rather than gunpowder, in underground barrels. The association between disease and explosives in the minds of local Natives drew from the conviction

---

[100] John Winthrop, *The Journal of John Winthrop: 1630-1649*, ed. Richard S. Dunn, James Savage, and Laetitia Yeandle (Cambridge, MA: Harvard UP, 1996) 105.

[101] Matthew Mayhew, *A Brief Narrative of the Success Which the Gospel Hath Had among the Indians* (1694; Early American Imprints, Series 1, no. 701) 15 (emphasis original). Cf. Mather, *Magnalia* II:426-427.

that the Europeans' ability to kill long-distance with guns and with disease derived from the same source of supernatural power. Some Indians believed that the English and/or their God controlled epidemics and could use them as weapons, as Massasoit's request to unleash lethal contagions against the Narragansett indicates: "he came in solemne manner and intreated the governour that he would let out the plague to destroy the Sachem, and his men, who were his enemies, promising that he himself, and all his posterity, would be their everlasting friends, so great an opinion he had of the English."[102] Clearly, leaders across the cultural divide had recognized the tremendous potential of diseases in shifting and reconfiguring power relations in early New England.

English rationalizations of disease-induced depopulation centered primarily, though not exclusively, on the notion of providence. Time and again, early commentaries were marked by a mixture of joy and awe over the ostensible fulfillment of religious expectations in the "New World." In 1629, *before* co-founding the Massachusetts Bay Colony, John Winthrop contributed to the doctrine of *vacuum domicilium* by claiming that, "God hath consumed the Natives with a miraculous plague, whereby the greater part of the country is left voide of inhabitants."[103] Defending the validity of the royal patent to settle in the

---

[102] Morton 245. The episode is also related in Bradford 99 and E. Winslow 10-11. The linkage between disease and weaponry is a foundational theme in the cultural contact and early interactions between the Natives and the English colonists. Thomas Hariot's late-sixteenth-century exploration narrative reports that Virginia Natives explained the mysterious afflictions with epidemics as having been caused by "invisible bullets" that the English had shot from their guns. Thomas Hariot, *A Briefe and True Report of the New Found Land of Virginia* (1588; Early English Books Online, STC 12785) 28-29. For a discussion of the notion of "invisible bullets" see, Stephen Greenblatt, *Shakespearean Negotiations: The Circulation of Social Energy in Renaissance England* (Berkeley: U of California P, 1988) 36-37; Joyce E. Chaplin, *Subject Matter: Technology, the Body, and Science on the Anglo-American Frontier, 1500-1676* (Cambridge, MA: Harvard UP, 2003) 29-33.

[103] "John Winthrop, General Observations: Higginson Copy," *Winthrop Papers* II, 120. This notion was echoed in a number of promotional tracts and settlement histories prepared by Puritan writers. In 1620, for example, the Reverend John Cotton published a sermon that similarly stresses the notion of *vacuum*

area against charges brought forth by Roger Williams, Winthrop asked five years later: "if God were not pleased with our inheriting these parts, why did he drive out the Natives before us? and why dothe he still make roome for us, by deminishinge them as we increase?"[104] For Winthrop and most Englishmen the perceived health disparities indicated that the colonists were better prepared to live in North America than the indigenous population, whose time and purpose in, as well as entitlement to, this region of the globe had expired. Epidemics were not only a central factor in preparing the land for English settlement, they also provided colonists with a language through which their relocation to New England could be grasped and legitimized. Cristobal Silva explains that "as epidemics physically clear the land, epidemiology creates a discursive framework for appropriating Native Americans within European civil law, for reifying that law as a reflection of 'natural' immunological processes, and for legally dispossessing them of their property rights."[105] For most English observers, the message contained in Native diseases and in apparent health disparities between indigenous people and Europeans seemed obvious: it was an outside,

---

*domicilium*: "Wherein doth this worke of God stand in appointing a place for a people? [...] when he makes roome for a people to dwell there. [It is] a principle in Nature that in a vacant soyle, hee that taketh possession of it, and bestoweth culture and husbandry upon it, his Right it is." John Cotton, *Gods Promise to His Plantation* (1620; Early English Books Online, STC 5854.4) 3-5. Cf. Edward Johnson, *Wonder-Working Providence of Sions Saviour in New-England* (1654; New York: Scholars' Facsimiles and Reprints, 1974) 17; White, *Planters Plea* 25. The conviction that the epidemics constituted evidence of God's providence was not particular to Puritan writers; Anglican observers such as John Smith, Thomas Morton, and Ferdinando Gorges also explained the land-clearing diseases in religious terms (cf. Salisbury 3; Kupperman, *Settling* 32). For the ideological bases of Puritan occupation of Native land, founded on English law and religious conviction, see Chester E. Eisinger, "The Puritan Justification for Taking the Land," *Essex Institute Historical Collections* 84 (1948): 131-143.

[104] "John Winthrop to John Endecott, 3 January 1634," *Winthrop Papers* III, 149.

[105] Cristobal Silva, "Miraculous Plagues: Epidemiology on New England's Colonial Landscape," *Early American Literature* 43.2 (2008): 267.

higher authority and not human agency that depopulated the area so that a chosen people could claim and cultivate it in the name of God and Crown. This confluence of civil, theological, and medical narratives conveniently assuaged the English of their responsibility for Native American mortality: the discourse of "medical providentialism" offered an interpretive grid within which Native epidemics could be deemed expected, tolerable, and justified.[106]

Yet, the realities of disease proved more ambiguous and complex than hoped for and demanded more elaborate explanations. If, for instance, God was indeed looking favorably on the colonial endeavor in the "New World," why did He allow the death of almost half of the *Mayflower* passengers during the first winter after reaching Patuxet/Plymouth? If the providential hand of God had really set aside and cleared land so that the Protestant project could proceed, why did so many English settlers continue to suffer from fevers, fluxes, smallpox, and a host of other illnesses after reaching New England? While their own diseases had profound mental effects on the colonists, inducing periods of gnawing doubt about their personal and communal piety and salvation, the errand as such was never (officially) questioned, in part because New England Natives continued to disappear whereas the colony as a whole made steady progress. In addition, despite their own illnesses, the first English colonists were certain that the navigational error that brought the *Mayflower* to Plymouth, instead of its intended destination, the mouth of the Hudson River, was a clear sign of providence that could not be mitigated by selective suffering. Also, English settlers argued retrospectively that if God had allowed the survival of all *Mayflower* passengers (many of whom were non-Puritan adventurers), then the shortage of food during the first winter might have caused the end of the whole mission. God's disease intervention, therefore, constituted a disguised blessing: fewer colonists meant more food for the survivors and hence illness facilitated the ultimate growth

---

[106] For the notion of medical providentialism, see Walter W. Woodward, *Prospero's America: John Winthrop, Jr., Alchemy and the Creation of New England Culture, 1606-1676* (Chapel Hill: U of North Carolina P, 2010) 163-182.

and prosperity of the Plymouth Colony.[107] As William Woodward has convincingly argued with regard to the continuation of collective illnesses during the Great Migration,

> Ironically, New Englanders' brief episodes of seasoning mortality served to amplify rather than undermine colonial Puritans' belief in their favored providential medical status. Those settlers who had the most reason to doubt medical providentialism either died from their sicknesses or became disillusioned and returned to England. Those who remained interpreted their avoidance of or recovery from illness as an intentional providential blessing. Many New Englanders came to think that the seasoning mortality had been a divine winnowing of godly wheat from fallen chaff, which set the stage for intensification of medical providentialism among the godly.[108]

For some early New England commentators, however, the providential narrative, according to which God had foreordained English settlement in North America and was facilitating it by inflicting the Native population with disease, proved difficult to maintain. For instance, Rhode Island founder Roger Williams pointed out that illness affected American Indians and English colonists alike and concluded that

> the plague and other sicknesses were alone in the hand of the one God, who made him and us, who being displeased with the English for lying, stealing, idleness and uncleanness, (the Natives' epidemical sins,) smote many thousands of us ourselves with general and late mortalities.[109]

---

[107] Mather, *Magnalia* I:54.

[108] Woodward 167-168.

[109] Roger Williams, *The Letters of Roger Williams*, vol. 6, ed. John Russell Bartlett (Providence: Publications of the Narragansett Club, 1874) 17. Williams' challenges to Puritan orthodoxy, which caused his ostracism from the Plymouth Colony in 1634, in part rested on his firm belief in the common humanity of English and Natives: "Nature knowes no difference between *Europe* and *Americans* in blood, birth, bodies, &c. God having of one blood made all mankind." Roger Williams, *A Key into the Language of America* (1643; Early English Books Online, W2766) 53.

According to this disease narrative, God does not necessarily favor the English over the indigenous. Instead, Williams emphasizes the common humanity of both groups, prone to retribution by their creator. Interestingly enough, though, despite the implied equality before God, Williams posits moral deviance as a disease that spreads *from* the Natives *to* the English and in doing so clings to the notion that the indigenous population of New England is culturally inferior. In a similar vein, John Eliot, missionary to the local Algonquians also recognized a common susceptibility to divine-sanctioned illnesses in both groups:

> a great sicknesse epidemical, did the Lord lay upon us, so that the greatest p[ar]t of a town was sick at once, whole familys sick young & old, scarce any escaping English or Indian. [...] This visitation of God was exceedingly strange, it was suddaine, & generall: as if the Lord had imediatly sent forth an angel, not with a sword to kill, but with a rod to chastize.[110]

Contrary to the dominant narrative of medical providentialism, which pointed merely to epidemiological differences between the settlers and the Natives, Williams's and Eliot's accounts express a sense of helplessness vis-à-vis God's sovereignty rather than His sustained preferential treatment of the colonists.

Convinced that English settlers and their Algonquian neighbors shared similar fears and anxieties about life under hazardous conditions, some settlers nursed sick Natives (which later contributed to the further glorification of the New England Pilgrims).[111] Other colonists expressed in written form their sympathy for their suffering neighbors, who had

---

[110] "Rev. John Eliot's Records of the First Church in Roxbury, Mass.," *The New-England Historical and Genealogical Register* 33 (April 1879): 237-238. Cf. Bradford 260.

[111] Not all colonists helped their sick Native neighbors because it constituted an act of Christian charity. In fact, some English settlers throughout the seventeenth century demanded payment from the Indians for the provision of health services and thereby often indebted Native people to a point where they had had to concede part of their lands. Jean O'Brien, "We Shall Remain," PBS Series, "Episode One: After the Mayflower," 2010, transcript, 15.

helped the newcomers to survive the first winter. William Bradford, for instance, laments that the speed and breadth of the first wave of epidemics (1616-1619) allowed neither time nor energy "to bury one another" and hence calls the collective demise of the local Natives "a very sad spectacle to behold."[112] When his own group was faced with an infectious illness, Bradford struck a similarly contemplative and compassionate tone, stating that "it pleased God to visit *us* then with death daily, and with so general a disease that the living were scarce able to bury the dead, and the well not in any measure sufficient to tend the sick."[113] Aside from undermining the dominant providential narrative according to which God showed his preference for the Puritans by afflicting (only) Native people with lethal diseases, these statements illustrate a shared sense of helplessness at a time when medical practice could do little to cure major afflictions. In addition, Bradford's words give voice to the recognition of shared suffering and of preserving human dignity in times of disease.

A few chapters further into *Of Plymouth Plantation*, Bradford graphically depicts how the skin of smallpox-infected Natives, covered with pustules and scabs, stuck to the mats on which they slept: "a whole side will flay off at once as it were, and they will be all of a gore blood, most fearful to behold. And then being very sore, what with cold and other distempers, they die like rotten sheep."[114] Here, the horrors of disease cause a temporary shift from Puritan plain-style aesthetics to a

---

[112] Bradford 87. The sight of multitudes of Algonquian corpses lying above ground left a deep impression on all Christian observers. Time and again, the sight of denied burials and horrific body images informs the tropes of early colonists' disease narratives. Roger Williams, for instance, writes: "I have often seene a poore House left alone in the wild Woods, all being fled, the living not able to bury the dead, so terrible is the apprehension of an infectious disease, that not onely persons, but the Houses and the whole Towne takes flight." (*A Key* 188).

[113] Bradford 95 (emphasis added). Cf. Edward Johnson's description of how governor John Winthrop and Reverend John Wilson nursed Native smallpox victims in their homes (51-52).

[114] Bradford 270-271. Cf. Cotton Mather's use of "rotton sheep" in chapter six of this study.

more engaged and sensationalist narrative tone. The notion of "rotten sheep" functions as a metonymic symbol of diseased alterity, depicting the racial and cultural Other in dehumanized and decomposed terms. The Plymouth governor thus momentarily disavows the pastoral myth of America, replacing it with a much more gloomy narrative of the new environment. At the same time, Bradford's response to dying Indians echoes a dominant mode of human reaction to pandemics following the plague ("Black Death") that had ravaged Europe in the fourteenth century, when "Death was no longer considered a departure or a passage, but was seen rather as an end, as decomposition."[115]

The author's linkage between the plague and Native epidemics, as well as his melancholic lament of indigenous suffering illustrate that sympathy marked a Puritan duty and doctrine, especially when the hand of divine providence was perceived as acting upon someone else. The Plymouth governor emphasizes how sympathy was transformed into pity, which enabled solidarity and fostered the social good, across cultural boundaries. However, such an approach is not based on disinterested benevolence but is rather part and parcel of the colonial endeavor itself. Bradford's short illness narratives exemplify how epidemics both problematized and cemented colonial definitions of cultural difference and socio-religious responsibilities. Hence, one needs to take Kathleen Donegan's insightful observation that "catastrophic testimony becomes a key vehicle for representing and recuperating the aporia of being colonial" a step further.[116] Bradford's depiction of

---

[115] Agrimi and Crisciani 196. For a comprehensive account of the pervasiveness of, and responses to, death in early America, see Matthew Dennis, "Death and Memory in Early America," *History Compass* 4.1 (2006): 384-401. Bradford's discourse of catastrophe also shows how the history of the living was driven by the dead. For New England colonists, disease-induced mortality became both an opportunity for, and a problem of, settlement because the image of dead bodies in the wilderness resonated typologically with Numbers 14.35: "in this wilderness they shall be consumed, and there they shall die." Bradford resounds this notion twice in *Of Plymouth Plantation* when his most forceful hyperbole for describing epidemics is that both Algonquians and English colonists "were scarce able to bury the dead" (95, 271).

[116] Donegan 25.

Natives suffering from smallpox, on the one hand, expresses an unsettling sense of doubt about the gruesome effects of the colonial endeavor. On the other hand, by reaching out in sympathy to the sick Other, the governor reinforces notions of health and cultural disparities between the two leading groups in early New England, emphasizing Algonquian degeneration and Puritan compassion and charity. The depiction of disease-ridden Natives thus establishes a larger pattern, to be continued for centuries, according to which indigenous people function as ambivalent objects of disgust, abjection, pity, and patronage in order to aid the cause of Anglo-American progress.

Next to compassion, attending afflicted Natives was also politically motivated. The most prominent example occurred in 1623, when Edward Winslow helped Wampanoag sachem Massasoit to overcome an illness (most likely typhoid). Energized by the desire to maintain a vital alliance with tribes that could ensure the prosperity of Plymouth colony, Winslow decided to honor a culturally entrenched Native healing ritual by visiting a sick tribal member and sitting by his bedside. After a cursory examination, the English colonist scraped Massasoit's swollen and furred tongue and fed him soup and sassafras tea, which caused a quick recovery of the leader. Asked to treat all members of the tribe, Winslow reluctantly consented and scraped the mouths of other Natives, finding it "much offensive [...], not being accustomed with such poisonous savours," yet necessary to serve his overall purpose.[117] This display of medical expertise by the English leader proved significant for Native-Anglo relations because, as Alfred Crosby claims, "[i]n an era which was, for the Indians, one of almost incomprehensible mortality, Winslow had succeeded where all the powwows had failed in thwarting the influences drawing Massasoit toward death. The English could not only persuade a profoundly malevolent god to kill, but also *not* to kill."[118] One can argue further that with God seemingly on their side,

---

[117] E. Winslow 30.

[118] Crosby, "God" 42 (emphasis original). For a recent biography, which focuses on Winslow's political activities, see Jeremy Dupertuis Bangs, *Pilgrim Edward Winslow: New England's First Diplomat* (Boston: New England Historic Genealogical Society, 2004). Kelly Wisecup has even argued that "Winslow incorporated Native medical philosophies and imitated shaman's practices" (19),

colonists were able to help Native people *because of*, rather than despite, their belief in providence. In short, assured that God had selected them for settling New England, colonists would not have to fear contamination from helping disease-ridden Algonquians. As Woodward has pointed out, "[g]iven the degree to which person-to-person contact was considered a risk factor for contagion during epidemics, the readiness of the English to assist the natives highlights their faith in medical providentialism."[119] However, when considered in conjunction, it seems that Bradford's and Winslow's understanding of a common humanity of suffering, regardless of its motivation, also challenged the dominant providential reading of Native diseases, because by practicing and expressing compassion, both leaders implicitly conceded partial responsibility for the demographic upheaval that had been unfolding before their eyes. Aware that their arrival coincided with epidemics, colonists such as Winslow and Bradford stressed human agency and Christian charity over passive acceptance of what appeared to be divine punishment for indigenous paganism, idleness, and failure to cultivate the land.[120]

Only a few colonial observers challenged the discourse of medical providentialism by attributing Native diseases solely to natural causes, such as an unhealthy diet, a poor environment or a lack of physical strength.[121] The latter explanatory approach relied in part on views of corporeality that were significantly different from modern concepts of the body. In general, English colonists believed in monogeneticism, the

---

an assertion that I find somewhat overstated because it is not backed sufficiently by evidence.

[119] Woodward 169.

[120] Martha L. Finch, *Dissenting Bodies: Corporealities in Early New England* (New York: Columbia UP, 2010) 30-46.

[121] The notion that Native diseases were not necessarily due to divine providence, but may have had natural causes such as the Indians' dietary choice, thus shifting the blame toward a failure within Indian social and cultural formations, can be found, for instance, in Wood, *New England's Prospect* 102, 111. See also, David S. Jones, *Rationalizing Epidemics: Meanings and Uses of American Indian Mortality since 1600* (Cambridge, MA: Harvard UP, 2004) 18-19.

notion that all people originated from the same stock (Adam and Eve) and hence shared certain physical properties. As one result, early New England settlers did not regard the indigenous population as *racially* inferior; the discursive and material subordination of Native Americans resulted from evaluating what seemed obvious cultural, social, national, and adaptive differences that disease, among others, made visible.[122] Virtually all early disease narratives in New England shared the stigmatization of the Other as sick and, conversely, the sick as Other. Biological, cultural, and/or religious deviance often went hand-in-hand and was hence conceived as constituting illness. By the same token, a sick person, regardless of his or her geographic origin, bore the stigma of Otherness, of deviance from the social, cultural, or religious norms brought to the American strand by the first waves of English settlers.

As the demographic tide in New England turned in the course of the seventeenth century, the "space for creative interpretation"[123] of Indian epidemics found in some early commentaries (e.g., by Winslow, Bradford, and Williams) decreased in favor of providentialism. After English colonialism had been firmly established in the "New World," one historical account after another interpreted the virtual collapse of the Algonquian population across the North American continent as an indication of God setting aside land so that a new and better society might prosper. Daniel Gookin's 1674 report, for example, recalibrates the history of colonization by asserting that "divine providence made way for the quiet and peaceable settlement of the English in those nations,"[124] a settlement that is not only ordained by God but also devoid

---

[122] Joyce E. Chaplin, "Natural Philosophy and an Early Racial Idiom in North America: Comparing English and Indian Bodies," *The William and Mary Quarterly* 54.1 (1997): 229-233, 244-246; Kathleen M. Brown, "Native Americans and Early Modern Concepts of Race," *Empire and Others: British Encounters with Indigenous Peoples, 1600-1850*, ed. Martin Daunton and Rick Halpern (Philadelphia: U of Pennsylvania P, 1999) 79-100.

[123] Jones, *Rationalizing Epidemics* 51.

[124] Gookin 8. Gookin's account echoes Gorges' 1658 justification of settlement which became possible, even necessary, after "a great and generall plague, which so violently rained for three years together that in a manner the greater part of that Land was left desert without any to disturb or appease our free and

of English violence in Gookin's view. In a similar vein, Cotton Mather, repeating the interpretive tropes of earlier observers in 1702, attributes depopulation by epidemics to Native transgressions of God's laws. Recalling how in the winter of 1622-1623 a French captive prophesized the demise of indigenous people by divine punishment, Mather explains that "[t]hose infidels then blasphemously replyed, 'God could not kill them;' which blasphemous mistake was confuted by an horrible and unusual *plague*, whereby they were consumed in such vast multitudes, that our first planters found the land almost covered with their unburied carcases [...]."[125] The Boston minister's reading is typical of retrospective English rationalizations of Indian epidemics in the way it places responsibility for annihilation squarely within their cultural norms and religious behavior ("blasphemous mistake"). The implication that disease was introduced by French Catholics and not by English Protestants, whom Mather euphemistically refers to as innocent "planters," renders visible a mode of explaining and justifying settlement based on divinely sanctioned health disparities between the regenerate and the unregenerate. By thus interpreting epidemics in providential terms, observers such as Mather anticipated a particular proto-American response to disease that differed from other European colonial narratives. For example, in the report of the French missionary Hierosme Lalemant, who reflects on contacts with the indigenous population of Canada during the early seventeenth century, one reads:

> no doubt we carried the trouble with us, since, wherever we set foot, either death or disease followed us. [...] where we were most welcome, where we baptized most people, there it was in fact where they died the most; and, on the contrary, in the cabins to which we were denied entrance, although they were sometimes sick to extremity, at the end of a

peaceable possession thereof, from whence we may justly conclude, that GOD made the way to effect his work according to the time he had assigned for laying the foundation thereof" (77).

[125] Mather, *Magnalia* I:51 (emphasis original). The incident related by Cotton Mather had become an often-told story by the end of the seventeenth century and was included in a number of English reports. Cf. Morton 131-132.

few days one saw every person prosperously cured. We shall see in heaven the secret, but ever adorable, judgments of God therein.[126]

Although few French colonists would deny the righteousness of their conquest of North America, Lalemant's comment, in contrast to most English observers, draws a causal connection between colonization, disease, and indigenous depopulation that is lacking in most English reports. In addition, it is most troubling for the Jesuit observer that those Natives apparently saved by Christianity were more prone to disease than those who retained their indigenous religious views and practices. In hindsight, the comparison of English and French voices reveals once more how the social meanings of epidemics in colonial times had complex and plural levels and how Native diseases failed to lend themselves for a monolithic, deterministic explanation.

In the New England colonies, however, a comparatively homogenous rationalization of the land-clearing epidemics was deemed necessary in order to integrate the staggering morbidity and mortality rates among indigenous people into the worldview of the settlers. For the English, collective self-assurance about their colonial endeavor under the guise of providence was motivated by more than theological necessity; it combined science, religion, and politics into a powerful narrative for justifying the origins and developments of colonialism in North America. The initial and retrospective invocations of divine providence marked a crucial hinge within an evolving national narrative: they served to disavow culpability for the decline of the Algonquian population and to defend the legitimacy of English, and later Anglo-American, land claims. Although such a criticism of the English/American adherence to medical providentialism seems warranted from a twenty-first-century perspective, one should keep in mind that for those who lacked today's scientific insights, attributing the sudden decline of Native Americans and the increasing life expectancy

---

[126] Hierosme Lalemant, *The Jesuit Relations and Allied Documents: Travels and Explorations of the Jesuit Missionaries in New France, 1610-1791, Vol. 19 (Quebec, 1640)*, ed. Reuben G. Thwaites, trans. Finlow Alexander, et al. (Cleveland: Burrows, 1898) 93.

of the settlers to providence seemed as logical and self-evident as its current postcolonial critique.

In looking back at the initial depopulation of early New England, twentieth-century scholarship discards the providential narrative but often maintains the notion that Native Americans were genetically and/or environmentally susceptible to disease. According to the theory of "virgin-soil epidemics," popularized by Alfred Crosby in 1976, the immunological impecuniousness of indigenous populations, as well as the inadequacy of their cultural systems in dealing with devastating pandemics, was responsible for the demographic catastrophe that preceded and accompanied European colonialism in the Americas.[127] While Crosby's approach deserves credit for highlighting some of the factors that contributed to the decline of Native populations, it is far from exhaustive and remains problematic. For instance, the virgin-soil model erroneously assumes that indigenous communities were disease-free before the arrival of the Europeans; "virgin-soil," aside from sexualizing Native bodies and land (ready to be penetrated by the colonists), insinuates further that the "New World" was not only devoid of diseases but also of people; in addition, the concept links genetic disadvantages with cultural immaturity and, in doing so, presents an image of the Natives' complete and irreversible helplessness.

The dominance of the "virgin-soil epidemics" model in American historiography is further criticized by David Jones, who asserts that it tends to substitute the earlier notion of theological predetermination with biological determinism. Both concepts fail to assign adequate responsibility to European activities in the Americas and stress, instead, the *inevitable* demise of Native people. Jones argues that Europeans did not unleash deadly pathogens coincidentally, but that they "triggered the conditions that made them so destructive."[128] This is an insightful point

---

[127] Alfred W. Crosby, "Virgin Soil Epidemics as a Factor in the Aboriginal Depopulation in America," *The William and Mary Quarterly* 33.2 (1976): 289-299.

[128] Jones 4. David Arnold makes a similar argument, explaining that Crosby's model "overlooks the Europeans' capacity to devise structures of exploitation and control that would turn even environmentally hostile lands to their own advantage and profit" (9).

because it attributes a degree of agency and culpability to English settlers that is largely absent from the master narrative of providence and from virgin-soil theories, in which the demographic collapse is attributed to something inherent in, or missing from, Native bodies and/or behavior. Jones's claim overlooks, however, that Europeans, as far as we can discern today, lacked the knowledge to spread or contain disease, especially smallpox, in early New England. His speculation that some desperate early colonists practiced a precursor of biological warfare by claiming dominion over disease in order to force Native people into submission fails to withstand empirical scrutiny and thus cannot serve as proof for his assumption that settlers recognized their direct responsibility for the epidemics.[129]

Because Native genetic susceptibility to disease is difficult to prove and often considered akin to racial theories, scholars have increasingly stressed post-contact cultural and environmental factors to explain the devastating effects of European pathogens on the Amerindian population. Accordingly, the introduction of European plants and animals, Native malnutrition, and increasing trade activities have to be considered as important factors in explaining the velocity and sustenance of epidemic diseases in the early colonies.[130] One also has to take into account the interactions between disease and social forces in causing high mortality rates among Algonquian populations. For example, as we have seen, already a relatively small number of infected persons could disrupt the system of care and food provision. It is hence difficult, if not impossible, to evaluate how many Native people died as a direct cause of insufficient immunity and how many contracted lethal

---

[129] Jones, *Rationalizing Epidemics* 59.

[130] The notion of environmental factors facilitating European imperialism and colonialism around the world is particularly stressed in Jared Diamond's *Guns, Germs, and Steel: The Fates of Human Societies* (New York: Norton, 1997). Cf. David Jones' careful assessment of the literature on virgin-soil epidemics which leads him to assert that "the analyses clearly show that the fates of individual populations depended on contingent factors of their physical, economic, social, and political environments." David S. Jones, "Virgin Soils Revisited," *The William and Mary Quarterly* 60.4 (2003): 705.

diseases due to socio-cultural shifts or spiritual and environmental stress in the wake of European colonization.

* * *

Native and English disease concepts and healing practices showed certain similarities as well as incompatible differences. In very general terms, both indigenous and imported theories of disease relied on an interrelation between natural and supernatural causes. Both New England groups adhered to the view that many illnesses were brought about and could be alleviated by divine intervention and hence afforded priest-healers (the shaman and the minister-physician) a prestigious position within their respective social orders. Both functionaries combined spiritual treatments of illness with rational practices, applying plants and various medicinal techniques to extract the cause of disease from the human body. Aside from assigning a healing role to individuals who had expert knowledge in medicine, English and Native cultures shared a sense of suffering and of responding to illnesses. A comparison of indigenous and European medical approaches also reveals how societies reacted differently to certain diseases and how certain deviances in the role and function of medicine impacted cultural and political processes within, and interactions between, both groups. Unable or unwilling to fully understand the cosmology underlying Native therapeutics, colonists by and large regarded animistic healing practices as devil worship. As one consequence, they categorized spiritualistic medical approaches as irrational or pagan and divorced them from natural therapeutics.

After English men and women began to colonize North America on the heels of an epidemiological disaster, Native bodies and destinies emerged in the European consciousness as signed by disease. In the wake of epidemics, seventeenth-century New England witnessed a dramatic demographic transition that was marked by a decline of American Indians and a rise of English colonists simultaneously. Communicable diseases proved more important than guns in facilitating this demographic revolution. While Algonquians were able to adopt European weaponry to resist encroachments, they were unable to turn the tables of disease against the newcomers. Epidemics thus played a crucial role in the colonization of North America: they forced Indian people to abandon their villages, produced a shift from a gift to a commodity economy, and coerced Natives into adopting a culture that based its superiority, among other things, on health differences.

From a Native perspective, the Other (i.e., Europeans) was already present in the indigenous body before settlers arrived in sustained numbers. Unaware of Europe's microbial presence in indigenous blood and of the specificity of their biological advantages, most settlers, regardless of their religious faith, employed the notion of divine providence in order to rationalize the events that preceded their arrival and that continued unabated during the first decades of colonization. This dominant explanatory approach to early epidemics entailed far-reaching social and cultural consequences throughout U.S. history, for instance, by feeding into notions of Manifest Destiny and the Vanishing Indian. In fact, America's redemptive purpose in the present and future, prefigured in writings by European explorers, was only fully revealed as the English couched disease in providential terms and thus elevated the significance of their colonizing endeavor to both national and cosmic proportions.

For most English settlers, the trauma of disease that they shared with the Algonquian population at least in part, acquired a foundational and emancipatory status. They now had gained, in Cotton Mather's words, "a whole world before them to be peopled."[131] In the eyes of most colonists, epidemics destroyed much of what had existed before arrival, gave rise to a new state of becoming, and functioned as an apt illustration of heavenly judgment for moral inadequacies and transgressions. As a manifestation of "divine" or "sovereign violence"—to adopt literally what Walter Benjamin calls the "pure power over all life"[132]—epidemics demarcated God's *omni*potence from human

---

[131] Mather, *Magnalia* I:78.

[132] Walter Benjamin, "Critique of Violence," *Reflections: Essays, Aphorisms, Autobiographical Writings*, trans. Edmund Jephcott, ed. Peter Demetz (New York: Harcourt, 1978) 297. Cf. Giorgio Agamben, *Homo Sacer: Sovereign Power and Bare Life*, trans. Daniel Heller-Roazen (Stanford: Stanford UP, 1998), whose highly contested argument about concentration camps as a paradigm of the modern era significantly builds on Benjamin's notion of *das bloße Leben* ("the bare life").

*im*potence and differentiated the elect from the heathen. Such a reading of disease was immediately problematized, however, by the fact that the colonized Other's seeming impotence vis-à-vis lethal epidemics marked, at the same time, the impotence of the colonizing Self. Looking into the dark forests of New England, many colonial observers inadvertently had to come to terms with the reflection of their own susceptible bodies and of a common humanity that caused them to tend to infected Natives, a symbolic gesture, often without much success. By adhering to the ideal of Christian charity, some colonists contested a strict providential explanation of disease ecology of early New England. They thereby produced a conflict of interest between humanitarian responses to illness and the discourse of medical providentialism that inherently denied the efficacy of human intervention in disease affairs. As a result, the plurality of English reactions to epidemics, the *grands* and *petits récits* of illness, along with medical practices that pragmatically integrated knowledge from a cultural group stigmatized as pagan, constituted a counter-productive "infection" of religious orthodoxy both from the inside out and the outside in.

Early Native epidemics furthermore had significant and lasting effects on the everyday conceptualization of disease and medicine in seventeenth-century New England. Having witnessed God's intervention in health affairs, who seemed to have selectively sent contagion to almost all Natives, colonists became convinced that the American landscape constituted an exceptional theatre for divinely sanctioned afflictions and cures. Hence, medical providentialism, ostensibly at work during the early years of settlement, shaped the course of New England culture and society by instructing individual colonists how to deal with illnesses conceptually. As the following chapter will show in further detail, seventeenth-century settlers placed greater emphasis on attributing disease to God's immediate involvement than most of their European compatriots, for whom, in accordance with the Galenic tradition, the divine had encoded its medical power and wisdom in creation and thereafter had largely abstained from an intervention in human health affairs.

# 2. Writing Cures: John Winthrop Jr.'s Epistolary Healing Networks

One of the points discussed in the previous chapter is that New England's minister-physicians could only meet part of the public demand for healers. Out of necessity, therefore, other men of learning assembled and applied medical knowledge for the advantage of their communities. A particular case in point is politician, colonial planner and organizer, amateur alchemist and scientist, John Winthrop Jr. (1606-1676), who was particularly admired by New England colonists for his extensive medical expertise and his willingness to apply his knowledge for the health of settlers from all walks of life. His interest in medicine not only benefited many colonists but also increased Winthrop's power and influence: his medical and scientific talents marked a personal asset that many communities recognized and aimed to employ for themselves. As medical expert, experienced overseer of building new settlements, and son of the famous Massachusetts Bay Colony leader, John Winthrop Jr. was the ideal candidate for political leadership. He was hence elected governor of Connecticut in 1657 and again from 1659 until shortly before his death.

Aside from his many public roles, John Winthrop Jr. was an avid recipient and conveyor of scientific knowledge. His publications include essays and letters sent to the Royal Society in London relating information on the natural environment, husbandry, astronomy, and medicine.[1] In addition, historians and archivists have retrieved a

[1] Alasdair Macphail, "John Winthrop, Jr.," *American Colonial Writers, 1606-1734*, *Dictionary of Literary Biography*, vol. 24, ed. Emory Elliot (Detroit: Gale, 1984) 363-364. Until the 1980s, scholars believed that Winthrop had authored a number of books on alchemy under the pseudonym of "Eirenaeus Philalethes" (Peaceful Lover of Truth), who was said to be an English citizen living in North America. We know now that the author was actually the alchemist and scientist, George Starkey, whose books were revered by intellectuals across Europe,

fascinating body of letters written by and to John Winthrop Jr. that offer extensive insights into the range of medical knowledge and illness narratives in colonial America. Throughout his life, Winthrop sustained a lively correspondence with alchemists, medical practitioners, and scientists in Europe, thereby building a network of knowledge exchange that helped him secure a spot on the founding roll of the Royal Society. His membership allowed him to witness and participate in the formation and development of scientific agendas and methods, especially in the fields of agriculture, astronomy, chemistry, and medicine. The knowledge gained from his correspondence with European adepts consistently served his colonial constituents. Winthrop's interest in the practicability of scientific discoveries ensured that he applied what he had learned in his Connecticut hometowns, especially in New London and Hartford.

Perhaps even more fascinating than his communication with Samuel Hartlib, Robert Boyle, George Starkey, and other sages of mid-seventeenth-century Europe are the medical request letters sent to John Winthrop by colonists from all over New England. Seeking advice in times of often severe medical conditions, these letters offer unusual insights into the modes of conceiving and representing illness in early America. Like few other sources, the patient letters reveal how the elite and the common people of New England conceptualized and communicated their physical conditions to someone who was not only a respected and well-versed medical practitioner but also a person of exceptional power and influence. The present chapter hence focuses on the structure, form, and contents of selected medical letters written mostly during the 1650s and 1660s. The following analysis of a broad

including Isaac Newton. Starkey was born in Barbados and attended Harvard College from 1643 to 1646 and afterwards practiced chemical medicine and studied alchemy with Winthrop before moving to England in 1650. The debate about the identity of Philalethes can be traced in Ronald S. Wilkinson, "The Problem of the Identity of Eirenaeus Philalethes," *Ambix* 12.1 (1964): 24-43; George H. Turnbull, "George Stirk, Philosopher by Fire," *Publications of the Colonial Society of Massachusetts* 38 (1949): 219-251; William R. Newman, *Gehennical Fire: The Lives of George Starkey, an American Alchemist in the Scientific Revolution* (Cambridge, MA: Harvard UP, 1994) 1.

array of patient narratives seeks to carve out the differences in the discursive and textual registers that common colonists, on the one hand, and members of the cultural elite (ministers and officials), on the other, employed to write about their illnesses. The letters illustrate how illnesses often caused the correspondents to discard conventions of courtesy, humility, tone, and style otherwise common in epistolary practices at the time. These deviances from formal guidelines often led to a striking realism of the illness descriptions. Further, the patient letters sent to Winthrop also reveal a sense of humanity that is, at times, lost in popular and scholarly portrayals of New England colonists, whose seeming obsession with their own spiritual estates and that of all others around them has been noted time and again.

The younger John Winthrop's first sustained engagement with medicine occurred after his enrollment at Trinity College, Dublin, at the age of sixteen. Little is known about his precise course of studies, except that he was exposed to new books, maps, and "a human 'sceliton,' thoughtfully clothed in 'taffety hangings.'"[2] As a representation of hidden secrets, forbidden knowledge, and inexplicable superstitions, the veiled skeleton marks an apt metaphor of Winthrop's fascination with medicine and alchemy throughout his lifetime. His devotion to the art and science of medicine further increased after 1625, when he lived with his relatives, Thomas and Priscilla Fones, who owned an apothecary shop in London. Aside from learning about the curative properties of certain herbs, plants, and roots, the future colonial New England leader took a growing interest in the preparation of alchemical medicaments, a field of medical inquiry and application that had been popularized by the writings of Paracelsus and his disciples. As Louis G. Kelly has noted, most London apothecaries were devoted Christians (and many adhered to the Puritan faith) but "made no secret of their intense interest in the occult, often advertising themselves as astrologers. As alchemists, they practised their profession within a complex of religious and political ideas that saw no boundary between religion, physical science, and

---

[2] Quoted in Robert C. Black, *The Younger John Winthrop* (New York: Columbia UP, 1966) 21.

medicine."[3] These principles, along with Winthrop's observation of the rigid and hierarchical medical system in England, influenced his career in medicine and laid the foundation for his discontent with the entrenched cultural homogeneity and religious orthodoxy in mid-seventeenth-century New England.

Another medical guide for John Winthrop Jr. was his father, who passed on his knowledge and, more importantly, taught him that medicine complemented the work of a devoted Christian willing to help an ailing humanity and of an effective leader aiming to gain the trust and support of his followers. Winthrop Sr. maintained a communication network with physicians in the Atlantic world and readily made use of his expertise for the benefit of his Bay Colony constituents. The extent of the elder Winthrop's medical practice lacks documentation; however, the fact that he asked his son to send or bring material that could be used for medical applications indicates that his abilities were in great demand, especially during the early years of the Massachusetts Bay Colony, when many colonists necessarily developed an interest in medicine, given the scarcity of learned physicians at the time.[4]

---

[3] Louis G. Kelly, "London Apothecaries as Early Christians: Renewing the Covenant," *Healing in Religion and Society, From Hippocrates to the Puritans*, ed. J. Kevin Coyle and Steven C. Muir (Lewiston: Mellen, 1999) 163.

[4] In the spring of 1631, after the first dismal winter in the "New World" had drawn to an end, Governor Winthrop requested "Conserue of red roses, and mithride" ("John Winthrop to John Winthrop, Jr., 28 March 1631," *Winthrop Papers* III, 21). The demand for "conserve of red roses" indicates that settlers were suffering from respiratory disorders and dysentery, among many other diseases; mithride, a concoction of several ingredients, was used to treat various forms of poisoning. Winthrop, Sr. also asked for "nitre;" however, from the letter it remains unclear whether Winthrop's plans for using saltpeter were military (i.e., for making gunpowder), alchemical (i.e., for making medicaments), or for other purposes. Later, Winthrop's order list included "Paracellsus plaister" and "indian bezoar," a hairball from the stomach of a cat, which was often used in mystic healing practices. "John Winthrop to John Winthrop, Jr., 6 November 1634," *Winthrop Papers* III, 175. For the elder Winthrop's medical activities, see also "John Endecott to John Winthrop, Sr., January 1635/36," *Winthrop Papers* III, 221-222; Lawrence Shaw Mayo, *The Winthrop Family in America* (Boston: Massachusetts Historical Society, 1948)

The younger John Winthrop also developed his medical expertise by conversing with New England physicians such as Dr. Giles Firmin, who came to America in 1632 and moved to Ipswich in 1638, where he had been granted land and practiced medicine, before returning to England in 1647. In a letter to the elder John Winthrop, Firmin expressed the typical difficulties of practicing medicine in a developing environment, which forced healers to procure alternative sources of income. "I am strongly sett upon to stydve diuinitie," Firmin informs the Bay Colony leader, "my studyes else must be lost: for physick is but a meene helpe."[5] Since Firmin and Winthrop Jr. resided at Ipswich at the time, one may reasonably assume that they exchanged knowledge on medical theory and practice, not least because Firmin is credited with having delivered the first anatomical lecture in colonial North America.[6]

Winthrop became an adept in the state of the art of medicine during his journey to Europe in 1642, where he was introduced as a student of medicine and met a number of continental medical experts, among them Johannes Tanckmarus, doctor of medicine and member of a group of German mystics, Paul Marquart Schlegel, professor of anatomy and surgery at Hamburg, with whom Winthrop exchanged American specimens for European minerals, and Jacob Golius, a Dutch orientalist, who traded views and knowledge on Hermetic philosophy and medicine

48; Henry R. Viets, *A Brief History of Medicine in Massachusetts* (Boston: Houghton, 1930) 21.

[5] "Gyles Fyrmin to Governor John Winthrop, 26 December 1639," printed in Thomas Franklin Waters, *Ipswich in the Massachusetts Bay Colony* (Ipswich: Ipswich Historical Society, 1905) 508-509.

[6] For Firmin's place as first anatomical lecturer in the history of American medicine, see Henry R. Viets, *A Brief History of Medicine in Massachusetts* (Boston: Houghton, 1930) 37. Oliver Wendell Holmes provides an insightful fictional rendition of how Firmin taught medicine by practical instruction during the day and by anatomical lectures at night, using "the body of some poor wretch who had swung upon the gallows" and which was "by the light of flaring torches hastily dissected by hands that trembled over the unwonted task." Oliver Wendell Holmes, *Medical Essays. The Writings of Oliver Wendell Holmes,* vol. 9 (Boston: Cambridge UP, 1891) 279.

with Winthrop.[7] The elaborate network of personal communication which Winthrop had built and maintained since his first return to England in 1634 offered not only access to knowledge that was crucial for providing medical care to colonists but also established a sense of belonging to the "civilized" world. Throughout his correspondence with European intellectuals one finds a number of jubilating remarks concerning the possibilities of bridging the distance between a quaint and fragile existence in his colonial home and the bustling seventeenth-century world of science, commerce, and culture. In fact, Winthrop claimed that Western cultural superiority relied significantly on literacy and writing, stating that "Our barbarians in this America cannot enough admire this device [letters; M.P.], when they see messages conveyed on paper as if aloud."[8]

In 1643 John Winthrop (it remains unclear whether the elder or the younger) received a letter from an English physician, Dr. Edward Stafford, containing a broad scope of pragmatic medical advice. Stafford offers mostly botanical recipes, taken largely from John Gerard's well-known handbook *Great Herball, or General Histoire of Plantes* (1597), for a host of common illnesses at the time, including madness, epilepsy, hysteria, urinary diseases, jaundice, fractures, smallpox, the plague, poisoning, scrofula, and gunshot wounds. Stafford also provides some professional guidelines for amateur physicians, among them occasions for bloodletting, the importance of diet and fasting, principles of

---

[7] Winthrop's participation in the transnational community of elite knowledge exchange depended on his ability to read and write in the major languages at the time. "Augustinus Petraeus to John Winthrop, Jr., 9 March 1643," *Winthrop Papers* IV, 368-369, indicates that Winthrop was highly respected among German and Dutch chemists and physicians and had at least a reading knowledge of German. "John Winthrop, Jr. to Jacob Golius, 20 November 1639," *Winthrop Papers* IV, 155-156 and "Paul Marquart Schlegel to John Winthrop, Jr., 30 January 1652," *Winthrop Papers* VI, 170-173, exemplify Winthrop's Latin communications with European scholars. Cf. "Johannes Tanckmarus to John Winthrop, Jr., 28 October 1642," *Winthrop Papers* IV, 361-362. A typical college graduate at the time would have been fluent in English, Latin, Greek, and Hebrew.

[8] "John Winthrop, Jr. to Johannes Tanckmarus, 10 November 1650," *Winthrop Papers* VI, 83.

purging, the ethics of compensation, and the importance of sustained treatments. The letter represents a learned person whose approach to medicine is almost exclusively drawn from Galenic humoralism and Hippocratic ethics.[9]

In later years, John Winthrop Jr. communicated closely with leaders of the iatrochemical movement in England, especially with Samuel Hartlib and Kenelme Digby, who nurtured his intellectual interests, offered practical methods and techniques, and kept him up to date on the medical debates between proponents of Paracelsian alchemy and Helmontian medical chemistry, on the one hand, and of traditional Galenic medicine, on the other.[10] In addition, his "Old World" correspondents introduced him to a number of other influential representatives of scientific knowledge in England and Europe. During his journey to London (1661-1663) to renew the Connecticut charter, for instance, Winthrop became acquainted with William Brereton, Sir Robert Moray, Henry Oldenburg, Robert Boyle, Elias Ashmole, and Dr. John Wilkins, among others, and these meetings often resulted in sustained communications after his return to New England. Winthrop assiduously related his intellectual preoccupations and observations about life in the "New World" to his interlocutors across the Atlantic. As one result, his reputation among European correspondents was unmatched by any English colonist at the time. Although he failed to generate new scientific knowledge, some erudite men rumored that the Connecticut leader had successfully concluded the alchemical search for the alkahest, a sought-after material for facilitating the transmutation of metals and for producing a panacea. Others praised his ability to observe, record, and comment on various aspects of natural philosophy pertaining to North America, while still others recognized his reputation as an innovative and effective physician.[11] His election in 1662 as one of

[9] "Dr. Stafford to John Winthrop, 6 May 1643," *Proceedings of the Massachusetts Historical Society*, Series 1, Vol. 5 (1860-1862): 379-383.

[10] Cf. "Sir Kenelme Digby to John Winthrop, Jr., 26 January 1656," *Collections of the Massachusetts Historical Society*, Series 3, Vol. 10 (1849): 15-19.

[11] Cf. "Samuel Hartlib to John Winthrop, Jr., 16 March 1660," *Proceedings of the Massachusetts Historical Society*, Third Series, Vol. 72 (1957-1960): 45. Hartlib served as a hub of scientific information exchange at the time and was

115 "Original Fellows" of the Royal Society in London came as a natural consequence.[12] Winthrop attended the first meetings of the society, and, in 1664, was selected to serve as the "Chief Correspondent of the Royal Society in the West." The letters that he exchanged with about thirty other Fellows, from the beginnings of the Royal Society until his death, suggest that Winthrop was more interested in sharing and receiving information about natural curiosities and astronomy than about chemistry and medicine.[13] Members repeatedly urged Winthrop to compile a natural history of New England so as to nourish their scientific aptitudes but also to further develop the colonies for the economic and political benefit of the recently restored Crown.[14] Winthrop, aware of the importance of this knowledge and the tightening of colonial control it entailed, cleverly postponed a comprehensive guide

hence an important interlocutor for Winthrop, who received books, alchemical rumors, news about common acquaintances, and about political developments in Europe from Hartlib. In the extant Hartlib-Winthrop correspondence between 1659 and 1661, Winthrop devotes considerable writing space to possible treatments for Hartlib's bladder stones, which the Connecticut physician had not encountered during his medical practice. Aside from speculating on the efficacy of mineral water and possible surgical intervention, Winthrop reports that he sent a barrel of cranberries and of corn for easing the pain and discomfort of Hartlib's ailment. "John Winthrop, Jr. to Samuel Hartlib, 25 August 1660," *Proceedings of the Massachusetts Historical Society*, Third Series, Vol. 72 (1957-1960): 49-58.

[12] Raymond Phineas Stearns, "Colonial Fellows of the Royal Society of London, 1661-1788," *Notes and Records of the Royal Society of London* 8.2 (1951): 196. For a concise overview of the beginnings of the Royal Society, see Meyrick H. Carré, "The Formation of the Royal Society," *History Today* 10.8 (1960): 564-571.

[13] See, for instance, "John Winthrop, Jr., to Henry Oldenburg, 25 July 1668," *Collections of the Massachusetts Historical Society*, Series 5, Vol. 8 (1882): 121-125, in which Winthrop offers rare comments on medical topics, warning against the internal use of mercurial medicaments.

[14] Henry Oldenburg, quoted in Henry Lyons, *The Royal Society, 1660-1940: A History of its Administration under its Charters* (Cambridge: The UP, 1944) 28.

to natural resources of New England by sending regular, yet selected, reports about his observations of the natural surrounding.[15]

His contacts with European medical and alchemical experts directed Winthrop's interests toward the evolving field of chemical medicine. Although he frequently administered herbal treatments such as powdered ivory, wormwood, anise, saffron, sassafras, aloe, and rhubarb, the mainstay of Winthrop's medical practice derived from alchemical procedures, often including saltpeter, antimony, mercury, tartar, copperas, white vitriol, sulphur, iron, and red coral.[16] Among his medical recipes was a powder called rubila, whose exact ingredients and measurements have been lost. In the mid-nineteenth century, Oliver Wendell Holmes speculated that it was comprised of a mixture of antimony, niter, salt of tin, and perhaps traces of powdered "unicorn's

[15] Winthrop's only significant report to the Royal Society (which was merely summarized in the *Transactions*) concerns the planting, harvesting, storage, and utilization of corn (maize). Fulmer Mood, "John Winthrop, Jr., on Indian Corn," *New England Quarterly* 10.1 (1937): 121-133. In 1741, the Royal Society dedicated a volume of the *Philosophical Transactions* (XL) to Winthrop, celebrating his "extraordinary Knowledge [...] in the deep Mysteries of the most secret *Hermetic Science*," which rendered him "esteemed and courted by learned and good Men" (n. p.; emphasis original). For a more detailed account of Winthrop's relation with the Royal Society, see Walter W. Woodward, *Prospero's America: John Winthrop, Jr., Alchemy and the Creation of New England Culture, 1606-1676* (Chapel Hill: U of North Carolina P, 2010) 262-273. For Winthrop's contribution to science, see Ronald S. Wilkinson, *The Younger John Winthrop and Seventeenth-Century Science* (Farringdon: Classey, 1975); Robert M. Benton, "The John Winthrops and Developing Scientific Thought in New England," *Early American Literature* 7 (1973): 272-280; Charles A. Browne, "Scientific Notes from the Books and Letters of John Winthrop, Jr., 1606-1676," *Isis* 11.2 (1928): 325-342.

[16] Winthrop adhered to the "Paracelsian compromise," meaning that he prescribed chemical cures but largely rejected Paracelsus' mystical and anti-Galenic approach to healing. See Ronald S. Wilkinson, "*Hermes Christianus*: John Winthrop, Jr., and Chemical Medicine in Seventeenth Century New England," *Science, Medicine and Society in the Renaissance*, vol. 1, ed. Allen G. Debus (London: Heinemann, 1972) 221, 229. Cf. Black 169; Woodward 160-162, 193-195. For the "Paracelsian compromise," see also Allen G. Debus, "The Paracelsian Compromise in Elizabethan England," *Ambix* 8 (1960): 71-97.

horn."[17] Rubila was used as a strong purgative and diaphoretic, and Winthrop's medical notebooks and letters indicate that he prescribed it for coughs, fevers, dropsy (edema), smallpox, measles, worms, and other afflictions. While some patients complained about the taste of the powder, rubila was among the most sought-after curatives in seventeenth-century New England, having gained a reputation as an American remedy superior to similar medicaments from Europe.[18] Although the colonists' demand for Winthrop's rubila is amply documented, there is no evidence that he distributed the recipe for the powder. To do so, he employed a number of trusted men and women in the colonies as unofficial medical surrogates who disseminated the medication on Winthrop's behalf and used it for their own medical services. Through this distribution service, he increased his popularity and political power, for each color-coded packet of medicine that reached the sick and proved efficacious advertised Winthrop as a caring colonial leader.[19]

[17] For the (assumed) recipe for rubila, see Holmes 335; "Wait Winthrop to Fitz-John Winthrop, 2 October 1682," *Collections of the Massachusetts Historical Society*, Series 5, Vol. 8 (1882): 429. In all likelihood, Winthrop did not invent rubila but seems to have adopted it from an unknown alchemical source. J. Worth Estes, *Dictionary of Protopharmacology: Therapeutic Practices, 1700-1850* (Canton, MA: Science History, 1990).

[18] "Roger Williams to John Winthrop, Jr., 22 June 1645," *Winthrop Papers* V, 30, writes: "I have books that prescribe powders etc. but yours is probatum in this Countrey." Until his death, Winthrop prescribed and distributed rubila to suffering colonists. See, for instance, "Daniel Clarke to John Winthrop, Jr., 7 August 1675," Beinecke Rare Book and Manuscript Library, Yale University. Walter R. Steiner, "Governor John Winthrop, Jr., of Connecticut, as a Physician," *Bulletin of the Johns Hopkins Hospital* 14 (1903): 301, argues that the powder was as close as Winthrop came to discovering the alchemical "elixir of life." Woodward explains, however, that "Rubila was not John Winthrop's most frequently prescribed medication, or even nearly so, but, because it was widely distributed by his sons after his death, many historians incorrectly assumed that it was Winthrop's primary prescription" (195).

[19] Woodward 199; Rebecca J. Tannenbaum, *The Healer's Calling: Women and Medicine in Early New England* (Ithaca: Cornell UP, 2002) 83.

In 1653, seven years after its foundation by John Winthrop Jr. the settlement of New London was in dire need of medical experts. Since the town, as most colonial outposts, failed to attract physicians in sufficient numbers, Winthrop began to apply his knowledge in alchemy and medicine for the benefit of the settlers and their Algonquian neighbors. His reputation as a successful healer soon spread beyond the town limits, as colonists from Connecticut, New Haven (then still a separate colony), Rhode Island, and Massachusetts increasingly addressed their medical needs to Winthrop. As we know from his unpublished medical notebooks, which he kept between 1657 and 1669, the younger Winthrop treated approximately 700 individuals during that time, often up to 12 patients a day, both in writing and in person. This is an astounding number considering that Connecticut's population amounted to roughly 5,000 at the time and that Winthrop practiced medicine concomitant to his gubernatorial duties.[20] His various health services, recorded in his notebooks and hundreds of extant medical request letters, not only tied in with a long tradition of Christian charity and practical divinity but also reflected a more secular, science-oriented understanding that a colony can only be built with sound bodies and minds.

## Medicine-by-Mail: Social and Cultural Implications of Long Distance Healing

Until recently, historians studying colonial American medicine have mainly focused on the lives of practitioners and/or on the efficacy of their treatment methods. This approach has tended to neglect the socio-cultural systems of meaning in which diseases were embedded. As Sander L. Gilman has shown in his comprehensive study of illness representations, "[l]ike any complex text, the signs of illness are read within the conventions of an interpretive community that comprehends them in the light of earlier, powerful readings of what are understood to

---

[20] Black 170. Richard Dunn estimates that about half of the colonial population in Connecticut sought Winthrop's medical advice. Richard Dunn, *Puritan and Yankees: The Winthrop Dynasty of New England, 1630-1717* (Princeton: Princeton UP, 1962) 83.

be similar or parallel texts."[21] When we apply this conceptual focus to the colonial American scene, Winthrop's medical correspondence offers new insights into the illness narrations by the people of New England. In fact, a study of medical letters sent to Winthrop by ministers, officials, farmers, artisans, housewives, and other representatives of colonial society opens an additional window on the practice and conceptualization of medicine in early America.

Throughout much of the seventeenth century, New England colonists depended on personal contacts, travelers, and a fragile postal system, largely run by Algonquian and Dutch couriers, to send and receive news about family, town, country, and the world. Due to the isolation of colonial settlements from each other and from the rest of the world, letters were an important medium of knowledge and information exchange. In the early days of the English colonies, however, the danger of raids by Indians or hostile seafarers, the possibility of bad weather, and the great distance between Europe and America, all contributed to making mailing letters a rather slow and precarious undertaking.

Letters also constituted an integral part of Winthrop's medical practice, offering means to convey recipes, advice, and solace for the sick and those treating them. Many surviving messages sent to and from Winthrop's various residences afford unprecedented insights into how early colonists appropriated, filtered, and shaped cultural conceptualizations of illness. In addition, Winthrop's long-distance consultation letters illustrate how one particular physician-alchemist transformed theoretical healing approaches, such as the Paracelsian notion of sympathetic attraction, into a form of medical practice appropriate for the challenges of life in early America.[22]

---

[21] Sander L. Gilman, *Disease and Representation: Images of Illness from Madness to AIDS* (Ithaca: Cornell UP, 1988) 7.

[22] For a recent study of communication processes in seventeenth-century New England, see Katherine A. Grandjean, *Reckoning: The Communications Frontier in Early New England.* Diss. Harvard U, 2008. William Decker lists the following central topics in American letter writing from the seventeenth to the nineteenth century: "spatiotemporal isolation, separation from family and friends, the invocation of a transcendental principle of enduring presence, dread of change in the intended recipient, anxiety over the miscarriage of incoming and outgoing mail, longing for reunion, and fear of death." William Merrill

To undertake a study of the socio-cultural implications and constructions of illness in colonial patient letters, it is useful to divide John Winthrop's medical communications into two groups: the correspondence with members of the political and theological elite in the colonies and letters exchanged with the New England lower and middling sorts and the laity. Although a differentiation between (letters by) professionals and the laity seems somewhat rigid and artificial, it offers an opportunity to demonstrate how Winthrop's knowledge exchange within a transatlantic community of savants influenced his treatment methods and how clerical interpretations of illness compared to those of the laity. This methodology, moreover, advances a "history from below" of colonial New England by comparing practical approaches to, and textual meaning-endowments of, illness by highly educated leaders and less learned, non-elite members of colonial American society.[23]

The main purpose of Winthrop's correspondence with members of the political, theological, and scientific elites, for whom I will use the shorthand "professionals," was to participate in, and benefit from, a network of knowledge that spanned across the Atlantic. Most of the letters exchanged between Winthrop and other professionals follow the interactional styles outlined in Angel Day's *The English Secretary* (1586) and other contemporary epistolary handbooks, especially with regard to formulaic and elaborate expressions of admiration, respect, courtesy, affection, humility, and/or request. In doing so, the interlocutors engaged in informational exchanges marked by general equality, common interests, implied obligations, and reciprocity. According to the protocols of early modern epistolarity, the stylistic expression of affection served to facilitate an exchange of intangible services (e.g., sharing knowledge, news, or networks) as well as of

Decker, *Epistolary Practices: Letter Writing in America before Telecommunications* (Chapel Hill: U of North Carolina P, 1998) 60.

[23] The methodological approach employed in the following sections takes its cue from Roy Porter, "The Patient's View: Doing Medical History from Below," *Theory and Society* 14 (1985): 175-198.

tangible material (e.g., specimens, books, or minerals) for the mutual benefit of the correspondents.[24]

While the advantages of epistolarity seemed self-evident to early modern intellectuals, the realities of mail delivery prior to the emergence of a state-run postal system were especially frustrating for men like Winthrop, who, living on the fringes of the known intellectual world depended on the exchange of goods and information. The unreliability of mail delivery left Winthrop and other correspondents guessing for months whether a letter had reached its destination. The certainty of geographic isolation hence caused a lingering uncertainty about belonging to an intellectual circle. Winthrop addressed this troubling circumstance at times in his correspondence, for instance when the Connecticut governor began a letter to Sir Robert Moray with the words:

> I had had sad & serious thoughts about the unhappinesse of the condition of a Wilderness life so remote from the fountains of learning & noble sciences,—the particular Ideas of some classic Heroes representing

---

[24] As Alan Stewart has shown, in the early modern world, letters "were the social glues that held firm friendships, alliances, and kinship ties between individuals at a distance." Alan Stewart, *Shakespeare's Letters* (Oxford: Oxford UP, 2008) 5. For a useful overview of letter-writing traditions in Europe, especially those represented by Erasmus and Angel Day, see Lynne Magnusson, *Shakespeare and Social Dialogue: Dramatic Language and Elizabethan Letters* (Cambridge: Cambridge UP, 1999) 61-90. For more comprehensive overviews on the practices and conventions of letter-writing in Renaissance and early modern England, see Gary Schneider, *The Culture of Epistolarity: Vernacular Letters and Letter Writing in Early Modern England, 1500-1700* (Newark: U of Delaware P, 2005); Susan E. Whyman, *Sociability and Power in Late-Stuart England: The Cultural Worlds of the Verneys, 1660-1720* (Oxford: Oxford UP, 1999) 3-12; James Daybell, *Women Letter-Writers in Tudor England* (Oxford: Oxford UP, 2006) 3-31; Jonathan Goldberg, *Writing Matter: From the Hands of the English Renaissance* (Stanford: Stanford UP, 1990); Roger Chartier, Alain Boureau, and Cécile Dauphin, *Correspondence: Models of Letter-Writing from the Middle Ages to the Nineteenth Century*, trans. Christopher Woodall (1991; Princeton: Princeton UP, 1997); Phillip H. Round, "Neither Here Nor There: Transatlantic Epistolarity in Early America," *A Companion to the Literatures of Colonial America*, ed. Susan Castillo and Ivy Schweitzer (Malden: Blackwell, 2005) 426-445.

nothing but sorrowes at the thoughts of their so great distance,—when I was greatly revived with the speciall favour of your honor's letter.[25]

This statement exemplifies how transatlantic intellectuals during the seventeenth century, like all letter-writers, employed the epistolary genre to overcome the geographic distance between addressor and addressee. For Winthrop, written correspondence, especially across the Atlantic, mitigated the realities of space, presence, and absence as much as they reified them. His experiences with delivery and non-delivery demonstrate how the construction of mental images, the fictionality of presence across distance in and through letters, marked a source of intellectual inspiration and sustenance as well as of emotional gratification and frustration, depending on whether and when an epistle reached its intended recipient.

In the colonies, the rise of Winthrop' medical and political reputation depended on the approbation of his healing services by the New England clergy. In light of the close intertwinement of theological and civil spheres, ministers functioned as important opinion leaders, whose influence could "make or break" a person, especially if s/he was a healer. One influential clerical supporter of the younger John Winthrop was John Davenport. The minister from New Haven Colony frequently consulted his Connecticut friend about matters of personal and public health and was so convinced of his medical expertise that he repeatedly attempted to persuade Winthrop and his wife to settle permanently in New Haven.[26] Davenport's medical correspondence with Winthrop illustrates how theological views on pathogenesis were translated into personal approaches to, and perspectives on, illness by one of the most orthodox New England clerics of the time. This is especially evident when Davenport writes about epidemics. In 1658, for instance, he interrupts his report on the symptoms of suffering colonists—"many are afflictively excercised, with grypings, vomitings, fluxes, agues and

---

[25] "John Winthrop, Jr., to Sir Robert Moray, 20 September 1664," *Proceedings of the Massachusetts Historical Society*, 16 (1878): 223.

[26] John Davenport to John Winthrop, Jr., 22 November 1655, John Davenport, *Letters of John Davenport, Puritan Divine*, ed. Isabel M. Calder (New Haven: Yale UP, 1937) 107-108.

feavers"—with a short prayer: "The good Lord prepare us for all changes, that under all changes of providences, we may have suitable changes of spirit, to honour, serve, and please God therein! Amen."[27] The repeated invocation of the word "change" in the letter can be read as an allusion to a number of transformations occurring in colonial New England society, in general, and in church policies, in particular. Davenport was deeply opposed to an extension of congregational membership beyond the realm of the visible saints and vociferously argued against the Half-Way Covenant, urging his fellow believers to remain on the course of orthodoxy.[28] Although none of his letters to Winthrop link the annual epidemics to on-going social and ecclesiastical transformations specifically, his narrative clearly implies a causal relation between disease, collective action, and "the afflicting hand of the Lord."[29]

Davenport's illness rhetoric differs, especially with regard to its degree of displayed literacy, from the bulk of patient letters Winthrop received during his career.[30] When the New Haven minister reports on

[27] Davenport to Winthrop, Jr., 4 August 1658, in Davenport, *Letters* 125-126.

[28] Formally introduced in 1662, the Half-Way Covenant marked a contentious compromise forged by New England ministers eager to counter declining church membership. It offered partial membership to the children and grandchildren of church members once they accepted the original covenant and led pious Christian lives. Significantly, Half-Way members did not have to give a public account of their conversion experience before the congregation in order to be accepted and allowed to partake in the sacraments. For Davenport's role and positions in the debate about church reform, see Isabel M. Calder, "A Biographical Sketch," *Letters of John Davenport, Puritan Divine*, ed. Isabel M. Calder (New Haven: Yale UP, 1937) 8.

[29] "Davenport to Winthrop, Jr., 4 August 1658," in Davenport, *Letters* 125. One year later, Davenport makes a similar allusion, when he interprets another epidemic as a divine intervention. See also, "Davenport to Winthrop, Jr., 6 December 1659," in Davenport, *Letters* 147.

[30] Scholars have estimated that roughly 60 percent of the English male population and about 30 percent of the female inhabitants of seventeenth-century possessed basic reading and writing skills, allowing them to at least sign their names. The percentage of colonists able to read (only) was significantly higher, although exact numbers are missing. Kenneth Lockridge, *Literacy in Colonial*

the progress of one of Winthrop's local patients who is suffering from an ocular disease, his description is comparatively detailed and elaborate: "from the ball of the eye groweth a carnous substance, which covereth the neathereye lid all over, and at the end of it, in the corner of the eye, by his nose, is a tumor of a pretty bignes."[31] Davenport's education, which obviously included some rudimentary instruction in medicine, enables him to suggest possible causes of the affliction in Galenic terms—"peradventure it is the chrystaline humor"—thus directing Winthrop's diagnosis and treatment.[32] When Davenport complains about one of his own afflictions, he supplements contemporary scientific discourse with religious references. He explicitly places the course of his health into God's hands. However, this does not mean that he abstains from accepting all the medical help he can muster. When Davenport seeks Winthrop's advice about his urinary tract problems, the description of his affliction again reveals that he has some state-of-the-art medical knowledge: he relates the color of his urine, writes as precisely but tactfully as possible about his bowel movements, while veiling the most intimate aspects of his condition in Latin. As his illness description unfolds, Davenport delineates the time and location of pain in his body, reports on his appetite, and relates how the weather affects his overall condition. In short, his patient letter attempts to anticipate the questions a physician might ask and seeks to answer them as if a personal consultation were proceeding.[33]

In one of the last letters he sent to Winthrop, Davenport writes about an affliction of his son, which the Connecticut governor had been treating both in person and in writing. His final statement encapsulates,

_New England: An Enquiry into the Social Context of Literacy in the Early Modern West_ (New York: Norton, 1974) 13, 38-39; Jill Lepore, _The Name of War: King Philip's War and the Origins of American Identity_ (New York: Vintage, 1998) 37, 54. For a more in-depth look at methods of learning to read in early New England, see David D. Hall, _Worlds of Wonder, Days of Judgment: Popular Religious Belief in Early New England_ (New York: Knopf, 1989) 31-43.

[31] "Davenport to Winthrop, Jr., 30 January 1657," in Davenport, _Letters_ 113.

[32] "Davenport to Winthrop, Jr., 30 January 1657," in Davenport, _Letters_ 113.

[33] "Davenport to Winthrop, Jr., 20 July 1660," in Davenport, _Letters_ 167.

perhaps like few others, the typical Puritan conceptualization of health and illness placed under the auspices of God's providence: "The good Lord pitty him, and rebuke the distemper, in mercy, and send forth his word and heale him: and guide you what course to præscribe for his helpe, and bless the same for his good, through Jesus christ! in whom I rest."[34] Here as elsewhere, Davenport acknowledges God's hand in the cause of the affliction and expresses central Calvinist tenets underlying the way to health. The appeal to God's mercy through prayer precedes the recognition that He has provided help not only through direct intervention but also through physicians as indirect divine means of healing. Davenport's carefully constructed letter furthermore underlines his conviction that medical knowledge and prescriptions must be bracketed by religion. Faith is the precondition of successful healing, and medical discourse and practices have to be kept within the boundaries of theological premises.

Davenport's illness epistles demonstrate also how professionals shared a degree of literacy and intellectual insight into disease etiology that surpassed that of the laity. Whether written by natural philosophers, theologians or other members of the intellectual elite of Europe and America, the patient letters, which Winthrop received from professionals, illustrate the ability to articulate thoughts, ideas, and observations about the world in a learned, insightful, and eloquent way and to express themselves in accordance with the stylistic and social etiquette of the time. Against this background, a comparison of Davenport's illness rhetoric, which exemplifies how religious leaders clothed their ailments in scientific and religious terms, with lay patient letters offers valuable insights into the scope and breadth of colonial New England illness narratives and exposes the effects of social positioning on language and style deployed in epistolary exchanges.

Patient letters shed light on illness conceptions and experiences like few other colonial documents. They convey the writer's pain and suffering, speculate on causes of illness, reflect (on) the previous course

---

[34] "Davenport to Winthrop, Jr., 1 May 1666," in Davenport, *Letters* 260. For an analysis of how Elizabeth Davenport intervened in her husband's letter-writing process, interjecting her own voice into the correspondence with Winthrop, see chapter three.

of life and, at times, on pending death, and seek solace and relief from the person addressed in the letter. Furthermore, as textual artifacts, patient letters illustrate how sensations, emotions, fears, desires, and expectations prompted by an illness are mediated by cultural codes and linguistic signs. These are in part drawn from a universal repertoire of conventions, and in part grounded in specific geographic locales, historic eras, individual preferences, and socio-cultural environments. In the early modern period, any letter about health and illness was contingent upon, and representative of, acceptable forms and contents of epistolarity. Although the formalities of letter writing, which New Englanders had imported from Europe, granted correspondents only limited room to invest them with subjectivity, letters in which the writer depicted his/her medical condition in relative detail necessarily entailed a revelation of the writer's physical and mental idiosyncrasies. Colonial illness letters, like few other pathographic genres at the time, dwelled in a dialectic space between private utterance and public discourse; they cast their object of representation—the writer's specific illness—in terms provided by cultural conventions. They assimilated these conventions for their own purposes and yet remained inextricably bound to them. In doing so, New England patient letters asserted and maintained a (however limited) degree of narrative authority and interpretative latitude that was energized by a polyphony and plurality of meanings concerning illness experiences.[35] Common epistolary descriptions of sickness ranged from a sentence fragment—"a desease much like the fluxe"—to elaborate, sermonizing accounts of how illness

---

[35] For useful studies on medical consultation letters in early modern Europe, see Micheline Louis-Courvoisier and Séverine Pilloud, "Consulting by Letter in the Eighteenth Century: Mediating the Patient's View?," *Cultural Approaches to the History of Medicine: Mediating Medicine in Early Modern and Modern Europe*, ed., Cornelie Usborne and Willem De Blécourt (New York: Palgrave, 2004) 71-88; José Pardo-Tomás and Alvar Martínez-Vidal, "Stories of Disease Written by Patients and Lay Mediators in the Spanish Republic of Letters, 1680-1720," *Journal of Medieval and Early Modern Studies* 38 (2008): 467-491; Hubert Steinke and Martin Stuber, "Medical Correspondence in Early Modern Europe: An Introduction," *Gesnerus* 61 (2004): 139-160; Martin Dinges and Vincent Barras, eds., *Krankheit in Briefen im deutschen und französischen Sprachraum. 17.-21. Jahrhundert* (Stuttgart: Steiner, 2007).

figures within God's providential plan for humanity.[36] In addition, the
writers of the patient letters represented the social, cultural, and
economic spectrum of mid-seventeenth-century New England. While
some writers were barely literate, others portrayed themselves as well
versed in the social etiquette and eloquence required in epistolary
manuals of post-Renaissance England.

In a time and environment where health was precarious and disease
constantly imminent, passing references to one's own or one's family's
health and wishes for the well-being of the addressee marked an intricate
part of epistolary conventions and can be found in letters from all ranks
of the socio-economic order in New England. In many colonial epistles,
especially those exchanged between family members and close
acquaintances, at least an allusion to, if not more lengthy descriptions
about the state of health either of the addressed or the addressee, were
included. For example, when John Winthrop Jr. writes to his father in
1649, shortly before the death of the Massachusetts Bay Colony leader,
he reports: "You may be pleased to vnderstand that we are all (through
Gods mercy) in good health, both in our owne family & all our
plantation."[37] The wording of health reports and concerns varied among
correspondents, but the questions or statements about illness and health
point to the centrality of disease in the daily realities of colonial
America and, moreover, to the importance of treating illnesses both
physically and mentally. That is, references to health and sickness
tended to exceed the formulaic and often constituted a form of "writing
cure" undergirded by a conviction that God knew the thoughts and
prayers of his flock and would respond accordingly.

In addition to ubiquitous comments on, and/or wishes for, the health
of the writer or the recipient, colonists frequently used the epistolary
genre to seek medical consultation from family, friends, physicians,
ministers, and/or public officials. Most of these letters have been lost;

---

[36] "Hannah Gallope to John Winthrop, Jr., 12 April 1660," *Collections of the
Massachusetts Historical Society*, Series 5, Vol. 1 (1871): 98. Cf. "Samuel
Gorton to John Winthrop, Jr., 21 October 1674," *Collections of the
Massachusetts Historical Society*, Series 4, Vol. 7 (1865): 604-626.

[37] "John Winthrop, Jr., to John Winthrop, 17 January 1648/49," *Collections of
the Massachusetts Historical Society*, Series 5, Vol. 8 (1882): 39.

however, since the early nineteenth century, historians have searched for, found, and published a substantial number of medical advice letters sent to (and to a much lesser degree written by) John Winthrop Jr. Of the patient letters sent to Winthrop between 1645 and 1675, the overwhelming majority was written by men, reflecting the social relegation of women to the domestic sphere. Some colonists wrote on behalf of family members or neighbors, who apparently lacked the means, strength or courage to address their health needs to the Connecticut leader. Most patients were often already in a serious medical condition and many correspondents reported that they first sought remedies that were available in their vicinity before addressing Winthrop.

Lay patient letters sent to John Winthrop illustrate how common colonists perceived their bodies and how they made sense of various illnesses. Most New England patient letters by non-professionals were written in plain style rather than following the elaborate, oratory epistolary etiquette prescribed in guidebooks by Erasmus, Angel Day, and others. Winthrop's lay patient letters are especially insightful because they respond to Puritanism's demand for self-reflection and, at the same time, demonstrate means of self-crafting that one finds in few other textual genres. That is, by producing accounts of their illnesses, letter-writers create topoi that shape their identity in accordance with, and in deviance from, Puritan religious norms. Taken collectively, lay patient letters not only present instances of self-fashioning the writer's identity, they also position the recipient as a capable and helpful physician since the epistolary form, especially when linked with illnesses, prefigures the response to the request.[38]

Most of the ninety-five lay medical requests surveyed for this chapter share a structural pattern similar to most patient letters at the time: they begin with a standard salutation, which expresses the author's reverence for Winthrop's achievements, knowledge, and social status. In order to establish an interpersonal relationship necessary for relating

---

[38] For a more in-depth discussion of the performativity and self-awareness of identity constructions in European humanism, see Stephen Greenblatt, *Renaissance Self-Fashioning: From More to Shakespeare* (Chicago: U of Chicago P, 1980).

intimate details about their bodies, patients often refer to a previous meeting or exchange of services. Such references to the past also seek to arouse Winthrop's sense of obligation in the present. Most writers recognize the need to apologize for the boldness of expecting Winthrop's sympathy and for intruding in his life, which is only justified by the matter at hand: a severe illness. The main part of most letters is then devoted to a more or less elaborate description of the illness, followed by a plea for advice and direction, and a formulaic valediction. The complimentary openings and closings in most patient letters—a typical characteristic of English epistles—illustrate the cultural custom of recognizing the social position of the writer and the recipient, and show how both the New England elite and the laity were versed in cultural conventions of courtesy inherited from the Renaissance.[39] In addition, many medical consultation letters sent to Winthrop constitute self-referential textual artifacts on a number of levels. They draw attention to the act of composition (e.g., by apologizing for addressing Winthrop), convey the material conditions under which they were written (e.g., the social status or geographic location of the writer), hint at the possibility of failed delivery, and construct the self by expressing certain fears, desires, beliefs, expectations, and knowledge concerning the health and sickness of the author.

The decision to pen a medical request letter to John Winthrop Jr. especially after he became governor of Connecticut in 1657, entailed leaving the private sphere and entering a semi-public realm. That is, the expression of intimacy signified an adoption of authority over interpreting the body and its afflictions, and, at the same time, submitted the writer to the authority of a person who was both healer and leader. In a letter to Winthrop, "the humblest citizen may dispatch a missive to the highest reaches of the political, social, or cultural hierarchy [...] bypass[ing] all intermediaries standing between ordinary public opinion and decision makers."[40] Because of the power asymmetries between the

---

[39] C. Dallet Hemphill, *Bowing to Necessities: A History of Manners in America, 1620-1860* (New York: Oxford UP, 1999) 17-31.

[40] Alain Boureau, "The Letter-Writing Norm, a Medieval Invention," *Correspondence: Models of Letter-Writing from the Middle Ages to the*

interlocutors, Winthrop considered it his duty to provide medical treatment, and colonists voiced their demands for healing accordingly. In early New England, as throughout the early modern Western world, the epistolary genre thus functioned as an index to social relations. As such, it was "a potentially dangerous form, since anyone writing a risk-taking letter (whether a request for a loan, an apology, or a declaration of love) must, if it is to succeed, accurately imagine the recipient's response both to the situation itself and the words and tone chosen."[41] This observation holds especially true for the medical needs addressed to Winthrop by members of the laity. By writing to a respected leader, and son of the revered founder of Massachusetts, colonists took certain risks, because the letters necessitated revelations of intimate details about the author's body, mind, soul, conduct of life, and interactions with others. Such a public rendering of private conditions inherently drew the sender out of the relative protection from colonial authority, often granted by a secluded frontier existence, and placed him/her in an exceptional position of vulnerability to the exercise of state-sanctioned biopower.[42] The vocabulary of illness in Winthrop's lay patient letters hence often sought to minimize the risks entailed in exposing one's physical and spiritual condition to a man of power by portraying sickness in functional terms and in accordance with Puritan plain-style rhetoric.

Most of the letters written to Winthrop by common colonists represent illness in colloquial terms. Language, the central constituent of culture, functions as a tool with which patients aim to translate disease into meaningful statements. Such a "translation" facilitates the manageability of illness and would hopefully trigger an efficacious treatment by Winthrop. Hence, the writer's education and degree of

*Nineteenth Century*, ed. Roger Chartier, Alain Boureau, and Cecile Dauphin (Princeton: Princeton UP, 1997) 24-25.

[41] John Barnard, "Keats's Letters," *The Cambridge Companion to Keats*, ed. Susan J. Wolfson (Cambridge: Cambridge UP, 2001) 120. Epistolary descriptions of the sick colonial body thus constitute what Lynne Magnusson has called, in a different context, "risk-filled speech-acts" (70).

[42] Michel Foucault, *The History of Sexuality Vol. 1: An Introduction*, trans. Robert Hurley (1976; New York: Random, 1978) 139.

literacy decisively guides the signs and modes of illness construction in the text. In describing their illnesses, most lay patients employ a realistic mode of delineating their afflictions, hoping to provide Winthrop with the best information about their conditions. Given the specific cause for writing, most correspondents attempt to replicate a personal doctor-patient encounter in the sickroom. They approximate a speaking voice and employ linguistic and tonal registers that express both the everyday and a sense of respect for the physician. For instance, in 1652 George Ward, a ship-carpenter from New Haven and member of John Davenport's congregation, orchestrates his affliction as follows:

> [...] About 10 or 11 yeeres agoe a litle before winter sett in I took a great cold upon an extraordinary heat in travell by occasion whereof I perceved an burning in my water being often provoked to Urine which growing on wrought a stopping in my making water with heate and payne after my water would passe from mee at unaware. By fitts I have more grievous payne than ordinary it may bee once or twict in a houer by my water stopping. The last yeere I had a soare fitt almost a month togeather, stopping almost every morning sorely payneing mee. This spring I had a sore affliction by a bastard plurisy which held mee sore a forthnight, and after a forenight more with lesse payne and ever since I have bin sore troubled with whitish slimemy viscous matter in my urine. I have often and espescially of late used what meenes I could but am not at all bettered. What God doth further requier mee to doe I stand bound to attend, and leave the issue with himself.[43]

In contrast to John Davenport's above-cited depiction of a similar medical condition, Ward's letter is more descriptive and less analytical, and thereby exemplifies how middling-sort and lay patients used different discursive and linguistic registers to ask for medical help. Nonetheless, similar to Davenport, Ward's illness narrative actively participates in the diagnosis, by suggesting the name of the disease ("bastard pleurisy"), and in the treatment, by pointing Winthrop toward

---

[43] "George Ward to John Winthrop, Jr., 15 June 1652," *Winthrop Papers* VI, 203.

possible medicaments (i.e., he already "used what meens I could").[44] This indicates that lay patients in the early modern English-speaking world were able to exercise some control over their treatment and were less dependent on the knowledge of medical experts for their recovery than most patients in Western societies today.[45] Moreover, by naming symptoms and relating them to someone known and revered for his medical expertise, Ward's representation of his bodily affliction can already be seen as part of the healing process. His efforts for a comprehensive depiction of his corporeal condition, including a brief summary of his case history, and his detailed, adjectival delineation of perceived sensations and excretions (e.g., "whitish slimemy viscous matter"), seem to indicate that Ward hopes to ameliorate his painful condition in and through writing. The therapeutic effects of such a representation of illness are especially evident when Winthrop responds by sending medicaments, providing directions for their application, and by offering words of advice and solace. Ward's patient letter shows, therefore, how many New England colonists believed in the curative power of words, particularly in conjunction with medicaments. Writing about one's illness seemed to flank recovery by attaching meaning to suffering and by knowing that someone "out there" cared and expressed his/her concerns and thoughts about healing in writing.[46]

---

[44] According to the *Oxford English Dictionary*, the term "bastard" here refers to "having the appearance of, somewhat resembling," meaning that Ward is not sure whether his condition would be termed "pleurisy" (designating pain in the chest or the side) in the medical parlance of his time. The "meens" used by Ward most likely refer to natural curatives derived from the "kitchen physic" commonly employed by women and lay healers (cf. chapter three).

[45] Andrew Wear, *Knowledge and Practice in English Medicine, 1550-1680* (Cambridge: Cambridge UP, 2000) 114. As Rebecca Tannenbaum explains in her study of seventeenth-century New England medical practices, "the relationship between patients and healers was much more egalitarian than it would later become, since most ordinary people had enough medical knowledge to make informed choices about their care and to judge critically the care they received" (6).

[46] The therapeutic effects of writing for colonial New Englanders are difficult to prove due to the lack of primary sources (i.e., most of the patient letters are one-time events and most of Winthrop's replies are missing). We know from the

One of the problems of this epistolary illness narrative is that Ward, like most patients in seventeenth-century New England, implicitly expects that Winthrop is able to decipher the signs that he employs to represent the experience of pain and suffering correctly. With regard to this authorial intention, Ward's request letter actually exemplifies the limits and inadequacies of a mere textual, language-based medical treatment, since the medium inherently precludes a holistic diagnosis because it has to omit the sights, sounds, and smells of illness. And even though the relationship between the experience and the reality of disease is characterized by a relation that is as unstable as that between linguistic sign and referent, a knowledgeable healer such as Winthrop, when interacting personally with a patient, could undertake various diagnostic processes, consult medical handbooks, and ask follow-up questions that are vital for procuring an efficacious treatment. Aside from the unbridgeable gap between the somatic and the semantic Ward's letter also indicates how the *mise en scène* of suffering provides the writer with an opportunity for self-fashioning. That is, his written etiopathology is unique in the sense that no other patient will likely represent the same symptoms and the experience of illness in the same way. By turning the idiosyncrasies of illness into narrative, the letter writer momentarily constructs a sense of presence and identity in textual space.

Other colonial letter writers express more explicitly how the chosen representational mode fails to do justice to their condition and, therefore, ask for a personal meeting with Winthrop. Besides negotiating a discursive space between language and reality, as well as between individual expression and public conventions, several lay patient letters

extended correspondence between Winthrop and Davenport, however, that the latter recognized the curative effects of "your former very loving lines" and one can reasonably assume that this notion was shared by many New England colonists. John Davenport to John Winthrop, Jr., 1 August 1660, John Davenport, *Letters of John Davenport, Puritan Divine*, ed. Isabel M. Calder (New Haven: Yale UP, 1937) 171. For a comparative perspective on the potentially therapeutic effects of writing about illness experiences, see Lisa Wynne Smith, "'An Account of an Unaccountable Distemper': The Experience of Pain in Early Eighteenth-Century England and France," *Eighteenth-Century Studies* 41.4 (2008): 466.

voice the author's concern over material space: the letter itself and the geographic distance it attempts to bridge. Despite the limited room for individual expression inherent in the epistolary genre, many patients aim to "embody" themselves in the letter—through the handwriting, the signature, and a specific representation of thought, voice, and personae—and thus to create a fiction of presence that mitigates the spatial distance between sender and recipient. In seventeenth-century New England, however, such an attempted bridging of distance soon reached the boundaries of practicability, especially when the content of communication involved illness. In Winthrop's case, patients frequently lament the inability of consulting with Winthrop in person and thus convey a sense of uneasiness about transforming a face-to-face meeting into a written correspondence.

Aside from language and geography, temporality marked a central constraint for the simulation of personal interactions in letter writing and particularly for Winthrop's epistolary therapeutics. The deferral of the communication through the medium itself—in mid-seventeenth-century New England, a letter from New Haven to Hartford, a distance of roughly forty miles, would take an average of three to four delivery days, depending on the carrier and weather conditions—entailed crucial consequences for writers seeking medical advice. In most cases, time was an essential factor in the treatment itself and with regard to the patient's condition; patients and their caregivers expected that the condition of the sick deteriorated while the letter was being delivered, answered, and returned. The various uncertainties involved in corresponding across space and time, the fear that the message would reach Winthrop too late or not at all, often caused a tone of heightened urgency. For example, John Davenport concludes one of his illness descriptions by noting: "Sir you see our need of a speedy answer, if it were possible, by some winged messenger, if an Indian could bring it sooner than Samuel can, I will pay him for his paines whatever you please to promise."[47] Some correspondents used non-verbal means to express the need for speedy medical help, for instance, by underlining the date of composition three times, thus emphasizing that a quick reaction by Winthrop was of utmost importance for the well being and

---

[47] "Davenport to Winthrop, Jr., 23 December 1660," in Davenport, *Letters* 188.

recovery of the patient.[48] These and other hastily written expressions of temporal constraints shed light on the intertwinement of material and rhetorical aspects of letter writing in early New England. They show how illness-related topics, including symptoms, anxieties, fears, and physical sensations, became intrinsic structural elements of the epistolary narrative itself, and how context and content shaped the form and narrative of a written communication that was essentially about matters of life and death.

Despite the linguistic and material restrictions that letter writing entailed for medical treatment, Winthrop's practice of medicine-by-mail was fully adapted to the life realities and cultural convictions of early Americans. As a consequence, it served as a welcome supplement to face-to-face interactions with local medical personnel. Long-distance consultations marked a practical, space-defying necessity and were, as such, undergirded by medical theories derived from Hermetic philosophy and by Christian tenets. Paracelsus' claim, outlined in his *Opus Paramirum* (1530-1531), that "[j]ust as the sun can shine through a glass and fire act through the walls of a stove, so bodies can send out invisible forces over distances while remaining at rest themselves," formed one conceptual foundation for various efforts to develop long-distance healing methods.[49] Alchemists such as Robert Fludd and Kenelme Digby believed that by applying a specific ointment to a sword or a lance, the wound it had caused could be healed across distances. This magical treatment, called "weapon salve," was based on the theory of sympathetic attraction, according to which various objects in the universe influence each other and can hence be manipulated by the alchemical sage for curative purposes.[50] Even more importantly, in order to gain public acceptance for long-distance cures, Winthrop's epistolary therapeutics complied with Christianity's emphasis on the possible

---

[48] See, for instance, the original manuscript of George Ward to John Winthrop, Jr., 15 June 1652, Countway Medical Library, Harvard University, BMS C.56.2.

[49] Paracelsus, *Paracelsus: Selected Readings*, ed. and trans. Nicholas Goodrick-Clarke, I. ix. 325 (Wellingborough: Crucible, 1990) 100.

[50] "Sir Kenelme Digby to John Winthrop, Jr., 26 January 1656," *Collections of the Massachusetts Historical Society*, Series 3, Vol. 10 (1849): 19; Carré 569; Woodward 196.

spiritual presence in the Lord. In accordance with Pauline epistles and related scriptural passages, Winthrop and his colonial patients implicitly asserted that bodily absence could be overcome by being "present in spirit" (1 Corinthians 5:3) through letters, thoughts, and prayers. The spiritual "presence in absence" helped to legitimize the medicine-by-mail system and to emphasize its potential to cure. In other words, by combining alchemical and Christian ideas about presence and absence, Winthrop sought and claimed absence not as an absolute condition grounded in a physical reality; rather, absence was seen merely as an incomplete presence, remedied by forging spiritual connections between healer and patient.

Yet, in a number of cases medical treatment through letters lacked tangible healing effects and, as a result, Winthrop visited the sick whenever possible. Patients also asked to relocate temporarily to his place of residence. The correspondence surveyed for this study show that, between 1653 and 1654, about ten patients were in constant residence at New London, and an additional five patients desired Winthrop's personal treatment. These numbers do not include those who had asked Winthrop in person, whose letters are lost, or who traveled to his home unannounced. Although details are missing, it seems certain that New London evolved into a medical town whose "hospital" was Winthrop's home, which also functioned as a medical library, treatment room, and "pharmacy of Aesculapius," as one observer raved in 1656.[51]

One of the most insightful examples of Winthrop's medical practice, involving both written and personal consultations, is the case of Lydia Odell. In November 1652, Richard Odell, then resident of Southampton, Long Island, penned an urgent request on behalf of his young daughter, Lydia. His salutation is unusually short, and without further ado, he addresses his daughter's condition: "Sir, I have mad bold to troble you with a few lines," Odell begins his request letter, stressing that "it hath pleased the Allmightie to laye his afflickting hand upon a child of mine by a disease which most do thinke to be the palsey." Odell's omission of formulaic features of seventeenth-century English epistolary

---

[51] Quoted in Harold Jantz, "America's First Cosmopolitan," *Proceedings of the Massachusetts Historical Society*, Third Series, Vol. 84 (1972): 19. Cf. Woodward 189-191.

conventions (i.e., he leaves out the usual expression of respect and reverence for the recipient) underlines the exigency of the medical case and indicates his conviction that exaggerated courtesies are mere barriers to, rather than necessary rhetorical resources for, exchanging medical information. Instead, the description of his daughter's paralysis is written in a tone of deep concern, certain to arouse pity and compassion in the reader: "she was nether able to stand nor speak and so shee hath continued till this Instant haveing lost the use of the right side from the head to he[r] foot."[52]

Winthrop's response to Odell's representation of the tragic dimension of human existence, especially when a young child is afflicted, is one of only few surviving medical advice letters addressed to the New England laity and is extant only because Winthrop had prepared a copy. The reply affords a number of insights into colonial medicine, Winthrop's relation to his patients, and some of the reasons for his popularity. It highlights some of the structural inadequacies of medical practice in colonial New England, especially the lack of apothecaries, who could provide and prepare necessary medicaments, and shows Winthrop's sustained understanding of, and engagement in, medical theories and their applications at the time. In addition, the letter proves him to be an empathetic physician who considers the case carefully. At the outset of his medical advice letter, he reminds his reader of the limits of epistolary therapeutics and the need to see the child in person, but also writes that "by your description I judge it to be a palsy, yet the cause of that diseas is often very differing for in some it is through too much drinesse in some too much moisture in some the cause is in the Nerves of the third conjugation of the braine sometymes in other nerves, in others it hath its originall in the marrow of the back bone."[53] It seems noteworthy how Winthrop takes up Odell's suggestion that his child's illness is palsy and offers an altogether different causal explanation. While Odell can only make sense of his daughter's illness

---

[52] "Richard Odell to John Winthrop, Jr., 16 November 1652," *Winthrop Papers* VI, 229.

[53] "John Winthrop, Jr., to Richard Odell, 27 November 1652," *Winthrop Papers* VI, 230-231.

by invoking the hand of God, John Winthrop places the etiology firmly in the hand of the emerging sciences.

Instead of merely asking Odell to send his daughter to New London, the physician elaborates probable diagnoses based on the written illness narrative. He then offers a number of possible remedies, but emphasizes that the efficacy of each depends on the actual cause of the child's condition. Medical historian Henry Viets has argued that the letter reflects Winthrop's adherence to Galenic medicine. Viets bases his argument on Winthrop's reference to the excess of humoral qualities ("too much drinesse"; "too much moisture"), his suggestion of a treatment of opposites (a coldness needs the application of heat), and his prescription of guiacum and sarsaparilla to induce vomiting.[54] Despite these references to Galenic remedies, however, some of Winthrop's curative suggestions are clearly drawn from Paracelsian medicine, among them the use of water (mineral baths) and medicaments derived from alchemical procedures. With regard to its representation of medical theory and practice, therefore, the letter actually outlines Winthrop's mixture of Galenic and Paracelsian approaches to healing.

In his response to Winthrop's list of suggestions, Richard Odell expresses his sincere gratitude for having received a medicament (most likely rubila) that has improved his daughter's condition. For a full recovery, Odell desires Winthrop's personal treatment and hence muses on the possibilities and difficulties of moving to New London. Since his wife is expecting another child and because someone would have to accompany his ailing daughter during her medical visit, he would have to relocate the whole family, a sheer impossibility given that the livelihood of a family such as the Odells depended on maintaining a farm. The postscript of the letter further relates to the difficult situation of frontier life: not only do the Odells have to worry about the health of their children, their decision concerning if and when to move to New London is also affected by geopolitical forces beyond their immediate control. The head of the family expresses his fear that virulent

[54] Viets 26.

skirmishes with the Natives or between the English and the Dutch will make the recovery plans for his daughter impossible.[55]

The final letter from Odell to Winthrop reveals yet another problem that illness posed for colonial families, especially poorer settlers: the inability to reimburse healers adequately for their services. Most colonists who sought Winthrop's medical advice did not offer concrete compensation for his services. It was commonly understood that medical expertise was not merely an acquired knowledge that could be sold, but rather a gift from God that the physician—based on Christian charity and compassion—should administer freely. Despite this cultural convention, many patients of John Winthrop Jr. promised services in the future or other means of compensating for his efforts. Odell, for example, offers Winthrop "an Ancer [i.e., a case or keg; M.P.] of whale Oyle and also som whalebone [...] as a token" of his gratitude and also promises unspecified services in the future.[56] In addition, he claims that he will acquire the necessary funds to ensure the medical treatment of his daughter. More importantly, Odell, as well as many other patients in colonial America, relegate payment to the spiritual realm.[57] The scarcity

[55] "Richard Odell to John Winthrop, Jr., Spring 1652/1653," *Winthrop Papers* VI, 270-271. In the follow-up letter it becomes clear that Odell managed to facilitate his daughter's visit to New London, although the practical arrangements remain unclear.

[56] "Richard Odell to John Winthrop, Jr., 26 May 1654," *Winthrop Papers* VI, 384. Lydia Odell's medical condition continued to concern Winthrop in the years following this exchange of medical letters with her father. On 22 May 1661, the Connecticut governor recorded the following note in his medical journal: "Odell Lidia 11 y[ears] Mr. Odell's daughter of Seataket upon Long Iland she was paraliticall in her leg & some on one side & was formerly with [one word blotted out] me at New London, hath now some strength & can go well &c., but hath now some kind of convulsion fits since a fright taken at Hempsted." John Winthrop, Jr., "Medical Account Books," Ms. (Hartford: Connecticut Historical Society) 507. I am grateful to Robert C. Anderson for alerting me to this reference and for sharing his insights on Winthrop's medical practice.

[57] "Richard Odell to John Winthrop, Jr., Spring 1652/53," *Winthrop Papers* VI, 270-271. Since cash was scarce in seventeenth-century New England, colonists often offered to pay Winthrop in wheat, honey, wampum (shells or beads used

of metal coinage in early New England energized mechanisms of informal credit exchange in all spheres of the economy and particularly in the field of medicine. During the seventeenth and eighteenth centuries, people on both sides of the Atlantic witnessed an increasingly mixed medical economy in which personal, intangible exchanges coincided with fiscal payments for healing services. Medicine hence marked a sphere of exchange that was not wholly monetized and subject to invisible market forces in the Friedmanian sense; rather, New England culture, in particular, shaped medical practice based on kindness, compassion, and the need to show fellowship with the afflicted.[58]

In return for his medical services, Winthrop not only received gratitude, religious blessings, and tangible compensation but, more importantly, he gained popularity and personal power. As Woodward explains,

> Being recognized as someone to whom God had granted special healing abilities was a significant status marker. In a culture that focused great attention on the spiritual connections between this world and the next and that saw the human body as a central metaphor defining the hierarchical organization of society (the body social), political authority (the body political), and the community of saints (the body ecclesiastical), the power to heal the body corruptible, especially by

as currency by local Native people) and other goods and services. By contrast, those (few) colonists who could afford reimbursement in specie hoped that their ability to pay in cash or silver would hasten Winthrop's reply in the matter. See, for instance, "Daniel Clark to Hugh Caulkins, 11 February 1653," *Winthrop Papers* VI, 246; "Daniel Clark to John Winthrop Jr., 17 March 1652/53," *Winthrop Papers* VI, 263-264.

[58] For a useful investigation of the medical marketplace in colonial America, see Ben Mutschler, "Illness in the 'Social Credit' and 'Money' Economies of Eighteenth-Century New England," *Medicine and the Market in England and Its Colonies, c. 1450-c. 1850*, ed. Mark S. R. Jenner and Patrick Wallis (New York: Palgrave, 2007) 175-195. For a more comprehensive study of pecuniary and non-pecuniary means of exchange in the early modern world, see Craig Muldrew, *The Economy of Obligation: The Culture of Credit and Social Relations in Early Modern England* (New York: Palgrave, 1998).

means of divinely blessed healing agents, provided a strong affirmation
of one's right to serve at the head of the social, political, or religious
hierarchy.[59]

This observation underlines a central argument of this study: colonial
medical practices were crucial in disseminating and shaping the course
and extent of power in early New England. By not insisting on monetary
payment and by claiming his medical service as part of his religious and
civil duties, Winthrop was able to increase his reputation, credibility,
and social influence that would later culminate in actual political
power.[60]

The Odell case also exemplifies how the bulk of Winthrop's
consultation letters provided colonists with access to the knowledge of
the world, especially with regard to the changing field of medicine. The
dialogic nature of Winthrop's medicine-by-mail fostered the
dissemination of contemporary cutting-edge treatment methods to and
among the colonial laity and, at the same time, afforded common New
Englanders a significant degree of visibility in colonial society. The
patient letters were, hence, more than means to an end; they offered
opportunities for the epistolary voice to constitute and construct itself in
a field of tension between cultural conventions and individual
subjectivity. As one result, any illness considered worth reporting
proved ambivalent for the lay correspondent, because it weakened
his/her bodily and often mental constitution and, yet, offered an
opportunity to strengthen his/her identity and recognition in and through
writing. Ironically, it was the portrayal of *suffering* that offered colonists
from all ranks of society a degree of initiative, autonomy, and
participation in shaping modes and means of grappling with health and
illness matters and, thereby, the course of culture in early New England.

---

[59] Woodward 200.

[60] Woodward points out that it was his reputation and power, in part gained
through his medical services, which afforded Winthrop enough latitude and
authority to resolve the witchcraft cases brought to his attention. As a
consequence, during his term as governor and while he was present in America,
no person accused of witchcraft was executed in the Connecticut Colony
(Woodward 210-252).

Interestingly enough, none of the lay letters surveyed for this study explicitly mentions the possibility of sin as a cause for the illness. This is especially surprising in the case of Lydia Odell. Preachers had long postulated, based on biblical exegesis, that sin was the cause of palsy; however, both Odell's medical request and Winthrop's reply include only few references to religious components of healing and none with regard to the relation between palsy and sin.[61] Against the backdrop of Puritanism's culture of confession, it seems striking that there are only few references to the patients' moral shortcomings or transgressions in the bulk of lay letters sent to Winthrop. While many epistles express how illness is caused and cured by God—George Ward, for instance, ends his illness description by stating that, "What God doth further requier mee to doe I stand bound to attend, and leave the issue with himself"—divine wrath or possible reasons thereof are rarely mentioned.[62] This seems to contrast with the official disease etiology to which colonists were subjected both in the churches and in private conversations with their ministers. Given the available documents, it is difficult to assess whether the majority of lay patients did not believe in the clerical explanations of illness or whether they concealed their moral transgressions from an influential and powerful person such as Winthrop because they feared that a confession of their inner estates would lead to official repercussions. It can be assumed, however, that among the many reasons for which Winthrop's medical services were in such a high

---

[61] At the time, palsy, along with epilepsy and convulsion, were widely regarded as caused by the devil, personalized demons, and/or witches. Charles Webster, *From Paracelsus to Newton: Magic and the Making of Modern Science* (Cambridge: Cambridge UP, 1982) 88; Martin Luther, *The Table-Talk of Martin Luther*. 1566. trans. William Hazlitt (1566; Philadelphia: The Lutheran Publication Society, 1868) 34.

[62] "George Ward to John Winthrop, Jr., 15 June 1652," *Winthrop Papers* VI, 203. Andrew Wear has shown in his study of Puritan conceptualizations of illness in England that "laymen less intensely devout [...] were less constant in their reliance on providential explanations [of illness]. It is almost as though the providential model of illness depended upon one's religious training and devotion." Andrew Wear, "Puritan Perceptions of Illness in Seventeenth Century England," *Patients and Practitioners: Lay Perceptions of Medicine in Pre-Industrial Society*, ed. Roy Porter (Cambridge: Cambridge UP, 1985) 76.

demand was the fact that he was not a minister-physician who would inevitably probe his patient's hidden thoughts and actions as a part of the curative process. When colonists addressed Winthrop, they knew that his diagnostic and prescriptive replies largely lacked theological and moral components but, instead, offered established and state-of-the-art approaches to healing—leaving the true cause of illness to the patient's private meditations.

This is not to say that lay medical request letters were completely devoid of religious references. In fact, the Odell letters aptly exemplify that New England colonists considered Winthrop and his medicines as a mediator and instrument of God on earth. The trust that colonists placed in his abilities derived from relegating human destiny to God's providence and sovereignty, especially in the case of illness. The explanatory framework for any illness implicitly recognized "[d]ivine wrath as the primary cause of an upsetting of elementary balance in the earth, causing the stars to send down the deadly poison" of disease.[63] Within the context of colonial New England culture, this notion, taken from the European occult tradition, was perceived as compatible with the belief in the omnipotence and providence of God; it subsumed astrology and medicine under religious doctrine and, in doing so, added an intellectual dimension to the healing of illnesses. New England healers and alchemists could employ this dimension in order to explain and justify their proto-chemical practices and processes.

Even though the patient letters sent to Winthrop from the laity contain few elaborate religious references, they often emphasize that the grace of God constitutes an essential prerequisite for the healing process. At some point in their narratives, most authors rationalize their illness by placing it within the realm of providence. A typical phrase in a medical request letter reads as follows: "it hath pleased the Lord to visite my wife with A soare paine one her backe."[64] The claim that an affliction "pleased the Lord" is more than a reflex invocation of God's inscrutable will and power. It acknowledges the belief in the omnipotence and providence of the Almighty and mirrors colonists'

---

[63] Walter Pagel, *Paracelsus: An Introduction to Philosophical Medicine in the Era of the Renaissance* (Basel: Karger, 1958) 189.

[64] "John Haynes to John Winthrop, Jr., 13 May 1653," *Winthrop Papers* VI, 296.

conviction that the true meaning of illness remains incomprehensible to human beings. Since religious doctrines urged the faithful to accept their place and situation in the world, the majority of Winthrop's lay patient letters refrain from complaining about inadequate or unavailable medical services. The call for medical help was not seen in contradiction to divine providence but as its logical extension. George Starkey, Winthrop's alchemical friend and colleague, sums up this notion, claiming that

> diseases and miseries, the fruits of sin, inflicted most justly from the righteous Judge, are yet curable by remedies which the Almighty hath created, for which end the Father of mercies and God of compassion hath also created the Physician, that he being an instrument of mercy, in the hand of a merciful Father, might make whole and binde up those whom the same God with his hand of justice hath wounded and broken.[65]

Thus, humanity is allowed and even held to improve its condition—after all, that was what the Puritan experiment in America was essentially about—and therefore, asking for practical medical help was deemed not only permissible but also vital for the success of the personal and collective advancement in North America.

As illustrated in the previous chapter, early Algonquian epidemics provided ample justification for the colonists' pronunciation of the sanctity of the New England way. Native diseases and deaths strengthened the belief in medical providentialism, which colonists had brought to the shores of America and which shaped the modes in which New Englanders conceptualized and dealt with illnesses on a daily basis. Medical providentialism expressed and fostered a central Puritan cultural notion, namely the sense of utter helplessness in an existence that was guided by God's omnipotence and design. This belief did not free human beings from making certain choices or from shaping their lives individually and collectively, but rather placed relatively narrow boundaries on human agency, particularly in matters of life and death.

---

[65] George Starkey, *Natures Explication And Helmont's Vindication, Or A Short and Sure Way to a Long and Sound Life* (London, 1657) 5.

Both the Bible and experience taught the godly that the human ability to influence health conditions was limited. Within these limits, most New England colonists who expressed their bodily conditions to Winthrop recognized that few members of their communities possessed a special healing ability that, in accordance with the belief in medical providentialism, emanated from the divine. Colonial leaders such as John Winthrop Jr. as well as most minister-physicians were regarded as intricate parts of God's providential health design and were conceived as potential tools trained and equipped by His power and wisdom to aid and protect those who believed in Him.

The New England belief in medical providentialism also fostered a preference of alchemical over Galenic healing methods. While Galen's "paganism" was often viewed with suspicion, American Puritans accepted the alchemists' claim that their medical prescriptions were spiritually empowered by divine guidance and revelations. Furthermore, in a culture that attached spirituality to all earthly and celestial matters, medicine "made by the fire" were inherently acceptable by the New England populace.[66] Most colonists believed in the efficacy of alchemically derived medicaments because the prescriptions, especially when they aimed at ejecting fluids and gases from the human body, suggested that a purified and blessed substance would expel spiritual and corporeal corruptions and thus facilitate healing. In short, alchemical medicine offered a natural correlate to the dominant theology: curing a sick body with medicaments gained from purifying natural substances by extracting its essence and rejecting its dross was regarded as essentially the same process as the salvation of a morally corrupt humanity through a purified religious system, which sought to separate the elect few from the unregenerate masses.

The belief that God played an active role in inflicting and alleviating illnesses was an overriding feature of Winthrop's medical universe, in theory and in practice. As one result, his medical services transcended mere personal doctor-patient relationships and also involved matters of public health. Even though evidence of legislation on, for instance, sanitary laws, are missing in the surviving Winthrop records, we know

---

[66] George Starkey, *Pyrotechny Asserted and Illustrated. To Be the Surest and Fastest Means for Arts Triumph over Natures Infirmities* (London, 1658) 14.

that during the epidemic of 1658 he followed the clerical notion of "the afflicting hand of the Lord" and supported an official day of "solemne humiliation" to rid the colony of illness.[67] And also in his extant personal correspondence God plays a central role as the source and means of all healing. In 1654, Winthrop writes to his son Fitz-John, who has been suffering from a severe and debilitating (though unspecified) illness. Instead of offering certain remedies drawn either from Galenic or Paracelsian medicine, Winthrop uses the occasion to instruct his son in the theology of healing prominent in New England at the time: "trust him with your life that gave you life and being, and hath only power over death and life, to whom we must be willing to submit to be at the disposing of his good will and pleasure. [...] In sicknesses vse those meanes that you can have and comitt your self for the successe to the Lord."[68] This reference suggests that Winthrop's medical work and his conceptualization of health and illness remained closely allied with contemporary religious approaches to medicine. When read in conjunction with his many letters expressing his interest in scientific developments of his day, his advice to his son also reveals that colonial intellectuals considered science and religion as mutually intertwined epistemological and practical spheres, rather than as contestants over interpreting and mending human corporeality.

* * *

Winthrop's medical career drew to an end in the late 1660s. In his professional correspondence, the final reference to medicine appears in 1668, when Winthrop informed the Royal Society about the efficacy and ingestion of *mecury dulcis* (mercurous chloride). His records of treating New England colonists end in 1669, indicating that his medical activities lessened toward the end of his life. In the early 1670s, he recommended his medical knowledge to his son Wait, who later became a well-known physician in the colonies, and instructed him about the effectiveness of rubila for treating measles, smallpox, and dysentery. It remains unclear

---

[67] Black 182.

[68] "John Winthrop, Jr., to Fitz-John Winthrop, 8 February 1654/55," *Collections of the Massachusetts Historical Society*, Series 5, Vol. 8 (1882): 43.

to what extent the decline of Winthrop's medical activities was due to old age or to the arrival of other medical practitioners in Connecticut. Robert C. Black argues that no younger physician was able to take Winthrop's place, with the exception of John Lederer who arrived in Connecticut in 1674 but returned to Hamburg within a year's time.[69]

A central argument of the present chapter is that medicine played a crucial role in advancing Winthrop's power. On the international scene, his membership in the Royal Society and his acquaintance with some of the major figures of the emerging scientific revolution provided a political leverage that was instrumental in securing a royal charter for Connecticut in 1662. The charter, in turn, increased his popularity and influence at home. In addition, on the domestic scene, the transfer of political power from the people to Winthrop occurred as part of a doctor-patient relationship whose features were both universal and place-specific. Almost everywhere, men and women of healing who are perceived as successful practitioners are revered and trusted because they perform a vital service for the advancement of the individual and the community. In colonial Connecticut, several factors amplified this relationship. The lack of surplus cash and produce made paying medical services impossible for many colonists. This led, on the one hand, to a scarcity of physicians. On the other hand, those with medical abilities were in high demand, especially because the steady rise of the colonial population caused an increasing number of sick settlers. In addition, since efficacious medical services could not be met through pecuniary means, the barter often consisted of unspecified services, i.e., the recovered patient or his/her family acknowledged a moral obligation to repay the healer by supporting him/her in the future. Thus, Winthrop was not merely following a Christian call for charity with his medical service but was also building a reliable network of support that could be activated for various purposes. Winthrop's payment, in lieu of money, often consisted of the transfer of trust from his abilities as a physician to his capacity as colonial leader. This investment in and of political power ensured Winthrop's elevated position within the colony and in New England as a whole and allowed him to influence, like few other

---

[69] Black 317-318.

individuals at the time, the cultural and political course of the colony he served and represented.

Aside from embodying the voluntary transfer of trust, allegiance, and power, Winthrop's patient letters also functioned as tools of control and influence in more subtle ways. Taken as a whole, the letters to the governor became part of what might be called, in reference to Foucault, "Puritan panopticism."[70] The sense of being watched constantly (by neighbor, world, and God) extended into epistolary practices, especially when a consultation letter was addressed to the seat of power in Connecticut. Even though these letters were written without an implied public readership, the author had to be constantly aware that what he or she was writing might have certain repercussions beyond the mere physical condition described in the letter. In addition, letter writing in the early modern period demanded the correspondent's adherence to a specific social etiquette. In many medical letters sent to Winthrop, the correspondent neglected the formalities of epistolary codes and, hence, seemed to express a lack of reverence for the social hierarchies of the time. On the one hand, patient letters presented a way for common colonists to subvert the clergy's authority of interpreting body conditions. Some letters, on the other hand, did not function as means of critiquing power; rather, the urgency of the letter's topic served as sufficient reason to circumvent the rules of writing, especially through the omission of formulaic courtesies and the recourse to the vernacular.

The case of John Winthrop Jr. furthermore demonstrates how space shaped the development of religious orthodoxy in colonial New England, and *vice versa*. Arguably, one of the reasons why the younger Winthrop chose to leave Boston and establish and advance new settlements outside the center of Puritan orthodoxy was that it allowed him to pursue his interests in occult thoughts and practices away from the surveillance of Boston divines and officials. While isolation proved advantageous for thoughts and practices that deviated from the religious norm, it also hindered the progress of Winthrop's philosophical and experimental inquiries. Despite his private book collection and improvised laboratory mentioned at the outset of this study, he lacked

---

[70] Cf. Michel Foucault, *Discipline and Punish: The Birth of the Prison*, trans. Alan Sheridan (1975; New York: Vintage, 1995) 195-228.

the material resources necessary for successful scientific endeavors. Expressing his frustration over his isolation from the intellectual centers of Europe, Winthrop closes a letter to Samuel Hartlib in 1659 with the words: "We are heere as men dead to the world in this wildernesse."[71] Inadvertently, the meaning of this statement is deconstructed by the medium. Winthrop answers and overcomes his frustration expressed in this sentence by the means with which he relates it, namely the letter itself. As this chapter has shown, the epistles sent to and from Winthrop's diverse residences demonstrate how an emerging society adapted European health concepts and curative approaches to the particularities of colonial existence. In doing so, they render visible the desires and urgencies involved in experiences of space, time, absence, and presence that constituted a particular feature of early American lives and illness narratives.

A common theme in virtually all patient letters surveyed for this study is their sustained attempt to cope with, make sense of, and reverse the lack of control over existence that a severe illness causes. Regardless of whether they were conceived as attempts to ward off an illness, guided by economic factors that precluded adequate treatment, or expressed a deep sense of helplessness and subjection to the will and providence of God, most consultation letters were energized by a quest for agency in matters of bare life otherwise confined by divine law. The frequent omission of references to health, aside from passing and/or formulaic remarks, in letters about official matters (e.g., trade, politics, Indian relations, land distribution) indicates that illness was conceived as an essentially personal affair.

One of the central insights drawn from Winthrop's patient letters is that instead of merely receiving and replicating theological doctrines, the laity mediated and negotiated official notions of disease etiology and treatment methods to serve both their bodily and mental needs. That is, the letters show how common colonists sought and found ways of reconciling what they heard in sermons about illness with their knowledge about disease that was mostly derived from the European folk tradition and the emerging medical sciences. The foregoing

---

[71] "John Winthrop, Jr. to Samuel Hartlib, 16 December 1659," *Proceedings of the Massachusetts Historical Society*, Third Series, Vol. 72 (1957-1960): 40.

comparison between illness representations by learned clergymen and their less educated parishioners supports David Hall's revisionist assumption that the relationship between ministers and common colonists of New England was marked by "a dialectic of resistance and cooperation."[72] The virtual absence of sin-related narratives in the majority of medical letters sent to a man of power reveals how the people of New England interpreted and judged a major event in their lives both in concurrence with the clerical notion of divine pathogenesis and in deviance and independence from it. By textualizing their illnesses in epistolary form, moreover, lay colonists often used their medical conditions as a subtle means of empowerment. Their bodily estates prompted practical decisions, in many cases without confessional references to the patient's religious transgressions. Thus, these medical request letters shed additional light on the social heterogeneity among New England colonists and help us to understand the broad scope of attitudes and patterns of medical treatment, consumption, and meaning-endowment in the seventeenth century Atlantic world.

[72] Hall 12. Historians of early New England culture and society, such as Perry Miller or Sacvan Bercovitch, have argued that the theology of the clergy and the laity were essentially the same. In more recent studies, however, including David Hall's, it is evident that they often tended to deviate significantly. Cf. Kenneth P. Minkema, ed., "The East Windsor Conversion Narratives, 1700-1752," *The Connecticut Historical Society Bulletin* 51 (1986): 10.

# 3. Scripting Medicine and Gender

Until the early 1990s, most historians discarded the roles of women in colonial medicine. It were men like Samuel Fuller, Giles Firmin, Thomas Thacher, John Winthrop Jr., and Cotton Mather who seemed representative of the early American medical system. Rather than suggesting the non-existence of female healers, most primary documents actually represent the exclusion of women from the publication scene and their relegation to the medical and social margins of colonial New England. In the wake of the social turn in American historiography of the late 1970s, scholars have re-visited old sources and discovered new texts such as personal account-books, diaries, and local court records that have helped to revise the notion of a male-dominated medical environment.[1] Since then, it has been impossible to overestimate the importance of women in early American medicine: when women gave birth, they were assisted by other women; when colonists fell ill, many first turned to a female member of the household, consulted women in the neighborhood, and only called a male doctor as a last resort. In addition, almost every rural household included a garden with a parcel for medical plants. In poorer families and/or those living in remote areas, a broad and effective "kitchen physic" was essential for securing the sustenance and success of individuals, families, and settlements and was practiced well into the nineteenth century.[2] Most women sowed,

---

[1] See, for instance, Rebecca Tannenbaum, *The Healer's Calling: Women and Medicine in Early New England* (Ithaca: Cornell UP, 2002); Patricia A. Watson, "The 'Hidden Ones': Women and Healing in Colonial New England," *Medicine and Healing. Annual Proceeding of the Dublin Seminar for New England Folk Life*, vol. 25 (Boston: Boston UP, 1991) 25-33.

[2] Albert Deutsch, "The Sick Poor in Colonial Times," *American Historical Review* 46.3 (1941): 564. Cf. Charles R. Lee, "Public Poor Relief and the Massachusetts Community, 1620-1715," *New England Quarterly* 55.4 (1982): 564-585.

tended, and harvested plants in their humoral gardens. They then dried, distilled, or processed these plants to produce more or less efficacious medicaments.[3] Most female colonists provided domestic medical services, treating minor illnesses and injuries, and watching over the sick, often for weeks. Others, such as Anna Edmunds, who practiced surgery and ran a private "hospital" in Lynn, Massachusetts, worked as professional healers, selling their nursing and doctoring skills to other colonists.[4] Women also functioned as keepers and disseminators of medical knowledge, often handing it down orally from generation to generation, occasionally supplementing it by recommendations from the many herbals, recipe books, and other guidebooks available in New England.[5]

In the social arena, the circumscribed life men accorded to women provided few outlets for intellectual discourse, free expression or debate. However, it is a repeated scholarly and popular fallacy that colonial

---

[3] A useful discussion of medical plants in colonial New England is provided by Ann Leighton, *Early American Gardens: "For Meate or Medicine"* (1970; Amherst: U of Massachusetts P, 1986) 123-138. See, John Josselyn, *New-England's Rarities Discovered in Birds, Beasts, Fishes, Serpents, and Plants of that Country* (1672; Early English Books Online, J1093) 52-84, for Native American plants discovered for English use; 85-91, for a list of seventy-seven plants the English imported and cultivated in their new habitat. Among common vegetables and grains, settlers grew barberry, bittersweet, burdock, buttercup, caraway, catnip, chamomile, dandelion, elcampane, live-forever, mullein, pennyroyal, peppermint, plantain, rose, spearmint, tansy, and yarrow, among others, for medicinal purposes. Nicholas N. Smith, "Indian Medicine: Fact or Fiction?," *Bulletin of the Massachusetts Archaeological Society* 26.1 (1964): 15.

[4] George Francis Dow, ed., *Records and Files of the Quarterly Courts of Essex County*, vol. II, 1656-1662 (Salem, MA.: Essex Institute, 1912) 226-228, 231. Rebecca J. Tannenbaum, "The Housewife as Healer: Medicine as Women's Work in Colonial New England," *Women's Work in New England, 1620-1920. Annual Proceedings of the Dublin Seminar for New England Folklife*, vol. 25 (Boston: Boston UP, 2003) 160-169.

[5] Among the most widely circulated books were George Baker, *The Newe Jewell of Health* (1576), Gervase Markham, *The English Housewife* (1615), Leonard Meager, *The English Gardener* (1683), and Thomas Tusser, *Five Hundred Points of Good Husband*ry (1557).

women were subordinate to men in all spheres of life. While it is true that female colonists were barred from participating in public affairs, and were thus denied access to the domains of power, their distinguished and influential position in the families and in New England meetinghouse culture needs to be taken into account when evaluating seventeenth-century gender hierarchies and the medical marketplace. As Laurel Thatcher Ulrich carefully argues,

> [a]ccording to law, women were civilly dead, subject to the authority of husbands and fathers. Yet the realities of daily life and the opportunities of a new world constantly undercut formal authority. Innocent gatherings of women became politically dangerous. Would-be rulers succumbed to the enticements of female dissenters. Wifehood became a model both for liberty and submission.[6]

Against this background of ambiguous social positionings of New England women, medicine afforded certain opportunities to create and enlarge female agency. While often seen as a benefit to society, female healing abilities on occasion also caused disadvantages for women, especially when they were rumored to meddle in black magic.

Since women were, with few exceptions, excluded from the colonial publication circuit, records about female medicine are scarce. As a consequence, one encounters similar difficulties in unveiling women's medical practices as with Native American healing techniques. In order to find clues about female healing practices and specifically female modes of coping with illnesses in colonial North America, scholars have

---

[6] Laurel Thatcher Ulrich, "John Winthrop's City of Women," *The Massachusetts Historical Review* 3 (2001): 22. For domestic gender roles, see Edmund S. Morgan, *The Puritan Family: Religion and Domestic Relations in Seventeenth-Century New England* (1944; New York: Harper, 1966) 29-64; Laurel Thatcher Ulrich, *Good Wives: Image and Reality in the Lives of Women in Northern New England, 1650-1750* (New York: Knopf, 1982). For an insightful analysis of the "indirect authority of Puritan women" in New England families and meetinghouses, see Amanda Porterfield, *Female Piety in Puritan New England* (New York: Oxford UP, 1992) 86-94. For women's roles and position in Puritan congregations, see David D. Hall, *Worlds of Wonder, Days of Judgment: Popular Religious Belief in Early New England* (New York, 1989) 117-165.

to resort to texts written by men or, by way of comparison, to English medicinal literature of the time. In the ensuing analysis of some of these texts, I want to stress the representational dimensions of these texts *about* women. To do so, it is useful to pay close attention to rhetorical strategies with which male writers fashioned certain images of women healers and gender-specific illnesses to a transatlantic audience. The central argument presented in this chapter is that gendered medical reports appear with particular frequency and intensity during moments of public crisis in New England culture.[7] These reports indicate that medicine played a salient role in the cultural scripting and meaning-endowment of the female body. In order to trace these illness representations, the arc of this chapter moves from elite women's healing networks, exemplified by the circle of medical experts surrounding New Haven minister's wife, Elizabeth Davenport, to the religious teachings and rebuttals of Anne Hutchinson, with a special focus on the official interpretation of her malformed birth, and ends with an investigation of documents that depict the role of physicians, midwives, and lay healers in seventeenth-century New England witchcraft accusations. Such an order of analysis appears useful to illustrate women's social positions and their underlying cultural reference systems, especially with regard to the role and function of medicine.

---

[7] One of Perry Miller's central arguments in *The New England Mind* is that Puritans conceived their American existence as both cause and expression of a constant crisis of the soul. While a sense of crisis was indeed immanent to Puritan thought, induced by the Calvinist doctrine of election, it became especially visible when it changed from a psychological state to political and cultural turbulences during which the newly established order was in danger of dismantling. The most prominent cases of existential public crisis included the Antinomian Controversy (1636-1638), the debate about the Half-Way Covenant (1662), Metacom's Rebellion/King Philip's War (1675-1676), the Salem Witch-Hunt (1692), and the Smallpox Inoculation Controversy (1721/22). Because the intersections between medical and gender issues became especially visible during the Antinomian Controversy and the Salem Witch-Hunt, the present chapter focuses mainly on these two events, omitting other important moments of social and cultural crisis.

Female Medical Networks: Bonding, Leading, Learning

In her book *The Healer's Calling*, Rebecca Tannenbaum provides new insight into colonial medical practices by investigating the multifaceted groups and functions of women healers. Many female members of the religious, civil, and mercantile elites had access to books and knowledge networks, which enabled them to build a medical expertise and to offer health services to their communities. More often than not, their medical practices were based on the same Galenic principles and prescriptions employed by educated, male physicians during much of the seventeenth century. Like their male counterparts, women healers diagnosed illnesses based on bodily signs, chose and prepared medications, and assessed the prospects of recovery. In addition to performing regular physician's tasks, they watched over and nursed the sick, assisted each other during childbirth, and often shared their medical knowledge in spaces of intimacy, when a small room in a colonial home was transformed into a sick or delivery room.[8]

Many "handmaids of the Lord," as Cotton Mather called women who operated in the shadows of their husbands, took up medicine as part of the culturally scripted roles and duties of their marital and social position: to provide spiritual and bodily care for the community in the name of God.[9] We know from scattered references in texts written by men that the wives and daughters of several influential New England theologians, e.g., Joanna (Rossiter) Cotton, Ann (Mountford) Elliot,

---

[8] For depictions of female networks of exchanging remedies, recipes, and medical advice, see Patricia Ann Watson, *The Angelical Conjunction: The Preacher-Physicians of Colonial New England* (Knoxville: U of Tennessee P, 1991) 32-33; Tannenbaum, *Healer's Calling* 29-34.

[9] Cf. Cotton Mather's observation of women's roles in colonial society: "There have been, and thro' the Grace of our God there still are, to be found, in many parts of these American Regions, and even in the Cottages of the Wilderness, as well as in our Capital city, those *Handmaids of the Lord*, who tho' they ly very much Conceal'd from the World, and must be called, The Hidden Ones, yet have no little share in the Beauty and the Defence of the Land." Cotton Mather, *El-Shaddai: A Brief Essay, on All Supplied in an Alsufficient Saviour* (1725; Early American Imprints, Series 1, no. 2669) 21 (emphasis added).

Hannah (Bradford) Ripley, Dorothy (Bulkeley) Treat, Abigail (Mather) Willard, and Elizabeth Davenport, either assisted their husbands' or fathers' healing efforts or became medical experts themselves. Their practice of medicine was not merely sparked by altruism or Christian duty but also, perhaps more importantly, informed by social and political motives. By serving as "handmaids of the Lord," female healers were, at the same time, handmaids of their fathers and husbands, and often aided in building or maintaining a positive reputation, one that would allow the men greater influence in social and congregational affairs. Conversely, this reinforcement of existing social hierarchies also enabled the empowerment of, for instance, a minister's wife, because during her medical visits she would often gain intimate knowledge of the spiritual, intellectual, and physical state of the community and could advise her husband on theological and civic measures accordingly. In addition, her access to information on local, regional, and world affairs from a broad array of sources and to networks of neighborly exchanges tended to elevate her own status and that of her family within the community. Ironically, epidemics provided particular occasions to enlarge a healing woman's social and cultural influence. As pathogens spread among the population, their paths were followed by healers whose bedside visits during times of epidemics offered further occasions for strengthening networks of information and influence. In this sense, epidemics constituted ambivalent states of exception that proved dangerous to the population, yet at the same time enabled the dissemination of social discipline in New England.

One revered female healer was Elizabeth Davenport, wife of the Reverend John Davenport of New Haven. The historical records are largely silent about her upbringing and education, but we do know quite a bit about Mrs. Davenport's medical knowledge and activities from her husband's correspondence with John Winthrop Jr. during the 1650s and 60s.[10] In addition to her proto-scientific medical training, the letters show her sharing recipes and knowledge with other leading women within and beyond the town's borders. Mrs. Davenport's healing abilities can be seen as equal to that of educated male physicians in the region, which allowed her to question the diagnosis and treatment of a

---

[10] Tannenbaum, *Healer's Calling* 73-74.

local doctor and, as seen in the previous chapter, caused John Winthrop Jr. to rely on her and other prominent colonial women for diagnostic information, new remedies, and as trusted distributors for his medical prescriptions.[11] Davenport's medical expertise, therefore, seems to have temporarily erased her gender-based position of social inferiority because her knowledge and reputation, in part fostered by Winthrop's trust in her abilities, equaled, and in some cases surpassed, that of male New England healers.

Many medical letters sent by Davenport constitute plurivocal illness narratives with the minister's wife dictating a report or request to Winthrop Jr. Such ventriloquial moments (i.e., when Mr. Davenport's authorial self recedes into the background to give voice to his wife) often appear in the letters' postscripts. In a letter written in August 1658, for instance, Davenport concludes as follows:

> My wife prayeth me to postscribe a word or two concerning our *maid* servant, about whom she had some speech with you. [...] She had paine in her leggs, with swelling, and paine in her back and head, with illnes in her stomack and grypings and stoppages, about a weeke before you came hither [...].[12]

Mr. Davenport writing on her behalf shows how the relegation of women to the private sphere and the cultural norm according to which men call a physician or midwife was maintained on a formal level. At the same time, the Davenport letters exemplify how these official social roles and relationships were subtly undermined through illness narratives. In the handwritten original of the correspondence cited above, Davenport reached the bottom of the page and had to rotate the sheet to include the medical postscript in the left side margin, positioned at a right angle to the main text. If we read this and other similar addenda as metaphors of women's relegation to the margins of the social

---

[11] See, for instance, "John Davenport to John Winthrop the Younger, 1 May 1666," John Davenport, *Letters of John Davenport, Puritan Divine*, ed. Isabel M. Calder (New Haven: Yale UP, 1937) 261-262.

[12] "Davenport to Winthrop, Jr., 19 September 1654," in Davenport, *Letters* 97 (emphasis original).

sphere, then Davenport's letters actually undermine this positioning because the postscripts treat topics that are as important as the religious and political issues discussed in the main body of the texts.

In addition to Elizabeth Davenport's marginalized voice in her husband's official correspondence, some letters are entirely about illnesses of family members. Here, gender ventriloquism encompasses the bulk of the letters, for instance, when Davenport seeks Winthrop's advice on her son's severe cold. The first epistolary report consists of a lengthy depiction of symptoms, a possible diagnosis, and previous treatments; the tone is rather detached, seeking to convey the most adequate illness description possible:

> He groaned in his sleepe, and tooke his wind short, hath a paine in his head and is, at present, somewhat dull of hearing, which we impute to winde in his head. He complaines of paine in his head, with coughing, and of winde in his belly and side. Coughing and winde are his greatest troubles, at present. He is stil very weake in his stomach, and spittes abundantly.[13]

Winthrop Jr. responded immediately by sending medicaments and directions. Since the patient's condition failed to improve noticeably, Davenport wrote another illness description only six days after the first. The author again relates his wife's treatment report, which includes a reference to a domestic recipe for purging the body as well as to Winthrop's "cure-all" powder (rubila). Both medicaments failed to improve the patient's health and as the Davenports reach their wits' end, the tone of the letter becomes increasingly emotional and desperate:

> He is so weake that he cannot turne him selfe and scarse stirr himselfe in his bed, but needes the helpe of others: and by reason of his paine, he is held, in his side, and where the paine is, with a man and a woaman, or with two woemen, one the one side and the other, his paine is so various and shifting, yet most under his short ribbes, or in his back.[14]

---

[13] "Davenport to Winthrop the Younger, 17 December 1660," in Davenport, *Letters* 185.

[14] "Davenport to Winthrop, Jr., 23 December 1660," in Davenport, *Letters* 188.

In contrast to the rather detached illness and treatment reports in the previous letters, mostly couched in short and direct sentences, this excerpt underlines the urgency of the situation through a panicky tone. The Davenports are searching for the right words to represent their son's pain, resulting in an unusual multi-clausal sentence that conveys a sense of suspension and helplessness vis-à-vis the bodily condition of young John Davenport. Yet, the pain of their son inherently precludes adequate representation and, hence, the experience of suffering translates into an emphatic loss of words, a void of signification that the writers attempt to fill by repeating the word "paine." In addition to marking a realistic report designed to prompt the physician's diagnosis and treatment, this letter highlights another function of colonial illness narratives: a means of coping with a bodily affliction by writing about it.

After concluding the report with the usual reference to divine guidance, the Davenports end on a hopeful note reporting how their son's nose began to bleed. The New Haven minister and his wife, following the prediction of a local female healer, choose to read this as a sign of imminent improvement, "her children having the cold and cough bled before they mended."[15] The verb "to mend" is central here because it indicates that the improvement of the physical condition is closely tied to spiritual reform and moral improvement. In short, the letter writers supplement and undergird more or less efficacious natural curative means with a continual alignment of human behavior to the word of God.

Throughout their correspondence, John Davenport remains the mouthpiece of the family in all affairs; yet, the consistent narrative interruptions by the medical voice of his knowledgeable wife illustrate both the possibilities and limits of larger cultural interventions of women in colonial affairs. The Davenport letters attest to what Tannenbaum has termed "a delicate balance between self-promotion and deference to structured male power."[16] By dictating illness descriptions, progress reports, and efficacy assessments to her husband, who is

---

[15] "John Davenport to John Winthrop, Jr., 23 December 1660," *Letters of John Davenport, Puritan Divine*, ed. Isabel M. Calder (New Haven: Yale UP, 1937) 189.

[16] Tannenbaum, *Healer's Calling* 88.

addressing Winthrop Jr., Elizabeth Davenport turns the letters into heteroglossic texts that reveal the cultural presence, impact, and authority of women and, at the same time, the persistence of gendered power asymmetries.

## Antinomianism and the Medicalization of Deviance

In colonial New England, two cultural spaces allowed women to suspend momentarily gendered power hierarchies: the church, where women were seen as possessing closer access to Christ as men, and the birth room, in which men were only peripheral figures.[17] During the seventeenth century, and in some isolated settings until the early nineteenth century, childbirth marked a domain controlled almost entirely by women. It was only in the course of the late eighteenth century that this hitherto gender-exclusive realm was slowly being appropriated by the newly-developing, male-dominated, and science-oriented obstetrics and pediatrics.[18]

Many seventeenth-century New England midwives were able to secure a high reputation, especially when their services extended from childbirth to general medicine. Because of her comparatively advanced knowledge of the human condition, a midwife was often the only learned medical expert, especially in remote locations, and was frequently called to treat injuries and minor or routine illnesses.[19] From a male perspective, the midwife remained an ambivalent figure. On the one hand, she was valued for her medical expertise that was central for sustaining the community as a whole. On the other hand, she had to be viewed with suspicion because what happened in her exclusively female

---

[17] See, Amanda Porterfield, "Women's Attraction to Puritanism," *Church History* 60.2 (1991): 198.

[18] For an engaging insight into the life and work of an early nineteenth-century midwife in New England as well as the appropriation of the delivery room by male physicians, see Laurel Thatcher Ulrich, *A Midwife's Tale: The Life of Martha Ballard, Based on her Diary, 1785-1812* (New York: Vintage, 1991).

[19] David Dary, *Frontier Medicine: From the Atlantic to the Pacific, 1492-1941* (New York: Knopf, 2008) 31.

space eluded men's knowledge and immediate control. As one result, while ministers' wives ranked at the top of hierarchy of female healers, midwives generally could engage less social and cultural authority.

Before the male take-over of control over female labor, colonial women, healers, and midwives gathered at the bedside to assist each other in the care for the birth givers. During many hours of waiting, watching, praying, and nursing, those present would inevitably share knowledge, gossip, and ideas with other women. In fact, as Tannenbaum explains, female medical gatherings often constituted pivotal cultural events in New England communities, because during these occasions, women

> were doing more than bringing comfort to the sick; they were enacting a social ritual as well. The ritual of the sickbed had the potential of serving several ends: it created bonds among the women gathered there; it created obligations between the healers and the healed; and it reinforced both social bonds and social hierarchies.[20]

The intimacy, pain, and, if the mother and the child were fortunate enough to survive, celebration after travail often forged special connections among women that extended beyond the birth room. In some instances, these special ties created lasting and empowering communal support networks; in others, the gossip and local news exchanged at the bedside turned women into enforcers of Puritan morality, often to the disadvantage of female "transgressors"; and in still others, they created semi-public forums in which women could discuss theological and political concerns.[21] On a number of occasions, child- and sick-bed conversations leaped into the broader social arena, entered into more formal structures of male-dominated authority and, in doing so, shaped the social, cultural, and political course of early New England.

---

[20] Rebecca J. Tannenbaum, "'What Is Best to Be Done for These Fevers': Elizabeth Davenport's Medical Practice in New Haven Colony," *New England Quarterly* 70.2 (1997): 276.

[21] Tannenbaum, *Healer's Calling* 21-36. Cf. Catherine Scholten, *Childbearing in American Society, 1650-1850* (New York: NYUP, 1985) 13-14; Ulrich, *Good Wives* 126-145.

The potency of informal public spheres created by transient and permanent female networks that revolved around birth and other medical issues became especially pronounced, and perceived as a threat to the larger socio-political order, during the free grace or Antinomian controversy of 1636-1638. This crisis in New England culture and politics centered mainly on the allegedly heretical thoughts and enunciations of religious dissenters, among them Anne Hutchinson, the wife of an influential Boston merchant and frequent participant in birth gatherings. Her social position afforded by her husband as well as her knowledge gathered during fifteen births of her own and during her attendance of numerous other deliveries, ensured her a position of respect and reverence among large parts of the female (and male) population of Boston shortly after her arrival in the colonies in 1635.[22]

New England Antinomianism has served as a popular and recurrent topic among scholars: it has been studied as a theological controversy significant for understanding the cultural course of the colony, as a turning point in women's participation and power in colonial society, and as an event that threatened to unravel the body politic. Medicine played an important role at the outset and in the aftermath of the crisis

---

[22] In the following, I view the events, actions, and words surrounding the Antinomian controversy through a medical lens. For a more comprehensive account, see Michael P. Winship, *The Times and Trials of Anne Hutchinson: Puritans Divided* (Lawrence: UP of Kansas, 2005). For other useful investigations of the free grace movement, see William K. B. Stoever, *"A faire and easie way to heaven:" Covenant Theology and Antinomianism in Early Massachusetts* (Middletown: Wesleyan UP, 1978). A study of the gender aspects is provided by Mary Beth Norton, *Founding Mothers and Fathers: Gendered Power and the Forming of American Society* (New York: Knopf, 1996) 359-400; Lyle Koehler, "The Case of the American Jezebels: Anne Hutchinson and Female Agitation during the Years of Antinomian Turmoil, 1636-1640," *William and Mary Quarterly* 31.1 (1974): 55-78. On the development of Antinomianism in England, see David R. Como, *Blown by the Spirit: Puritanism and the Emergence of an Antinomian Underground in Pre-Civil-War England* (Stanford: Stanford UP, 2004). For a study which considers the Antinomian controversy as a transatlantic rather than a mere local debate, see Jonathan Beecher Field, "The Antinomian Controversy Did Not Take Place," *Early American Studies* 6.2 (2008): 448-463.

and was especially linked to a distinctly female medical issue:
childbirth. When Hutchinson arrived in Boston and became a church
member, John Winthrop reports,

> shee began to go to work, and was being a woman very helpful in the
> times of child-birth, and other occasions of bodily infirmities, and well
> furnished with means for those purposes, shee easily insinuated her selfe
> into the affections of many, and the rather, because shee was much
> inquisitive of them about their spiritual estates, and in discovering to
> them the danger they were in, by trusting to common gifts and graces,
> without any such witnesse of the Spirit, as the Scripture holds out for a
> full evidence; [...].[23]

From the moment of her entry into Boston, it seems, Anne
Hutchinson was perceived by those at the center of colonial power as
operating in a conniving, intrusive, assertive, and persuasive manner,
using her medical skills to ensure entrance to the homes and minds of
colonists. Yet, Hutchinson was by far not the only Antinomian. Like
others she drew on the teachings of ministers John Cotton and John
Wheelwright, but became the most prominent proponent of a strain of
Puritanism eager to communicate the belief in necessary and immediate
relations with Christ. During the Antinomian controversy, Hutchinson
and others criticized and challenged the official alliance with the
covenant of grace and the covert practice of the covenant of works.
According to the latter pact between God and humanity, salvation from
sins and assurance about one's status among the elect could be prepared
for and was rendered visible through works (i.e., outside manifestations
of saving grace such as one's deeds, morals, words, health and/or
wealth). Antinomians, on the other hand, held that assurance of salvation
came directly from God during moments of spiritual enlightenment,

---

[23] John Winthrop, *A Short Story of the Rise, Reign, and Ruine of the
Antinomians, Familists & Libertines* (1644), *The Antinomian Controversy,
1636-1638: A Documentary History*, ed. David D. Hall (Durham: Duke UP,
1990) 263.

when He revealed Himself through certain scriptural passages or directly through "divine illuminations."[24]

In the months following her arrival, the doctrinal debate about how salvation could be ascertained evolved not so much during Sunday services but rather in conventicles at Anne Hutchinson's home as well as during births attended by Hutchinson and her closest followers, Mary Dyer and Jane Hawkins, two local midwives. Often accompanied by other female assistants from the community, a group of approximately twelve women (the number and constellation changed as members would take shifts at the bedside) were present at a given birth, often for several days and nights. The occasion itself was rarely a mere joyous one. Birth complications frequently required the collective expertise of the women. In some cases, mother and/or child died, causing grief among family members and witnesses. These tragic occurrences were often seen as godly punishments rather than a failure of a birth attendant, a view that secured the reputation of many midwives.

Anne Hutchinson and her followers realized that birth constituted a state of exception during which a woman was particularly susceptible to spiritual instruction. At the point when pain turned into agony, when life and death were especially close, the free grace message fell on fertile mental ground. Its emphasis on spiritual estates offered a route of escape from the physical condition of the birthing woman. The mother-to-be was reminded "to compare the feelings of pregnancy and labor to the breeding of the Spirit in their hearts."[25] The Antinomian promise that successful motherhood constituted a work unnecessary for receiving

---

[24] Edmund S. Morgan, *The Puritan Dilemma: The Story of John Winthrop*, 3rd ed. (New York: Pearson Longman, 2007) 129. According to the "legalists" or "Antinomians," one's behavior before or after having been justified (i.e., pronounced by God to have been freed from sin and chosen for eternal life) did not matter nearly as much as intense and instantaneous relations with Christ. Neither did faith. Antinomians claimed that faith was not a necessary precondition for salvation or a sign of sanctification (i.e., the inherent holiness in humans after God had pronounced their salvation), as long as Christ's message about one's spiritual estate was inherently and unshakably established in the believer.

[25] Porterfield, *Female Piety* 97.

divine grace, as well as the prospect of relief from gnawing doubts about the spiritual future, proved highly attractive for women who were either undergoing or witnessing these rites of passage.[26]

A faction of the Boston power elite, including John Winthrop, Thomas Shepard, and Thomas Dudley, as well as most ministers preaching at the periphery of the young colony, considered Hutchinson's conventicles and her theological views blasphemous and as producing negative social and political consequences. Antinomian teachings, they feared, would undermine the mutually agreed upon moral code and could thus disunite and threaten settler communities. One of the main problems for officials was that the Antinomian position took John Calvin's insistence on free and irresistible grace to its logical conclusion. If life were not seen as a constant preparation and inward search for Christ, as the dissenters claimed, then a main motivation for starting a new life in the "wilderness" would be lost. If works no longer prepared for salvation, Boston clergymen feared, then the physical improvement of the environment might as well cease. This, in turn, would have meant a severe threat to the colonial project itself. If, moreover, the Bible was no longer the sole guide to truth but subordinate to individual revelations, and if adherence to moral laws was no longer seen as sufficient for salvation (depending solely on free grace), then the gatekeepers and teachers of morality would lose their role and influence over the spiritual and social direction of the colony.

Aside from questions pertaining to religion, politics, and gender, the controversy actually ran much deeper. It evolved around the issue of epistemology: how do human beings arrive at truth when signs fail to represent meaning in a stable manner? It can hardly be overstated that the search for truth and assurance, engrained in Puritan ecclesiology and a central undertaking in the lives of many concerned settlers, led to an incessant quest for meaning behind natural and preternatural signs. This search also energized the Antinomian shift from letter to spirit, from scriptural knowledge and guidance to direct engagement with God and a theology based on a covenant of grace. This notion implied that believers could and would de-emphasize their worldly actions; since they no longer constituted signs of redemption, they lost importance.

---

[26] Porterfield, *Female Piety* 81-82; Hall, *World of Wonders* 241.

Winthrop and other colonial Bostonians geared up to defend the congregational way by re-claiming authority over signification processes. As a key player in the public examinations of, and controversy over, the actions and treatment of the Antinomians, Winthrop's public and private writings about the views and fates of the dissenters were aimed at winning the favor of religious and civil leaders in England, Old and New. As Winthrop is instigating and undertaking the prosecution and banishment of Anne Hutchinson, his personal relations present a different self, one that is on trial for deviating from the path of religious orthodoxy. In the spring of 1637, Winthrop confesses to his journal his personal flirtations with Antinomianism during the previous months. The retrospective confession portrays an individual who grapples with the promise of free grace, assurance of salvation, and immediate, emotional interaction with the divine, on the one hand, and with the contradictions between his public and private personae, on the other. His initiation into Antinomianism is, similar to other Winthropean religious revelations, prompted by illness: "I came to see more clearly into the covenant of free grace. First therefore hee laid a sore affliction upon mee wherein hee laid me lower in myne owne eyes then at any time before, and showed mee the emptiness of all my guifts, and parts."[27] While the writing subject considers illness as a token of the sanctity of Antinomianism, it soon has to realize that its error in reading the disease correctly. Winthrop attributes the misreading to his inability to discern the truth of God's message, rather than to a misguided sign by the sender. After a period of reflection, he realizes that "The Doctrine of justification lately taught here, took mee in as drowsy a condition,"[28] leading him to condemn Antinomianism in private and to further prosecute it in public. The emphasis on the "drowsy a condition" configures free grace theology as a momentary lapse of reason, a mental illness even, that can only be overcome by returning to "healthy" orthodoxy.

These journal entries help to understand more fully the governor's position toward Antinomianism during the court hearings of Newton/Cambridge in 1637. In Freudian terms one might say that

[27] John Winthrop, "Christian Experience," *Winthrop Papers* I, 159.

[28] John Winthrop, "Christian Experience," *Winthrop Papers* I, 160.

Winthrop's projection of his repressed Antinomian convictions on a culturally deviant midwife and self-styled prophet proved a hindrance during his attempted conviction of Anne Hutchinson in court and later in narrative space. In contrast to Hutchinson, who maintained and defended her beliefs in public, Winthrop's personal narrative, "Experiencia" envisions how the trial should have proceeded: the transgressor from the path of orthodoxy and proper religious and social conviction realizes the errors of the free grace position, repents, and returns to the mainstream of New England Puritanism.

Despite his private battle of conscience, Winthrop and other members of the patriarchal elite needed, under all circumstances, to avoid the impression that they persecuted compatriots such as Hutchinson and Wheelwright merely because of their dissenting beliefs. Such a repetition of William Laud's persecution would have been inacceptable and could have further weakened New England's political position. Always on shaky legal grounds from its inception, Massachusetts' late quarrels over charters, grants, and petitions that dealt with boundaries in, and jurisdiction over, land in North America afforded little room for political maneuvering on Winthrop's part. Instead, he had to uphold the impression, in action and in writing, that the treatment of the Antinomians was wholly justified by their words and ideas as well as by divine omens and portents.

Published in 1644, Winthrop's semi-fictional account of the free grace controversy, entitled *A Short Story of the Rise, Reign, and Ruine of the Antinomians, Familists & Libertines*, sought to convince compatriots in England of the necessity to ward off potentially heretic ideas veiled in a self-styled New Light theology. The text consists of a collection of sermons and court records that reflect Winthrop's specific point of view and interest during the controversy and that justify the ultimate banishment of Antinomians. Overall, the narrative seeks to blame the community's dissent and near break-up on Anne Hutchinson alone and thus downplays the roles taken by key male players during the controversy. For the second edition of Winthrop's text, Thomas Weld, one of Hutchinson's prosecutors during her civil trial in 1637, contributed a preface that was designed to give unity to Winthrop's rather incohesive assemblage of textual fragments. In this preface, Weld summarizes and refutes the main arguments postulated by the Antinomians and composes a fiery disputation with a clear message: the actions of the Boston magistrates and church elders who had examined and ostracized Hutchinson (and others) were justified in light of overwhelming intellectual, theological, and medical evidence.

At several instances Weld uses vocabulary taken from the semantic field of medicine to illustrate the contagious nature of the views of the Antinomians, spreading like an epidemic from one individual to another. He considers the followers of Cotton, Wheelwright, and Hutchinson as being "infected before they were aware, and some being tainted conveyed the infection to others: and thus that Plague first began amongst us [...]."[29] It seems likely that most colonists would have readily apprehended Weld's metaphoric linkage between medical and intellectual realms as well as between the body and the mind. Both sickness and health were, as shown previously, perceived as more than physical states. Hence, Weld's notion that there existed spiritual epidemics, which affected the condition of individual settlers and the colony as a whole, would not have encountered much opposition. Yet, when Weld equates the ways in which the Antinomians spread their ideas with the work of a medical practitioner, the limits of employing illness metaphors for propagandistic purposes becomes visible:

> They would not, till they knew men well, open the whole mystery of their new Religion to them, but this was ever their method, to drop a little at once into their followers as they were capable, and never would administer their Physicke, till they had first given good preparatives to make it worke, and then stronger & stronger potions, as they found the Patient able to beare.[30]

The metaphorical ties between Antinomianism and medicine remain incomplete here because the instructive work of the dissenters is related to the work of a physician, who normally treats a patient with the goal of *improving* his/her situation. Weld, in contrast, claims that the medicine of the free grace proponents causes a physical and spiritual deterioration of the patients. According to his argumentative logic and rhetoric of contagion, Antinomians first proceeded hidden from view and then

---

[29] Winthrop, *A Short Story* in Hall, *Antinomian Controversy* 202.

[30] Winthrop, *A Short Story* in Hall, *Antinomian Controversy* 206.

operated systematically, preparing their subjects for a foul-tasting medicine. A few pages further into his preface, Weld describes those dissenters who "administer their Physicke" in a more sensible light. Through vocal opposition against the Antinomians, ministers and officials were to "cure those that were diseased already, and to give Antidotes to the rest, to preserve them from infection."[31] Here, Weld retrospectively affords colonial officials significant latitude to govern and control human bodies and minds from infectious diseases—figural and literal.

The metaphorical linkage of contagious ideas with infectious illnesses resonated widely and vibrantly within the general conception of illness in early New England. Colonists held that sickness exceeded a mere natural cause and was, in essence, a spiritual affair. As shown in chapter one, people in the early modern period believed that illnesses could be induced by natural agents (miasma and contagion), but they were often initiated by divine (or satanic) interventions, moral transgressions, overwhelming doubts or impious thoughts. Since some illnesses were considered as having a non-material origin, ideas could not only spread like diseases, they could, moreover, induce a physical change in the afflicted.[32] This became especially evident when the opponents of Antinomianism learned that two of its female supporters, Mary Dyer and Anne Hutchinson, had given birth to abnormal fetuses during and shortly after the court and church trials against Hutchinson.

Despite the fact that Weld, Winthrop, and other colonists hesitated to draw conclusions from divine portents and prodigies—because providence was inherently mysterious and its deciphering considered futile and presumptuous—the Massachusetts governor and many of his colleagues sought to take control over the process of endowing bodily

---

[31] Winthrop, *A Short Story* in Hall, *Antinomian Controversy* 212.

[32] During Anne Hutchinson's 1638 church trial, John Cotton, who had previously sided with the Antinomians, reversed his position, accused his former devotee of heresy, and compared her doctrines to "a Gangrene" and "a Leprosie" that "infect farr and near, and will eate out the very Bowells of Religion." Cotton's betrayal of his former admirer, follower, and defendant is further underlined by his explicit agreement with Hutchinson's opponents who used similar disease-infused language (Hall, *Antinomian Controversy* 373).

signs with meaning by resorting, once again, to medical providentialism. Only three years after the "miraculous plague," which had killed approximately ninety percent of New England Natives, sparing most of the English colonists, God had intervened again and pointed His finger of medical providence in a seemingly clear direction. He had not remained impartial during the controversy, Winthrop and Weld explained repeatedly in *A Short Story*, but had revealed obvious signs of his favor for those New England settlers that followed official theology.

In Weld's preface and Winthrop's report, the premature and disfigured fetuses ("monstrous birth") delivered by Mary Dyer and Anne Hutchinson are configured as providential signs that play a central role in re-claiming moral and theological righteousness. Dyer had worked as a midwife in Boston and surrounding settlements and, along with Jane Hawkins, became part of the inner Hutchinsonean circle.[33] In October 1637, Dyer gave birth to a stillborn, malformed fetus, which was secretly and illegally buried. Five months later, on the day of Hutchinson's church trial, which sealed her banishment through excommunication, rumors of the concealed birth led to the exhumation and semi-public examination of the corpse. Winthrop retrospectively describes Dyer's female stillbirth in considerable detail: "it had no head but a face, which stood low upon the brest, as the eares (which were like an Ape) grew upon the shoulders. The eyes stood farre out, so did the mouth, the nose was hooking upward, the brest and back was full of sharp prickles, […] in stead of toes, it had upon each foot three claws […]."[34] After a thorough depiction of the non-human birth, Winthrop mentions strange behavior surrounding the delivery; for instance, that three persons were involved in hiding the dead fetus from public knowledge (in spite of a law that required all births and deaths to be reported to the authorities) and that all women attending Dyer's birth suddenly fell ill and had to leave the room. Winthrop provides no

---

[33] For a biographical account of Dyer's life and work, see Horatio Rogers, *Mary Dyer of Rhode Island* (Providence: Preston & Rounds, 1896). A critical assessment of Dyer's thoughts and actions is offered in Anne G. Myles, "From Monster to Martyr: Re-Presenting Mary Dyer," *Early American Literature* 36.1 (2001): 1-30.

[34] Winthrop, *A Short Story* in Hall, *Antinomian Controversy* 280-281.

interpretation of the parturition but the carefully placed clues—the birth
bed was trembling mysteriously, the afterbirth looked as strangely
deformed as the fetus, and the birth occurred on the same day that
Hutchinson lost her social and religious status—signal a reading in
providential terms that his culturally literate audience could easily
recognize and embrace.[35]

In Old England, deformed births had traditionally been regarded as
manifestation of the parents' moral deviance and in North America this
belief was coupled with religious interpretations and often seen as signs
of theological, intellectual, and personal failure.[36] As Valerie and Morris
Pearl point out,

> [m]onster and prodigy literature had been a huge genre, especially from
> the sixteenth century, drawing examples from the writers of antiquity,
> and had taken three main streams that sometimes intermingled: the
> anthropological, including [...] the wonders of nature; the somewhat

[35] Anne Schutte argues that Winthrop refrained from suggesting a providential
reading in his contribution to *A Short Story*. While Winthrop's language is less
explicit than Weld's in the book's preface, it nevertheless played upon the
cultural entrenchment of medical providentialism on both sides of the Atlantic.
Anne Jacobson Schutte, "'Such Monstrous Births': A Neglected Aspect of the
Antinomian Controversy," *Renaissance Quarterly* 38.1 (1985): 85-106.

[36] The notion that the physical features of a newborn baby coincided with the
ideas or imagination of the mother during conception or pregnancy was fairly
common in seventeenth-century England, even among learned and literate
healers, and was disseminated in guidebooks such as Jane Sharp, *The Midwives
Book. Or the Whole Art of Midwifry Discovered* (1671). Birth defects also
carried significant sexual connotations. It was widely believed that one of the
reasons for a woman's miscarriage was either her unusual sexual desire and/or
that she had mounted her husband during conception. The latter explanatory
approach had far-reaching symbolic resonances because the position during
sexual intercourse suggested that the woman had already placed, or desired to
place, herself above the man in both private and public settings. See Ulrich,
*Good Wives* 135-138, on the perceived relations between maternal behavior and
fetal development; for "monstrous births" in New England see, Hall, *Worlds of
Wonder* 72-74, 100-101; for the sexual connotations of birth defects, see Cheryl
C. Smith, "Out of Her Place: Anne Hutchinson and the Dislocation of Power in
New World Politics," *Journal of American Culture* 29.4 (2006): 442.

related classical stream stemming from the studies of Aristotle and Albertus as well as other medieval works; and the third, which saw monstrous births as portents or divine signs.[37]

Weld and Winthrop discarded the first two explanatory approaches and emphasized a providential reading of the "monsters." The rhetorical exploitation of Dyer's deformed birth for propagandistic purposes was further amplified after Anne Hutchinson's delivery of an equally providential fetus in 1638. From Winthrop's account we learn that the Antinomian leader delivered "several lumps of man's seed, without any alteration, or mixture of any thing from the woman."[38] Winthrop's depiction of the lacking corporeal shape of what was probably a hydatiform mole draws a line of distinction to his earlier sermon, "A Modell of Christian Charity," in which he outlines the ideal interfaces between the body human and the body social of the envisioned colonial settlements in Pauline fashion.[39] In contrast to Winthrop's vision of a tightly knit and orderly system of social discipline and control designed to sustain English colonialism in North America, Hutchinson's malformed birth stands for a social organization dreaded and rejected by the Bay Colony founder. Because it was "so confusedly knit together by so many several strings" that it lacked a discernible form and hierarchy, her birth suggested emergent chaos and anarchy rather than consistent order and uniformity of the body politic.[40] Furthermore, whereas Dyer's

---

[37] Valerie Pearl and Morris Pearl, "Governor John Winthrop on the Birth of the Antinomians' 'Monster': The Earliest Reports to Reach England and the Making of a Myth," *Proceedings of the Massachusetts Historical Society* 102 (1990): 32.

[38] John Winthrop, *The History of New England from 1630-1649*, vol. 1, ed. James Savage (Boston: Little, 1852) 326.

[39] John Winthrop, "A Modell of Christian Charity (1630)," *Collections of the Massachusetts Historical Society* 7 (1838): 31-48. Modeled on Paul's first epistle to the Romans, the main metaphor used throughout the speech is that of the body. Winthrop explains that Puritans in the "New World" are connected with each other through the body of Christ and in the church. Moreover, each member of the community is to function like a specific part of the human body, all working together and depending on each other to make the social entity survive and prosper.

[40] Winthrop, *History*, vol. I, 328.

female human-animal birth hinted at the social debasement and unsustainability of sinful and gender-marked ideas turned flesh, the absence of femaleness from Hutchinson's delivery is symbolic of women's virtual eradication from the community. Bryce Traister has asserted that "[s]imilar to the female withdrawal into the confined space of midwifery and the midwife's removal from overt patriarchal supervision, the monstrous birth metaphorically signals the female withdrawal from the anatomy of reproduction," and, one should add, from generating cultural meaning.[41] Hutchinson's lack of agency in choosing her church and place of residence extends into the textual realm as the Boston woman is barred from participating in the meaning-creation of natural occurrences and the inscription of the human and, especially, female body. Instead, Winthrop's account represents the attempt of the male authorities to regain power over signification processes that Hutchinson had seemingly wielded from them and harbored during her birth-gatherings and conventicles.[42]

Winthrop's attempt to reclaim his position as authoritative exegete in social, cultural, and political matters relied significantly on downplaying the inherent virtuality of Hutchinson's malformed fetus. If we feed Gilles Deleuze's notion of the "body without organs" back into Winthrop's description, the irreducible abstractness of Hutchinson's "lumps" becomes evident. Even though *A Short Story* configures the birth as an actual body, it remains a body without organs and as such—

[41] Bryce Traister, "Anne Hutchinson's 'Monstrous Birth' and the Feminization of Antinomianism," *Canadian Review of American Studies* 27.2 (1997): 145.

[42] Winthrop, *A Short Story* in Hall, *Antinomian Controversy* 215. The elaborate scholarly emphasis of the proto-feminist aspects of Hutchinson's actions (cf. Koehler; Smith) should be taken with caution, according to Michael Winship, who argues that twentieth-century readings often tend to depict the Antinomian crisis as a mere gendered conflict over agency and authority, even though one of Hutchinson's main line of defense centered on her full compliance with social roles and positions of women in society. Because her conventicles and child birth attendances were in keeping with English lay norms and female role ascriptions, Winship contends that "[f]or scholars to [...] focus on Hutchinson's gender, if at the expense of neglecting her considerable skills as a creative and polemical biblical exegete, takes the disavowal of her far past what Winthrop and his brethren attempted" (*Times and Trials* 116).

in Winthrop's eyes, seen through a Deleuzian lens—"is permeated by unformed, unstable matters, by flows in all directions, by free intensities or nomadic singularities, by mad or transitory particles."[43] By relating the de-organ-ized birth to a tumultuous and anarchic disorder threatening Massachusetts Bay, Winthrop not only draws a social analogy but also an ontological one, since the process of becoming human in a woman's womb is redefined as being non-human once the "monstrous birth" is visible to the outside world.

What is more, Winthrop's representation of crisis exposes a crisis of representation in New England culture. This crisis emerges with full force when Winthrop cites a report by Dr. John Clarke, one of Boston's most renowned seventeenth-century surgeons. Indebted to Baconian paradigms of scientific analysis, Clarke, after having visited Hutchinson and examined her miscarriage, concludes that, "if you consider each of them [i.e. the lumps; M.P.] according to the representation of the whole, they were altogether without form."[44] Clarke's proto-clinical report provides no clear indication of a providential interpretation of the "monstrous birth." Rather, the absent form of Hutchinson's delivery emphasizes the lack of accessible meaning. Contrary to Cheryl Smith's claim that Winthrop is deploying Clarke's report "to make [the] case against her scientifically sound," the doctor's narrative actually deconstructs the intention of its inclusion.[45] Winthrop, whose impatience with the physician's finding is underlined by his sending the doctor to re-examine the dissenter's hydatiform mole, ultimately receives no scientific fodder for his rhetorical battle against the presumed religious radicals. Instead of supporting Winthrop's condemnation of the Antinomians, the medical report of an indefinable and thus unreadable human tissue signals an emerging incompatibility between cultural and scientific voices in colonial New England. Equally important, Clarke's medical report included in Winthrop's work marks another ventriloquial moment that reveals a crisis in Puritan thought and writing. The providential approach to a medical case seeks to employ and control

---

[43] Gilles Deleuze and Felix Guatarri, *Thousand Plateaus*, trans. Brian Massumi (1980; London: Continuum, 2004) 40.

[44] Winthrop, *History*, vol. I, 327.

[45] Smith 447.

science—illustrated by Winthrop's paraphrasing rather than citing Clarke's report. In doing so, the account emphasizes not only the incompatibility of science and religion but also the former's emerging resistance to containment in the latter.

Because the medical report by Clarke and other evidence presented in Winthrop's narrative failed to fully lend themselves to a portrayal of Hutchinson's birth in providential terms, *A Short Story* was augmented by Thomas Weld's interpretative preface. In a text striving for narrative unity, the placement of Weld's explanation of the two miscarriages *before* Winthrop's account merits attention. For one, it indicates that Weld could rest assured that the story of the deformed births was already known. Also, he would have been well aware that his reading coincided with the dominant cultural interpretation of "monstrosity." Against the background of a pre-existing cultural coding of malformed births, Weld writes that

> God himself was pleased to step in with his casting voice, and bring in his owne vote and suffrage from heaven, by testifying his displeasure against their [i.e., the Antinomians'; M.P.] opinions and practices, as clearly as if he had pointed with his finger, in causing the two fomenting women in the time of the height of the Opinions to produce out of their wombs, as before they had out of their braines, such monstrous births as no Chronicle (I thinke) hardly ever recorded the like.[46]

Weld further sermonizes on how Hutchinson's miscarriage of thirty non-human lumps seemed a logical consequence and *representation* of her thirty-something doctrinal errors. For the author, the message contained in the deformed births was clear: according to the "loud-speaking providence from Heaven in the monsters," God punished Dyer and Hutchinson's transgressions by bringing about their miscarriages.[47] It is worth stressing that the reader never finds such explicit references to divine providence in the sections of the book written by Winthrop himself. Despite the fact that Winthrop's account is much less toned to

---

[46] Winthrop, *A Short Story* in Hall, *Antinomian Controversy* 214.

[47] Winthrop, *A Short Story* in Hall, *Antinomian Controversy* 215.

providence than Weld's preface, these words are Winthrop's as much as they are Weld's. When coming to the governor's report in the book, the reader is thus fully prepared to interpret the deformed births according to a cultural reservoir that the authors of *A Short Story* had found already present and that they merely needed to tap.

By relying on a cultural register that predetermined the meaning of providential portents, the two authors also aided in its sustenance and extension. Winthrop's contribution to the "monstrous birth" myth reveals, for instance, immanent connections between Antinomianism and witchcraft. These connections are based primarily on medical practice and knowledge and become particularly evident when Winthrop singles out Jane Hawkins, Boston midwife and open Hutchinsonean, as a person who has been "notorious for familiarity with the devil."[48] In the spring of 1638, Hawkins and her husband were expelled from the Bay colony and had to abstain from their seemingly dangerous medical practice. In the time between the official pronouncement of her banishment and the move to Rhode Island, Hawkins was "not to meddle in surgery, or physic, drinks, plasters, or oils, nor to question matters of religion, except with the elders for satisfaction."[49] In a similar vein, Winthrop associates Mary Dyer's medical practice with witchcraft:

---

[48] Winthrop, *A Short Story* in Hall, *Antinomian Controversy* 281. For an introduction to the careers of colonial New England midwives, including Jane Hawkins, see Henry R. Viets, *A Brief History of Medicine in Massachusetts* (Boston: Houghton, 1930) 14-40. For the proximity between midwives and witches as part of a larger cultural matrix in Renaissance and early modern Europe, see Thomas Rogers Forbes, *The Midwife and the Witch* (New Haven: Yale UP, 1966).

[49] David D. Hall, ed., *Witch-Hunting in Seventeenth-Century New England* (Boston: Northeastern UP, 1991) 20. A decade after Hawkins' banishment, another midwife, Alice Tilly, was imprisoned for malpractice. This time, more than two hundred women of Boston and Dorchester signed a petition in support of Tilly, which saved her from the gallows. Mary Beth Norton, "'The Ablest Midwife That Wee Knowe in the Land': Mistress Alice Tilly and the Women of Boston and Dorchester, 1649-1650," *The William and Mary Quarterly* 55.1 (1998): 105-134.

for it was known, that she used to give young women oil of mandrakes and other stuff to cause conception; and she grew into great suspicion to be a witch, for it was credibly reported, that, when she gave any medicines, (for she practised physic,) she would ask the party, if she did believe, she could help her, etc.[50]

In Winthrop's narrative of Dyer and Hawkins, medicine and religious beliefs are brought into close proximity, even complicity, as their healing practices are rendered as potentially harmful. Aside from revealing the high level of expertise and recognition of Hawkins' and Dyer's curative abilities, the conjunction between medicine and religion is charged with symbolism and radiates beyond the mere occasion and its reference in Winthrop's narrative. Voiced in careful and precise judicial language, the cultural interconnections between woman, healer, and religious troublemaker conceptualized socio-cultural deviance around medical practices. However, such deviance required a double coding of medicine. On the one hand, it had to be considered as a human practice sealed by God and geared at benefiting His servants; on the other hand, most colonists believed that curative procedures could easily be adjusted to meet more malign intentions. Healing techniques, especially when performed by women, were hence culturally configured as being potentially beneficial *and* harmful to humanity. Although none of the three prominent Antinomian midwives/healing women (Dyer, Hutchinson, and Hawkins) were officially charged with witchcraft, their words and actions were conceived as resting in a borderland between normalcy and deviance, God and Satan. For Winthrop, witchcraft constituted a subtext designed to absolve ambiguous cultural positions by discrediting the women's characters and by belatedly reconfiguring the free grace movement as diabolical.

Not all colonists shared Winthrop and Weld's interpretation of the deformed births, however. The latter's line of argument is contested in John Wheelwright's rebuttal, *Mercurius Americanus*, published in England one year after *A Short Story*. In his repudiation, the author

---

[50] John Winthrop, *Winthrop's Journal: "History of New England," 1630-1649*, vol. 1, ed. James Kendall Hosmer (New York: Scribner's Sons, 1908) 268. Winthrop also claims that Jane Hawkins had confessed to conversing with Satan (266).

refutes readings of the stillbirths as all too obvious signs of the divine. Winthrop falsely sought to "ingage, and magnifie Divine direction and derive this not known by him to be a truth," Wheelwright writes and thus claims that the Bay Colony leader fails to prove sufficiently the proposed links between the birth defects and God's disapproval of free grace propositions. Wheelwright, as a result, suggests that Hutchinson's condition would "require a most accurate physical inspection which I think his [i.e., Winthrop's; M.P.] learning will not reach."[51] This rebuttal posits Winthrop and Weld's medical providentialism as superstition and demands scientific examinations of the matter. As Anne Schutte has argued, though, Wheelwright's intentions were to discredit Winthrop rather than to suggest actual scientific inquiries.[52] In addition, for Wheelwright, the interfacing of the Dyer/Hutchinson miscarriages with divine favor revealed itself as an arbitrary ideological construct that Weld and Winthrop designed to incite (New) Englanders' support for the social, political, and cultural vision that energized the settlement of Massachusetts Bay.

Despite Wheelwright's charging, and in hindsight plausible, criticism, Winthrop's Hutchinsonization of the free grace controversy and his medicalization of female deviance set the tone for historical interpretations during the eighteenth century. Until the Great Awakening, New England commentators continued to follow Weld and Winthrop in inscribing deformed births as mental or behavioral errors onto the female body. The concomitant distortion of women's corporality and sexuality continued to correlate with a critique of female assertions of power and influence in the public arena. For instance, Cotton Mather's account in *Magnalia Christi Americana* picks up an earlier mode of interpretation by positing women as inherently more susceptible to spiritual instruction and delusion than men. While this often aids in bringing more people to Christ, Mather claims, it also entails a danger to social stability. The alleged special vulnerability of women is cleverly exploited by female religious dissenters, whose

---

[51] John Wheelwright, *Mercurius Americanus, Mr. Welds His Antitype, or, Massachusetts Great Apologie Examined* (1645; Early English Books Online, W1605) 6, 7.

[52] Schutte 105.

"poyson does never insinuate so quickly, nor operate so strongly as when *women's milk* is the *vehicle* wherein 'tis given."[53] The Boston minister proves a master of the rhetorical employment of parallels between cultural ideas and medicine in order to vivify his ideological message. Hutchinson serves as a metonymy for a gender-inherent mistake and, at the same time, her individual voice, conviction, and agency is eradicated by Mather. In addition to attributing moral and doctrinal errors to women as a whole, he readily appropriates Winthrop's hints at Hutchinson's proximity to witchcraft, describing her doctrines as "bewitch[ed]" and "cunning."[54] He furthermore marvels at the providential resonances of the deformed stillbirths, whose description he copies almost verbatim from Winthrop's various accounts. However, as much as Mather would like to underline Winthrop's medico-providentialist interpretation of the deformed births, his own medical and scientific education had taught him that such occurrences often have a natural cause, as will be shown in further detail in chapter six of this study. He, as a consequence, eventually distances himself from Winthrop's medical providentialism by writing that the births "were *lookt upon* as testimonies from Heaven," rather than claiming that they actually constituted divine signs.[55]

In sum, then, while the transformation of an intellectual strength into a gendered weakness had always been a favorite strategy of misogynists, this tool of exerting discursive power became especially pronounced and sustained with regard to the issues of truth and assurance during the

---

[53] Cotton Mather, *Magnalia Christi Americana; or, The Ecclesiastical History of New England,* Vol. II (1702; Hartford: Andrus, 1853) 516 (emphasis original).

[54] Mather, *Magnalia* II:517.

[55] Mather, *Magnalia* II:519 (emphasis added). A decade later, Mather further delineates his skepticism concerning providential readings of birth defects in a letter to the Royal Society. Although he makes no reference to the Dyer and Hutchinson cases, his observations on "monstrous births in my neighborhood" indicate that Mather has come to approach the phenomenon of strange bodies from a natural rather than a theological perspective. Cotton Mather to John Woodward, 3 July 1716, British Library, Sloane Ms. 3340, folio 280-282. See chapter six of the present study for a more detailed discussion of Mather's correspondence with the Royal Society between 1702 and 1724.

Antinomian crisis of 1636-1638. By medicalizing and feminizing deviant ideas and actions in their written retrospection, Thomas Weld and John Winthrop tried to recapture male exegetic agency that was otherwise denied to them by the cultural rendering of the birth room as a gender-exclusive space. In their view, the sprouting Antinomian seeds planted by Hutchinson had failed to blossom into a sustained movement and, instead, produced disfigured offspring that symbolized the failure of Antinomian ideas. In the hands of male commentators, Hutchinson's teachings became "a Leprosie" (Cotton); her tragic childbirth was interpreted as "God's punishment" (Mather); her skills as a midwife signaled "witchcraft" (Winthrop). These distortions relied to a great extent on medical issues, especially Hutchinson's combination of midwifery and spiritual instruction and the medical narratives surrounding her own and her co-worker's birth defects. By banishing Hutchinson and other Antinomians, the Massachusetts Bay Colony lost a leader for their community of women, a skilled healer and midwife, and a determined student of the Bible. What they gained instead was a "social disease" that grew out of increasing efforts at directing the minds and hearts of colonists to the official New England way: Hutchinson's banishment provided justification for more Bible study, more publications, more education, more sermons, and more intrusive monitoring of colonial bodies.

Medicine and Witchcraft

Next to the Antinomian controversy, witchcraft accusations constituted central indicators of social and cultural crisis in seventeenth-century New England. This crisis again involved the practice of midwives and "magic healers," who were accused of being in cahoots with the devil, and manifested itself in the corporeal state of mainly young women. During the winter of 1691/92, for instance, two young girls from Salem, Massachusetts, Betty Parris (age nine) and Abigail Williams (age eleven), began to show strange bodily symptoms: "These Children were bitten and pinched by invisible agents; their arms, necks, and backs turned this way and that way, and returned back again, so as it was impossible for them to do of themselves, and beyond the power of any Epileptick Fits, or natural Disease to effect," John Hale tells his readers in his retrospective account of New England witchcraft.[56] Neither his narrative, the first to take a critical stance toward the proceedings and convictions of the Salem Court of Oyer and Terminer (which ordered the execution of nineteen local and regional residents accused of witchcraft), nor the extant court records reveal a definite clue as to whether the fits, convulsions, seizures and other strange body movements and conditions of afflicted New England girls were fraudulent acts or caused by a physical condition that fell under the auspices of medicine. Hale's witchcraft narrative clearly rules out dissembling or natural causes and, in doing so, suggests, but fails to prove, that the girls were under a supernatural influence.

The above-cited bodily symptoms, which many colonists considered the result of satanic interventions, were restricted neither to Salem nor to young girls. In Cotton Mather's widely read pre-Salem witchcraft accounts collected in *Memorable Providences* (1689), for instance, the affliction of Philip Smith is particularly illustrative. This medical witchcraft narrative contains rhetorical strategies typical for the way in which colonists sought to rationalize bodily irregularities in supernatural terms. As part of a larger discourse designed to demonstrate the ubiquitous activities of witches in New England, Mather relates how Smith, one of the "pious and holy men" in the colony and among the leading men of Hadley, Massachusetts, suffered and died from a severe and inexplicable illness.[57] This narrative aims to provide evidence that the respected colonial leader was "murdered with an hideous Witchcraft," and that the person responsible for the crime was Mary Webster, who was put on trial before the Boston Court in 1683.[58] As Smith began to suffer from what appeared to be sciatic pain, he carried himself like a model Puritan: "As his *Illness* increased on him, so his *Goodneß* increased in him, the standers-by could in him see one

---

[56] John Hale, *A Modest Enquiry into the Nature of Witchcraft* (1697; Early American Imprints, Series 1, no. 1050) 24.

[57] Cotton Mather, *Memorable Providences, Relating to Witchcrafts and Possessions* (1689; Early American Imprints, Series 1, no. 486) 54 (emphases original unless stated otherwise).

[58] Mather, *Memorable Providences* 54.

ripening apace for another world; and filled not only with *Grace* to an
high degree, but also with Exceeding *Joy*."[59] Immediately following this
description of Smith's Jobean endurance, Mather suggests that a witch
caused the illness. This assumption allows him to proceed without
having to consider the medical plausibility of Smith's anamnesis; in fact,
it is precisely by representing a chain of illness events that is *not*
comprehensible from a scientific perspective that the claim of witchcraft
can be validated. Mather proceeds to relate how Smith's sciatic pain was
followed by speech delirium and by pricking pains all over his body.
Then, the narrative focus moves away from Smith's bodily condition
toward supernatural occurrences in his sickroom: a pot filled with
medicine mysteriously emptied; a bed momentarily caught fire; bizarre
noises and motions that occurred without an apparent source; the patient
is relieved of his pain and finally finds rest after his assistants have
interrupted the sleep of Mary Webster, the alleged witch. These strange
occurrences continued beyond Smith's death, when the jury examining
the corpse discovered that "[o]n his back, besides *Bruises*, there were
several *pricks*, or *holes* as if done with *Awls* and *Pins*."[60] In seventeenth-
century New England, most colonists would have recognized such
descriptions as clear signs of witchcraft and, in fact, Mather makes sure
that almost every thematic section—each covering a certain stage in
Smith's health developments—contains commonly readable witchcraft
referents. For example, Smith's post-mortem condition is ascribed to
interventions from the invisible world: the corpse continued to look and
feel lively—with "fresh blood seem'd to run down his Cheek in the
Hairs"—as if the witch or the devil were not satisfied by the patient's
death and therefore continued to haunt and abuse his body after his soul
had (ostensibly) ascended to heaven.[61] By thus attributing Smith's
illness to witchcraft, Mather cleverly deflects disease, etiology, and
responsibility away from both the thoughts and actions of the afflicted as
well as from the physicians of whom a remedy or at least an explanation
might be expected in such a case. Instead, he suggests that the cause of

---

[59] Mather, *Memorable Providences* 55.

[60] Mather, *Memorable Providences* 58.

[61] Mather, *Memorable Providences* 59.

illness lies under the sole authority and agency of the devil and his minions; and thereby under the authority of the churches. The medical narrative seeks to remind the reader that supernatural attacks can strike anyone at any time, and that, therefore, every colonist ought to seek assurance in Christ. For colonial intellectuals such as Cotton Mather, the relegation of illness to the realm of the supernatural was instrumental, even vital, for defending and maintaining a central aspect of Puritan cosmology: that godly providence and satanic interventions were common and expected events in the daily lives of New Englanders.

The Smith case exemplifies how illness and witchcraft were interconnected in seventeenth-century conceptions but allows only few insights into gender-specific aspects of colonial medicine and culture. When the frequent meeting points between healing and religion in early New England are seen through a gendered lens, a cultural fault line emerges between male physicians, who were called to alleviate and/or verify the causes of witchcraft, and female healers, who were often accused of witchcraft.

## Detecting Witches: Male Physicians

For most colonists the symptoms witnessed on the bodies and in the behavior of (mostly) young girls and women were of great concern. In order to rule out satanic intervention, the parents or masters of "bewitched" girls would usually call a local medical expert, in most cases a physician or a midwife. He or she would then examine the patient, administer a medicament if a natural cause was suspected, and often would return after a few days. If the symptoms persisted, as they did in many recorded instances, the medical examiner would rule out a natural cause and hand over the case to the local minister and/or the court.[62]

---

[62] See, for instance, Hall, *Witch-Hunting* 201-202; Richard Godbeer, *Escaping Salem: The Other Witch Hunt of 1692* (New York: Oxford UP, 2005) 17-18, 33-34. When describing the initial diagnosis of the first afflicted girls in Salem in his *Magnalia Christi Americana*, Mather rushes to the defense of the New England medical profession by carefully claiming that the people of Salem, rather than the examining physician, interpreted the girls' symptoms as a cause of witchcraft: "At length one physician gave his opinion that 'they were under

In many court hearings, physicians played an important role in either solidifying or invalidating witchcraft accusations. During legal proceedings, the case against the suspected witch was weakened if the seizures or fits were found to have a natural cause such as epilepsy; however, if the illness was deemed to be of magical or occult origin, a conviction was almost certain. Witch-hunters on both sides of the Atlantic based their beliefs about the interconnections between witchcraft and disease on *Malleus Maleficarum* (1486), a handbook for detecting witches written by two Dominican friars. In a 1616 treatise on witchcraft, the English medical doctor John Cotta advises his readers to consult a physician in doubtful cases because only he is able to identify "such diseases, as are truly and undoubtedly known and proved to have no consistence, or power of consistence, or cause in sublunary nature."[63] In contrast to Cotta's boastful confidence in the medical profession, experts had long been aware that fits, seizures, and convulsions could be due to natural causes and that, therefore, the task of deciding whether satanic influences caused certain diseases proved more difficult than Cotta suggested.[64] Boston minister Cotton Mather reports, for instance, how during the trials of Goody Glover, an Irish Catholic women accused of witchcraft in 1688, the court summoned "five or six Physicians one evening to examine her very strictly, whether she were not craz'd in her Intellectuals, and had not procured to her self by Folly and Madness the Reputation of a Witch." After hours of examining Glover, the physicians concluded that the accused did not suffer from a mental illness, "and Sentence of Death was pass'd upon her."[65] Here, as in many other New England witchcraft cases, male physicians played an important role in keeping the belief in, and the official treatment of, witchcraft alive throughout the seventeenth century.

---

an evil hand.' This the neighbors took up, and concluded they were *bewitch'd*" (Mather, *Magnalia* II:471 [emphasis original]).

[63] John Cotta, *The Triall of Witch-Craft, Showing the True and Right Methode of the Discovery with the Confutation of Erroneous Wayes* (1616; Early English Books Online, STC 5836) 74.

[64] Godbeer, *Escaping Salem* 138; Watson, *Angelical Conjunction* 24-27.

[65] Mather, *Memorable Providences* 3.

Some New Englanders, aware of new scientific publications that had reached Boston, attributed fits, seizures, and other symptoms to a combination of natural and supernatural influences. Cotton Mather and other colonists were familiar with witch trials in England at the time and, especially, with the opinions of Dr. Thomas Browne, who had testified in the 1665 trial at Bury St. Edmonds, England, that "the devil in such cases did work upon the bodies of men and women, upon a natural foundation, (that is) to stir up, and excite such humours super-abounding in their bodies to a great excess [...]."[66] According to Browne's humoral approach, the exact mechanism that interconnected the natural and the supernatural, especially in witchcraft accusations, remained inexplicable. One reason for New England physicians' general failure to diagnose the young women's fits and seizures as a medical condition was the lack of access to the latest research; knowledge of physical and mental causes underlying a variety of disease symptoms, provided most notably in George Gifford, *A Dialogue Concerning Witches and Witchcrafts* (1593), Edward Jorden's *A Briefe Discourse of a Disease Called the Suffocation of the Mother* (1603), John Cotta, *The Triall of Witch-Craft* (1612), and Robert Burton's *The Anatomy of Melancholy* (1621), had not been widely disseminated in the colonies. What is more, New England physicians lived and worked in a cultural environment that accepted and expected witchcraft as a reasonable phenomenon. As a consequence, any repudiation of supernatural causes in favor of natural ones was almost impossible to sustain intellectually and theologically until the end of the century. In both Old and New England, physicians who voiced their skepticism about the existence of witchcraft had to fear the reproach of heresy and medical incompetence. In addition, when physicians such as Dr. Oakes examined afflicted children and/or young women and came to the conclusion that "nothing

---

[66] H. L. Stephen, *State Trials: Political and Social*, vol. 1 (London: Duckworth, 1899) 228. For the English debate on witchcraft as the cause of disease, see Garfield Tourney, "The Physician and Witchcraft in Restoration England," *Medical History* 16.2 (1972): 143-155; Peter Elmer, "Medicine, Witchcraft and the Politics of Healing in Late Seventeenth-Century England," *Medicine and Religion in Enlightenment Europe*, ed. Ole Peter Grell and Andrew Cunningham (Burlington: Ashgate, 2007) 223-242.

but a hellish *Witchcraft* could be the Original of these Maladies,"[67] they had found a useful explanation for the inefficacy of their treatment methods. Had they detected a natural cause, they would have been expected to at least alleviate, if not cure the affliction. Ironically, then, by attributing a case in doubt to witchcraft, especially when kin and family had already predetermined this diagnosis, physicians could secure their social reputation as knowledgeable healers.[68]

As far as we know today, only few New England medical practitioners challenged the culturally dominant assumption that certain bodily signs or symptoms were indicative of bewitchment. A notable exception is found in a letter written by Dr. Nicholas Augur to John Winthrop Jr. in June of 1653. Augur served as a medical advisor at the New Haven court of magistrates during its investigation of witchcraft accusations and was so puzzled by the symptoms of ostensibly bewitched women that he sought Winthrop's advice. After having examined the afflicted for the first time, Augur's medical knowledge, which proved quite advanced for his time, offered no reasonable explanation for the women's strange fits and, even more curiously, for their sudden abatement after the suspected witch, Elizabeth Godman, had been called before the court. He writes:

> When I went to see them againe they tould mee they hoped now they weare cured for they found such an alteration in the stat of theire bodyes that they wondred at, which did Confirme them more in theire former feares and Jelesyes that it might arise from that suspected party, because they found themselves freed from all their pressures after her

---

[67] Mather, *Memorable Providences* 3.

[68] Paul Boyer and Stephen Nissenbaum, eds., *Salem-Village Witchcraft: A Documentary Record of Local Conflict in Colonial New England* (Belmont: Wadsworth, 1972) 53, 218; Tourney 153; Cf. Norman Gevitz, "'The Devil Hath Laughed at the Physicians': Witchcraft and Medical Practice in Seventeenth-Century New England," *Journal of the History of Medicine* 55.1 (2000): 29; Christian Deetjen, "Witchcraft and Medicine," *Bulletin of the Institute of the History of Medicine* 2 (1934): 173.

examination, which bee fore they could not; I shall waite to see what the issue of things shall bee.[69]

The last sentence of this excerpt is especially noteworthy because it expresses Augur's doubt about the obvious implication of the women's illness and recovery report, namely that their affliction was caused by Godman's interaction with satanic forces and was lifted once she had been brought under the auspices and control of the officials.[70] Augur's refusal to adhere to this culturally guided interpretation of the women's illness symptoms appears concomitant to his skepticism about scientific explanations. His education in medicine, which in all likelihood included contemporary works by medical skeptics of witchcraft such as Jorden and Burton, informs him that the fits "had binne Histericall, or an Inlett into an Epilepsie," but provides no clue about their abrupt disappearance.[71] As a result of the apparent inefficiency of both cultural and scientific explanatory approaches, the New Haven physician decides to wait, seek advice from other experts, and continue his observations. By doing so, Augur may not only have saved Elizabeth Godman from the gallows but also proved to have internalized a scientific ethos that was still relatively novel at the time: that conclusive knowledge, especially when used in decisions about the life or death of a human being, must be gained through skeptical observation and rational evaluation of facts.

[69] "Nicholas Augur to John Winthrop, Jr., 17 June 1653," *Winthrop Papers* VI, 301.

[70] The observation that healing set in as soon as the accused was brought under official control is no singularity in New England witchcraft records. In Salem, for example, deponents claimed that their illness subsided once Martha Carrier had been arrested for practicing witchcraft. In the testimony of Benjamin Abbott, we learn that he had been suffering from excruciating pain and "was brought unto death's door, and so remained until Carrier was taken, and carried away by the constable; from which very day, he began to mend, and so grew better every day, and is well ever since." Cotton Mather, *The Wonders of the Invisible World* (1692; Early American Imprints, Series 1, no. 657) 134.

[71] "Nicholas Augur to John Winthrop, Jr., 17 June 1653," *Winthrop Papers* VI, 301.

New England physicians were not only called to examine fits and seizures of those claiming to be bewitched but also to assess other signs of possible satanic intervention. Most notorious were certain marks and teats in sensual areas of the body of the suspected witch (e.g., on her hips, breast, vagina or under her armpits), which were believed to signal allegiance with the devil. According to folklore, the witches' teat was used for suckling so-called familiars or imps, who appeared in the shape of a human being or an animal and who aided the witch in her malevolent endeavors. Eunice Cole, for instance, who was tried for witchcraft in Salisbury, New Hampshire in 1656 reportedly had "under one of hir brests [...] a blew thing like unto a teate hanging downeward about thre quarters of an inche longe not very thick," and Mercy Disborough, a healing woman from Fairfield, Connecticut, on trial in 1692, had "on her secret parts growing within the lep of the same a los pees of skin and when puld it is near an inch long somewhat in form of the fingar of a glove flatted."[72] In order to detect the witches' mark, accused women were often examined by midwives and/or respected women of a given community, who afterwards testified in court. A rare written record of such an examination survives from the trial of seventy-one year old Rebecca Nurse, who was among the first group of Salem women charged in the summer of 1692. The court ordered a body search of Nurse and of three other accused women, which was undertaken by nine local midwives. Four hours after the female examiners had "discovered a preternatural excrescence of flesh between the pudendum and anus, much like to teats, and not usual in women," the court ordered the group to carry out a second examination. This time, the women reversed their previous judgment and reported that, "instead of that excrescence within mentioned, it appears only as dry skin without sense [i.e., without sensation]."[73]

What is particularly interesting about these two medical reports is that eight of the nine midwives who examined the body of Rebecca

---

[72] Quoted in John Demos, "Underlying Themes in the Witchcraft of Seventeenth-Century New England," *The American Historical Review* 75.5 (1970): 1323; Quoted in John M. Taylor, *The Witchcraft Delusion in Colonial Connecticut* (New York: Grafton, 1908) 44.

[73] Boyer and Nissenbaum 31.

Nurse signed their names by using a mark. That they were unable to give their signature attests to their illiteracy and, therefore, to a medical instruction received orally rather than through books. This meant that the midwives could evaluate the excrescence only based on their culturally conditioned experience rather than on new advances in anatomical studies. It is also important to stress that the court selected midwives for being trustworthy and impartial medical experts. Yet, they were not granted true autonomy in diagnosing the witches' mark, because both examination reports had to be signed and thus authorized by John Barton, a local surgeon, who himself was absent during the actual body search. The authorization by Barton enacts, seals, and enshrines the disempowerment of women in colonial society in a particularly vivid mode. His signature at once grants women cultural influence, allowing them to participate in the discovery of truth and, at the same time, manifests a misogynist belief in the incapacity of female New Englanders to assess truth accurately. In the case of Rebecca Nurse, the reversal of the first examination, which established the former "teat" as a piece of dry skin, failed to save the defendant's life. The refusal of the Salem court to consider the second medical report both denied women's empowerment and tied in with a larger judicial trend that became evident on both sides of the Atlantic by the end of the seventeenth century. As Richard Weisman explains, "[o]fficial reliance upon the witch's mark exposed the court to a form of criticism it was ill equipped to oppose, the task of systematically distinguishing natural from supernatural excrescences placed the trial of witchcraft within the hostile jurisdiction of medical authority."[74]As a result, other forms of evidence, including the notorious spectral evidence, were used by New England courts to convict Rebecca Nurse of association with Satan, a verdict which proved fatal: she was hanged in Salem on 19 July 1692.

In some instances, the role of physicians in witchcraft cases continued even beyond death. When the court ordered a post-mortem examination of witches and those having claimed bewitchment, physicians and surgeons inspected the bodies of the dead in order to confirm or repudiate a potentially lethal disease and also to justify

---

[74] Richard Weisman, *Witchcraft, Magic, and Religion in 17th-Century Massachusetts* (Amherst: U of Massachusetts P, 1984) 101.

retrospectively a court's sentence. Among the most vivid documentation of a coroner's inquest is Dr. Bryan Rossiter's 1662 investigation report of eight-year-old Elizabeth Kelly of Hartford, Connecticut, who had died after suffering from what appeared as typical symptoms of bewitchment. The synopsis of the medical examination, submitted to the Hartford Court as evidence of witchcraft, deserves to be cited in entirety because it aptly illustrates the congruities and discrepancies between cultural and scientific approaches to body meanings during the second half of the seventeenth century.

> These 6 particulars underwritten I judge preternatural—upon opening of John Kelly's child at the grave I observed[:]
> 1. whole body, the musculous parts, nerves, and joints, were all pliable, without any stiffness, or contraction, the gullet only excepted: Experience of dead bodies renders such symptoms unusual.
> 2. From the costall ribs to the bottom of the belly in the whole latitude of the womb; both the scarfskin and the whole skin with the enveloping or covering flesh had a deep blue tincture; w[he]n the inward part thereof was fresh, and the bowels under it in true order, without any discoverable peccunry, to cause such an effect or symptom.
> 3. No quantity or appearance of blood was in either vortex or cavity of belly or breasts but in the throat only at the very swallow where was a large quantity, as that part could well [contain] both fresh and fluid, no way [congelated] or clotted as it come[s] from a vein opened that I stroke it out with my finger as water.
> 4. There was the appearance of pure fresh blood in the backside of the arm, affecting the skin as blood itself without bruising, or [congelating].
> 5. The bladder of gall was all broken and curded, without any tincture in the adjacent parts.
> 6. The gullet or swallow was contracted, like a hard wishbone that hardly a large pease could be forced through.[75]

[75] Hall, *Witch-Hunting* 154-155. Ministers such as Cotton Mather had no objections against dissections if they helped to determine the cause of death. For instance, his diaries report the post-mortem examination of his sister and his children, suggesting that autopsies were common procedure, although not for educational purposes, in colonial North America. Watson, *Angelical Conjunction* 135-143. For a study of post-mortem examinations in seventeenth-century New England, see Paul F. Mellen, "Coroners' Inquests in Colonial

Rossiter's medical report illustrates important facets of the intersections between medicine and culture in colonial New England. First, similar to Clarke's report on Anne Hutchinson's miscarriage in Winthrop's *A Short Story*, Rossiter's text illustrates a Baconian approach that is based on close examination and deductive reasoning. The author starts from the premise that the child's symptoms had supernatural causes and then proceeds to provide observations whose meaning is already predetermined by the first sentence. However, in the description of the symptoms, the medical expert fails to prove how his observations relate specifically to the intervention of witchcraft. Second, the diction of the report is laced with medical terms in such a way that it *dissembles* scientific authority to a non-medical, yet learned audience. That is, Rossiter's engagement with medical and anatomical discourse conveys a sense of expertise needed to decide on the contested issue of the workings of witches. Yet, this expertise remains performative rather than representational because the text stages a scientific rhetoric that self-referentially draws attention to its absence of scientificity. Third, the first symptom of the medical narrative, the lack of *rigor mortis* of the corpse, is judged as abnormal based on the examiner's experience, instead of published anatomical methods. The author then lists five other conditions that he deems unusual and, in doing so, implies that they, too, constitute signs of witchcraft, rather than indications of his lacking knowledge or scientific research on a particular body part or condition.[76]

Rossiter's medical narrative illustrates how cultural meanings clashed and, at the same time, interacted with scientific renderings of the human body. The official exhumation and opening of Kelly's corpse sought to remove a corporeal opacity that was both culturally significant and signifying. However, as the report aptly demonstrates, the erasure of the body's symbolic meaning as (also) a metaphysical body and the concomitant transformation of the physical body into an object of scientific analysis remain unattainable endeavors. In other words,

---

Massachusetts," *Journal of the History of Medicine and Allied Sciences* 40 (1985): 462-472.

[76] Cf. Gevitz 17; Sanford J. Fox, *Science and Justice: The Massachusetts Witchcraft Trials* (Baltimore: Johns Hopkins P, 1968) 53.

Rossiter's medical narrative cannot but recast a multiply coded human body. Remaining within the Puritan cosmology of meaning, where it functions as a site of contestation between cosmic forces, Kelly's corpse is simultaneously drawn into a discourse and into a practice that consider flesh in increasingly materialistic and rational terms. Rossiter's text strives to integrate these conflicting systems of meaning-endowment by employing science as a tool for proving something that already is religiously and culturally predetermined. In short, medical discourse is used to validate certain preconceptions about changes in the human body. Because of its performativity, which negates the professed intent of the text to prove the presence of witchcraft through medicine, Rossiter's report fails to conclusively establish an interpretative hierarchy of either theology or science. Instead, by mimicking anatomical procedures and medical discourse, the examination and its report open the human body to objectification and de-individualization in a way that actually counters Puritan dogmas of corporeal sacredness, depravity, and idiosyncrasy.[77]

## Representing Witches: Female Healers

The susceptibility of healing women to charges of familiarity with the devil marked another prominent feature of the intersections between medicine and witchcraft in colonial New England. Midwives could, as discussed above, carve out spaces of social and cultural influence by acquiring recognition and respect in New England communities. At times, however, their services also rendered them and other healing women more vulnerable to slander and malpractice lawsuits as well as to accusations of witchcraft than other colonists, as we have seen in the cases of Anne Hutchinson, Jane Hawkins, and Mary Dyer. Among the many healing women who were cited before a New England court to defend themselves against accusations of witchcraft were Anna

---

[77] Robert Blair St. George, *Conversing by Signs: Poetics of Implication in Colonial New England Culture* (U of North Carolina P, 1998) 116-119, 198-202; Barbara Duden, *The Woman Beneath the Skin: A Doctor's Patients in Eighteenth-Century Germany*, trans. Thomas Dunlap (Cambridge, MA: Harvard UP, 1991) 10.

Edmunds, Katherine Harrison, and Elizabeth Morse. One of the witnesses in Morse's case was Elizabeth Titcomb, who deposed that after the accused had touched her friend, Susanna Tappan, she

> continued ill, and an itching and pricking rose upon her body. Which afterwards came to such a dry scurse, that she could scrape it off as it were scales from an alewife, and that side which she was touched in was most out of frame, and she is smitten in the lower parts of her body after the same manner that she had testified against the said Morse what she heard her speak: and from that time she hath continued very ill, but little from her bed, and hath not been able to go abroad ever since to the public meeting.[78]

Such testimony exemplifies how female healing abilities were seen as an important component in configuring witchcraft as a socio-cultural transgression. Since illness was broadly conceived of as sanctioned by God as well as by Satan, some healers were suspected of employing black magic and other occult practices that relied on invoking the devil and his minions. The ubiquity of illness in New England, the demands it created for medical care providers, the lack of affordable and efficacious medical provisions, as well as the uncertainty about one's future on earth and after death, all contributed to a popular interest in the skills of "cunning folk," who practiced ancient folk techniques for the purpose of divination and healing and from whose ranks some of the accused women came.[79]

---

[78] Hall, *Witch-Hunting* 247-248. For Katherine Harrison's case, which stood at the center of the Connecticut witch craze of 1662-1665, see Carolyn Langdon, "A Complaint against Katherine Harrison, 1669," *Bulletin of the Connecticut Historical Society* 34 (1969): 18-25; Hale 21-24.

[79] It remains impossible to reasonably estimate how many New England women (and men) actually employed magic in their healing efforts. Richard Weisman suggests that "[a]t least one third of the pre-Salem suspects either claimed or actually practiced magical skills" (86). These skills, i.e., fortune-telling and healing, built on the employment of charms, amulets, spells, divination and/or mysterious concoctions and potions, and were highly sought-after services in seventeenth-century New England. Cf. Watson, *Angelical Conjunction* 29-31; Richard Godbeer, *The Devil's Dominion: Magic and Religion in Early New*

Despite the widespread, and often commonsensical, co-presence of magic and religion, particularly in isolated regions of New England, occult healing rituals at times aroused the suspicion of pious settlers who claimed to recognize behavioral and bodily signs as satanic. For a number of devout colonists who rejected all forms of magic, the mere audacity to predict if and when someone would fall ill and/or recover was proof enough that witchcraft was at hand. Time and again, as extant New England court records illustrate, the culturally defined borders between healing as a helpful and a hurtful ability—medicine as *beneficium* or *maleficium*—proved highly permeable. As one result, while most female healers, including midwives, were able to practice without persecution, even if their methods included occult elements, some were singled out for "entertaining Satan," especially if their practices caused a sudden and inexplicable illness.[80]

The rationale for the selective accusation of women healers is as difficult to extract from the historical records as the explanation of witchcraft as a socio-cultural phenomenon. One reason for the disproportionate number of witchcraft accusations among female healers is that women, in general, and women healers, in particular, functioned as planes of projection of evil in the world. When the devil was perceived as launching yet another attack on the godly kingdom erected by New England Puritans, women were likely subjects and scapegoats, especially when natural explanations for what might have been symptoms of an illness were lacking. A particular glimpse into colonial motivations for singling out female medical practitioners is provided in the case of Margaret Jones, one of the first New England women sentenced to death for having practiced witchcraft. In June of 1648, the line of prosecution followed by the Boston magistrates rested on the kind of evidence that would later be used in a number of witch trials. Jones was found guilty of using a "malignant touch" that caused

*England* (Cambridge: Cambridge UP, 1992) 41. For magical healing practices in post-Reformation England, see Keith Thomas, *Religion and the Decline of Magic: Studies in Popular Beliefs in Sixteenth and Seventeenth-Century England* (1971; New York: Penguin, 1982) 177-211.

[80] John Demos, *Entertaining Satan: Witchcraft and the Culture of Early New England* (New York: Oxford UP, 1982) 81-84.

"deafness, or vomiting or other violent pains or sickness," her herbal remedies had "extraordinary, violent effects," and the symptoms of her patients (and especially those who refused to take her medicaments) were "beyond the apprehension of all physicians and surgeons."[81] The court's argument both reflected and shaped cultural beliefs according to which deviations from ordinary medical practice were attributed to witchcraft. Such deviations were, however, difficult to define and co-existed within a fluent cultural spectrum of healing that included acceptable and inacceptable medical practices.

In a similar vein, the trial of Rachel Fuller of Hampton, New Hampshire, who was charged with witchcraft in 1680, relied primarily on the deposition of Mary and Sarah Godfrey, who claimed that the accused had visited their house to treat a sick child. As she entered, her face smeared with molasses, she "spat in the fire. Then she, having herbs in her hands, stood and rubbed them in her hand and strewed them about the hearth by the fire." She then left the house, telling Goodwife Godfrey that her child would be well soon. The witnesses continued that they "saw Rachel Fuller standing with her face towards the house, and beat herself with her arms, as men do in winter to heat their hands, and this she did three times; and stooping down and gathering something off the ground in interim between the beating of herself, and then she went home."[82] Even for colonists unfamiliar with medicine's state of the art, such a ritual would have suspiciously looked like pagan folk healing. The description of her curing ceremony includes references that one

---

[81] The Jones case was exemplary of other witchcraft indictments because the alleged occult medical practices were supplemented by fortune-telling, previous social marginalization of the accused, and the presence of a "witch's teat." John Winthrop, *Winthrop's Journal: "History of New England," 1630-1649*, vol. 2, ed. James Kendall Hosmer (New York: Scribner's Sons, 1908) 344-345. Cf. William F. Poole, "Witchcraft at Boston," *The Memorial History of Boston, including Suffolk County Massachusetts, 1630-1880*, vol. II, ed. Justin Winsor (Boston: Osgood, 1881) 133-136. The notion that human touch could produce either healing or illness was common during the seventeenth century. For instance, scrofula, a skin disease also known as "King's Evil," was believed to be cured by the touch of the monarch.

[82] Hall, *Witch-Hunting* 193.

might also read as cross-cultural: painting her face dark brown, using herbs in a ritual rather than a direct application, and beating her body could either stem from Algonquian powwow rituals or from English folk healing (or a combination of both). Either one constituted a deviance from officially acceptable healing methods in colonial New England. Similar to other women, "Rachel Fuller ended up an accused witch not just because she was a healer, but for a combination of factors: her magical practices overstepped the bounds of the acceptable; she already had a reputation as a witch; and perhaps most important, her healing failed spectacularly."[83] In the end, the Hampton court did not find the evidence against Fuller sufficient for a death warrant, which indicates that healing practices alone, even if they were suspicious and failed, were not enough to justify a conviction.

Another possible explanation for the disproportionate number of accusations of female healers lies in their competition with male physicians. Due to the illiteracy of most female medical practitioners, as well as to their social relegation to public silence, there exist no written account that outlines and develops intellectual positions or practical approaches to medicine—only a few court records offer glimpses into the professional disputes between the two groups of medical practitioners. Ann Burt of Lynn, Massachusetts, for instance, had arrived in New England in 1635 and epitomized the typical female lay healer who practiced medicine with some success and at times included quasi-magical techniques into her curative repertoire. Accused by suspicious neighbors and disappointed patients, Burt was officially charged for practicing witchcraft in November 1669. Among the witnesses testifying against her was Phillip Reade, a physician who traveled between colonial outposts in northeastern Massachusetts to offer his medical and apothecary services. During his itinerancies he often met local healing women and, as Tannenbaum asserts, "[g]iven Reade's abrasive personality and fragile ego, it is plausible that he did in fact see women like Burt as dangerous competitors, and seized the opportunity to

---

[83] Tannenbaum, *Healer's Calling* 44. Cf. Samuel G. Drake, *Annals of Witchcraft in New England* (Boston: Woodward, 1869) 150-156.

eliminate them."[84] If this character assessment is accurate, then Ann Burt's witchcraft trial probably indeed was a welcome opportunity for Reade to rid himself of a competitor for patients and, hence, income. His testimony after having investigated Sara Townsend, one of Burt's accusers, demonstrates yet another link between medicine and witchcraft in colonial New England:

> the said Sara Townsend being in a more sadder condition he [i.e., Reade] had no opportunity to examine her condition but did plainly perceive there was no natural cause for such unnatural fits. But being sent for the fourth time and finding her in a meet capacity to give information of her aggrievance cause of her former fits she told me the above said Burt had afflicted her and told her if ever she did relate it to anyone she would afflict her worse [.][85]

This deposition is especially noteworthy because the physician arrives at a medical diagnosis without a prior examination. The quickly passed medical judgment suggests that Reade was convinced that his authority as an educated male physician carried enough weight to sway a New England court without having to provide substantial evidence. From the point of view of the circuit physician, his mere statement that "there was no natural cause," followed by the naming of Burt in the following sentence, actually *makes* witchcraft, turning the accused into a witch during the moment of utterance.

---

[84] Tannenbaum, *Healer's Calling* 131. This was not the only time Reade accused a New England woman of witchcraft. In September 1680 he filed a complaint and presented evidence to the County Court of Salem that supposedly proved Margaret Giffords' familiarity with the devil. Notable here is the persistence with which Reade returned to the Ipswich Court, ready to present evidence against the accused. For Reade's medical practice and character, see Andrew V. Rapoza, "The Trials of Phillip Reade, Seventeenth-Century Itinerant Physician," *Medicine and Healing: Annual Proceedings of the Dublin Seminar for New England Folklife* (Boston: Boston UP, 1992) 82-94. See also, Carol F. Karlsen, *The Devil in the Shape of a Woman: Witchcraft in Colonial New England* (New York: Vintage, 1987) 141-144.

[85] Hall, *Witch-Hunting* 186. Cf. William E. Woodward, ed., *Records of Salem Witchcraft*, vol. II (Roxbury, 1864) 263.

As the preceding observations have illustrated, witchcraft and medicine were closely intertwined in the cultural scripts that English colonists imported to the "New World." This intertwinement had far-reaching and often negative consequences for women who sought to apply their healing knowledge for the benefit of their communities. Aside from their practical, everyday consequences, both witchcraft and its persecution based on medically sanctioned evidence must also be considered in more abstract terms: as indicators of socio-cultural pathologies inherent in, and produced by, Puritan theology and ideology.

## The Illness of Witchcraft

Colonial officials and contemporary scholars studying witch-hunting in New England have long attempted to link witchcraft phenomena to medical conditions. One remaining mystery in American historiography is the exact cause of the physical symptoms that a number of New England girls were displaying in the second half of the seventeenth century and that their contemporaries interpreted as instances of witchcraft. Linnda Caporael, for instance, has claimed that the girls suffered from ergotism, or ergot poisoning. According to this assumption, a poison stemming from fungi-infected rye and other cereals caused the girls' behavior and produced delusive thoughts, speeches, and actions. In their response, Nicholas Spanos and Jack Gottlieb refute that ergotism matches the symptoms described in the witchcraft literature and argue instead that the girls "were enacting the roles that would sustain their definition of themselves as bewitched and that would lead to the conviction of the accused." In contrast, Laurie Carlson postulates that epidemic encephalitis lethargica (or sleeping sickness) caused the symptoms that led to the Salem witch hysteria in 1692.[86] These and other attempts to interpret deviant behavior exemplify

---

[86] Linnda R. Caporeal, "Ergotism: The Satan Loosed in Salem?," *Science* 192 (2 April 1976): 21-26; Nicholas P. Spanos and Jack Gottlieb, "Ergotism and the Salem Village Witch Trials," *Science* 194 (24 December 1976): 1391; Laurie Win Carlson, *A Fever in Salem: A New Interpretation of the New England Witch Trials* (Chicago: Dee, 1999). Caporeal and Carlson's studies detract responsibility for the witch hysteria away from the girls by citing medical

an approach that seeks to diagnose illness symptoms retroactively by studying *written* material.

New England records rarely reveal hints at natural causes behind phenomena associated with witchcraft. Some medical experts, for example, Dr. Augur suggested that it "had binne Histericall, or an Inlett into an Epilepsie," and with this diagnosis he anticipated later (and still valid) theories of the psychopathology of social and cultural deviance.[87] Other New England physicians, such as those investigating Mary Glover in Boston and pronouncing her *compos mentis*, recognized that what seemed to be signs of witchcraft could also have been symptoms of "madness." Contrary to the great confinement in Europe, when, beginning in mid-seventeenth century, the insane were imprisoned along with the poor and other social delinquents, community treatment of people with mental illness was common in the colonies; physicians were rarely consulted nor was there a specific institution where the mentally ill could be treated or detained.[88] Although New England colonists knew to distinguish "madness" from other afflictions, they continued European conceptual linkages of madness with poverty, idleness, and transgression. John Winthrop, for instance, configured gender deviance in terms of "madness" when he remarked how the wife of Connecticut governor Edward Hopkins had devoted "herself wholly to reading and writing, and had written many books." This transgression of a woman's calling as domestic keeper had, for Winthrop, resulted in a "sad

influences that make them appear much less conniving and manipulative than in Spanos and Gottlieb's account.

[87] "Nicholas Augur to John Winthrop, Jr., 17 June 1653," *Winthrop Papers* VI, 301.

[88] As Lawrence Goodheart explains, "[b]oundaries between supernatural and secular explanations in describing those who were different were not distinct." Lawrence B. Goodheart, "The Distinction between Witchcraft and Madness in Colonial Connecticut," *History of Psychiatry* 13.52 (2002): 434. Larry Eldridge adds that Puritanism "encouraged a relatively kind and incorporating attitude toward the mentally disturbed." Larry Eldridge, "'Crazy Brained': Mental Illness in Colonial America," *Bulletin of the History of Medicine* 70.3 (1996): 385.

infirmity, the loss of her understanding and reason."[89] Aside from expressing the undeniable misogyny of early American culture, such a couching of a behavioral error in terms of "madness" was rather commonplace in New England, as a number of short and passing references in letters, reports, treatises, pamphlets, and other textual productions indicate.

Throughout the Salem witchcraft crisis, as well as in its aftermath, two of the most vocal guides in deciphering the providential significance of the events were Increase and Cotton Mather. In giving cultural orientation through their sermons and essays, the two offered passing nods at the lack of scientificity among physicians, which often led to false diagnoses of bodily symptoms as witchcraft. While the elder Mather warned about the inadequacy of the New England medical establishment, writing in 1684 that, "sometimes the Devil hath laughed at the physicians, who have thought by medicinal applications to dispossess him," his son anticipates explanations that stress ill-guided human minds as the source for the bewitchment by demon spirits: "And it has been too Common a Thing, for People under the Invasion of this Malady [epilates; M.P.], to imagine a *Witchcraft* in the Case; And anon perhaps the Folly proceeds unto the Accusation of a poor, mean, ill-loved old Woman in the Neighborhood. *Away, Away*, with such Idle Fancies."[90]

While early New England certainly had its share of the mentally ill, little is known about the specificities of their condition. Some court records suggest that insanity may have been the reason for behavior that resembled symptoms of witchcraft. For instance, Ann Burt is said to have commanded one of her patients to believe "in her god," so she could "cure her body and soul: but if she told of it she should be as a distracted body as long as she lived: and further that her husband did not

[89] Winthrop, *History*, vol. I, 216.

[90] Increase Mather, *An Essay For the Recording of Illustrious Providences* (1684; Early American Imprints, Series 1, no. 372) 20-21; Cotton Mather, *The Angel of Bethesda*, ed. Gordon W. Jones (Barre: American Antiquarian Society and Barre, 1972) 153 (emphasis original). Cotton Mather is referring to nightmares (*epialtes*), which at the time were considered as being caused by demons or witchcraft.

believe in her god and should not be cured and that her maid did believe in her god and was cured[.]"[91] This passage, with its mysterious and repeated reference to *her* god in implied distinction to *their* God, provides a useful glimpse into how colonists associated certain religious behavior with deranged thought, speech, and action. This was hardly a novel or isolated occurrence. In early modern England, "madness" was defined as a mixture of mania and melancholia, resulting either from a humoral imbalance, a divine or satanic intervention, or both known and hidden natural causes.[92] Often brought in close proximity with "madness," excessive spiritual and, at times, religious excitement and enthusiasm had long been defined "as a diabolical contagion, spread by witches, demoniacs and heretics" and was viewed with suspicion and classified as a disease by every Christian denomination.[93] Critics ranging from English Puritan-hunter Archbishop William Laud to Sigmund Freud have pointed out that Puritans' overabundant religious zeal and fanatic culture of introspection placed immense mental strain on the believer and thus led to (or constituted) a form of insanity. Moreover, scholars have argued that Puritans' incapacity to distinguish between natural and supernatural influences in their lives stemmed from a delusion that was not caused by Satan but rather by a psychopathological state that their religious views inevitably induced.[94] As part of the increasing medicalization of "madness" after the eighteenth century, the perception of certain occurrences as signs of witchcraft was often explained as a reality distortion in the minds of

[91] Hall, *Witch-Hunting* 188.

[92] John Sena traces the early modern English conviction that the putrification of the melancholic humor, coupled with certain religious opinions and practices, negatively affected the human brain and could be harmful to a person's mental ability. According to some anti-Puritan observers in Elizabethan England, "[m]elancholic vapors [...] were responsible for generating delusions and apparitions so powerful that their possessors felt they came from heaven." John F. Sena "Melancholic Madness and the Puritans," *The Harvard Theological Review* 66. 3 (1973): 300.

[93] Roy Porter, "Mental Illness," *The Cambridge Illustrated History of Medicine*, ed. Roy Porter (Cambridge: Cambridge UP, 1996) 278-303; 282.

[94] Roy Porter, *Flesh in the Age of Reason* (New York: Norton, 2003) 306.

individuals and/or of the community of religious devotees as a whole. It was claimed that this distortion resulted from conversion neurosis, a psychological disorder caused by a distressing anxiety about one's salvation. Michael MacDonald explains that,

> psychiatrists argue [...] that conversion neurosis characteristically occurs among adolescents, particularly adolescent girls, and that it is a kind of defence that originates in repression. They distinguish between a 'primary gain' that the patient achieves by repressing disturbing sexual urges, and a 'secondary gain' that she enjoys by virtue of her illness and the response of others to it.[95]

In historical hindsight, both the person accused of witchcraft and the accuser have been reconfigured as deluded and deranged and, thus, as medical cases. Similar to the view engrained in Renaissance culture that witchcraft spread among persons who associated with Satan, the rationalizing of witchcraft in the wake of the Enlightenment maintained that it, now conceived as a mental disorder, was contagious because its host was a specific religious conviction. Such a view undergirded the late nineteenth-century interpretation of the Salem witchcraft hysteria by George M. Beard, who explores the girls' affliction as symptoms of insanity.[96] A century after Beard, Michel Foucault unfolds a larger genealogy of cultural signification processes in Europe that established mental and behavioral normalcy by concomitantly defining its other, madness, in medical terms. As part of these larger shifts in the definition of mental infirmities, which took place in the course of the seventeenth century, witchcraft and "[t]he old rituals of magic, profanation and blasphemy [...] passed from a domain filled with their effective power to the domain of unreason, a place of mere illusion, where they became guilt-laden markers of insanity."[97] Recent psychoanalytic studies of the

[95] Michael MacDonald, Introduction, *Witchcraft and Hysteria in Elizabethan London: Edward Jorden and the Mary Glover Case*, ed. Michael MacDonald (London: Routledge, 1991) xxxiii.

[96] George M. Beard, *The Psychology of the Salem Witchcraft Excitement of 1692* (New York: Putnam, 1882).

[97] Michel Foucault, *History of Madness*, ed. Jean Khalfa, trans. Jonathan Murphy and Jean Khalfa (1972; London: Routledge, 2006) 96.

events at Salem, which take their cue from witchcraft's "passage to pathology" (Foucault) during the early modern period, suggest that the symptoms were caused by a combination of conversion neurosis, projection, psychosomatic disorders, and communal post-traumatic stress; mental conditions that in some cases (e.g., paranoid hysteria) are considered as being as communicable as somatic diseases.[98]

The continuation of psychopathologizing social and cultural deviance in New England highlights the cultural frames that have surrounded definitions of "madness" and witchcraft and, similarly, of religion and medicine. Instead of static entities, these frames have been comprised of highly mobile and flexible discursive practices that usually serve the powers that be. When, for example, in the wake of the scientific revolution, the frames shifted to include witchcraft and witch-hunting as the product of mental disorders, religious enthusiasm was attacked for obstructing the rise of science through recurring lapses of reason. After assigning all forms of magic and the occult (including alchemy and witchcraft) to *un*reason, the eighteenth-century transatlantic world witnessed a lasting redefinition of social relations, epistemic hierarchies, cultural formations, and of nothing less than humanity's place in the cosmos through the establishment of scientific principles and practices.

A somewhat different medical linkage between illness and witchcraft has been suggested by John Demos, who notes that epidemic diseases (along with other harmful events, such as fires, floods, droughts, crop failures or sea wrecks) often preceded witchcraft accusations and trials by one or two years. Indeed, it seems tempting to connect the communal

---

[98] Foucault, *Madness* 96; Mary Beth Norton, *In the Devil's Snare: The Salem Witchcraft Crisis of 1692* (New York: Knopf, 2002) 3-13; 295-308, outlines the possible connections between mental illness and witchcraft. Hansen's diagnosis interprets the court records as indications of clinical hysteria that stemmed from a deeply engrained cultural belief in the reality of witchcraft. Chadwick Hansen, *Witchcraft at Salem* (New York: George Brazillier, 1969). John Demos (*Entertaining Satan* 193, 209-210, 276) suggests that psychological conditions (e.g., anxiety, repressed emotions, identity problems, and role conflicts) were responsible for the girls' physical symptoms. Cf. Edward Bever, "Witchcraft Fears and Psychosocial Factors in Disease," *The Journal of Interdisciplinary History* 30.4 (2000): 573-590.

distress caused by witchcraft to epidemics. For instance, the New England-wide smallpox epidemic of 1644-1646 and the Boston yellow fever outbreak in 1691 preceded significant outbreaks of witch-hunting. In both instances, the clergy interpreted the events as signs of God's wrath and imminent withdrawal of His favor from the New England saints. According to Demos' argument, epidemics and other portents, instead of granting assurance, rather imbued in colonists a sense of panic about God's seemingly imminent withdrawal of favor from the elect. This panic then led to a widespread search-and-destroy mission of all that was conceived as evil in the world, especially when it seemed as strikingly evident and as seemingly easy to eradicate as in the witchcraft cases. Although there existed a discernible regularity in the intersection of epidemics and witch-hunts, it remains impossible to draw a definite chain of causation since not all epidemics were followed by outbreaks of witchcraft; nor were all cases of witchcraft preceded by epidemics.[99]

A more sustainable connection between medicine and witchcraft takes recourse to the realm of metaphor. Demos' claim that, for many New England communities, "a suspected witch worked both to deflect hostility from other targets and to concentrate blame, like a boil on the body that pulls in toxic fluids. To bring the suspect eventually to trial was, in effect, to lance the boil and release its toxicity," positions witchcraft as a process of cleansing the community of its sinful parts.[100] Similar to excommunicating members whose thoughts and/or actions were considered as deviant from religious orthodoxy (as, for instance, in the case of Anne Hutchinson), witchcraft prosecutions constituted a form of social surgery, an operation during which a malignant part of the body politic was removed so that the larger entity could achieve healing.[101] Continuing the medical metaphorization of abnormal behavior, one might claim that witchcraft constituted a social malady that needed to be purged before a new epistemological paradigm, and as a result a new cultural and political order could be established. During

---

[99] John Demos, *The Enemy Within: 2,000 Years of Witch-hunting in the Western World* (New York: Viking, 2008) 125-126; Demos, *Entertaining Satan* 370.

[100] Demos, *The Enemy Within* 48.

[101] Martha L. Finch, *Dissenting Bodies: Corporealities in Early New England* (New York: Columbia UP, 2010) 167.

this cathartic process, which emerged fully in the late seventeenth century with the writings of John Locke, specifically, and continued with increasing force during the eighteenth century, the field of medicine underwent a lasting shift from accomplice to critic of witchcraft and witch-hunting. In most colonial New England cases, theological and medical experts worked collaboratively in evaluating certain illness signs as stemming either from demonic possession, disease, or fraud. The role of the physicians in failing to detect witchcraft as a pathological condition is in part indicative of a general lack of confidence in the healing and diagnostic abilities at the time. The emancipation of the trade from the interpretative power of the clergy had not yet begun by the time New England witch-hunting reached its peak and abrupt end in 1692. With the growing advances and dissemination of medical knowledge in Europe, colonial physicians would soon gain more confidence in their profession and challenged the authority of the church concerning matters of the human body. As became evident during the Boston smallpox inoculation debate of 1721-1722 (see chapter six), the redefinition of witchcraft as a sign of supernatural intervention into a medical condition was driven by, and signaled, a larger societal transformation toward secularization, the dawning Enlightenment, and toward a potentially explicable and manageable universe.

* * *

The medical narratives surveyed for this chapter confirm Laurel Thatcher Ulrich's observation of "the centrality of gender to struggles over social order in the first decades of Puritan settlement."[102] The textualization of seventeenth-century healing practices by women, whether in personal writings, official reports or court records, emphasizes the relegation of women to the margins of the social. The textualizations also highlight female attempts to carve out spaces of enunciation and empowerment. Whether Elizabeth Davenport's medical voice expressed in her husband's letter, the elder John Winthrop's descriptions of Anne Hutchinson's birth room gatherings *cum* religio-

---

[102] Ulrich, "City of Women" 20.

political instructions, or the written attempts of objectifying female social deviance in records of witch-hunting: the rhetoric of medicine functioned as a means of containing but also, albeit to a lesser degree, of producing female agency. Female illness narratives furthermore shed light on the interfaces between religion and science as well as between culture and politics in colonial New England. Whether medical letters, reports on deformed childbirth, or descriptions of alleged witch-doctresses, textualized medical conditions or practices constituted political events that were endowed with meaning by the cultural environment in which they occurred.

In such an environment, healing proved a double-edge sword (or, rather, scalpel) for many women. On the one hand, medical practice provided opportunities to gain and exert cultural authority that was denied to most other colonial women; on the other hand, the elevated social position that came with (successful) healing was reserved for men and hence created gender ambiguities that contributed to the particular vulnerability of healing women to legal retributions. Whereas John Winthrop Jr. and other members of the elite could engage in occultism and mysticism in a relatively safe physical and cultural environment, most laymen and especially laywomen rumored to engage in popular versions of the occult had to fear persecution by neighbors and officials. The examples of Elizabeth Davenport, Anne Hutchinson, Rachel Fuller, and other medical women illustrate, therefore, the presence of healers on both sides of a magico-religious spectrum in colonial New England. They were overrepresented among the faithful and the "cunning folk" and thus, in seventeenth-century parlance, were seen as handmaids of the Lord *and* the devil. This ostensible binary created more ambiguities than civil and religious leaders asked for because the possibility of interpreting female medical practices as either beneficial or harmful produced uncertainties that resonated in and with a larger cultural field circumscribed by Puritanism, the emerging sciences, and the remnants of occult and folk traditions.

Female illness narratives underline furthermore how the cultural continuum between acceptable and inacceptable healing practices in "an era when science and religion co-mingled in supernatural awe," tended to polarize around theological conventions, especially during moments of crisis in colonial New England society.[103] Antinomianism and witchcraft were more than expressions of a community in peril; they marked a crisis of the relationship between official religion, medical practice, and popular culture in New England. At the same time, and even more important for the purpose of this study, both culturally constructed deviations from orthodoxy entailed crises of representation, moments in which the medicalization of deviance, designed to wield elite political power and exert cultural influence, turned out to be self-defeating rather than self-serving. Such moments of crisis in representing New England medicine occur, for example, in ventriloquial writings, in inconclusive metaphoricity, and in slips in argumentation— instances when sickness exceeds textual representation. The inescapable incompatibility of illness and modes of representation is poignantly evoked in Joshua Moody's report to Increase Mather about the alleged bewitchment of four young girls in Boston. He writes: "then they roar out, Oh my head, oh my neck and from one part to another *the pain runs almost as fast as I write it*."[104] What links this medical report to Elizabeth Davenport's illness narratives, and thus highlights a central argument developed in this chapter, is the realization that the experience of pain and suffering and its textual representation can not be fully synchronized.

---

[103] Goodheart 437.

[104] Hall, *Witch-Hunting* 266 (emphasis added).

# 4. Conversion and the Rhetoric of Disease

The previous chapter has revealed the ambiguous role of medicine during moments of crisis in colonial New England, especially during the Antinomian controversy and the Salem witchcraft trials. Questions of health and illness also shaped colonists' *personal* crises that were induced by existential concerns about their present condition and the future estates of their soul. In light of what Max Weber called "the unprecedented inner loneliness of the single individual" in Puritan America—produced by the doctrines of predestination, human depravity, and helplessness, and amplified by life in an environment perceived as hostile, steeped in sin, and far removed from the centers of "civilization"—the question whether someone would be saved after death reigned prominently in virtually every pious colonist's thoughts and actions.[1] The primary spiritual goal of Puritans on both sides of the Atlantic was the conversion from a life of sin to an inward experience of God's saving grace (justification) and its outward manifestation in behavior and speech (sanctification). Conversion, seen as a means of preparing for salvation, could only come about through intense and continual self-examination. Constituting the central spiritual experience for English Protestants, the conversion of the heart through knowledge of the divine and the self was considered not necessarily as a single event of divine intervention but as a process of personal change and growth over time that was brought about by God's gradual entrance and intervention in the life of the sinner. Conversion, in other words, marked an intricate part of a life-long spiritual pilgrimage during which a person, guided by providence and Scripture, discovered sin, repented, doubted, prayed, combated temptations, attended sermons, and

---

[1] Max Weber, *The Protestant Ethic and the Spirit of Capitalism*, trans. Talcott Parsons (1920; New York: Scribner's Sons, 1958) 104.

conversed with ministers and fellow believers in preparation for eternal bliss.[2]

Since the full scope of God's will and intentions was considered inscrutable, knowledge about a person's membership among the elect could never be conclusively determined. Puritan divines held, however, that a believer could receive glimpses into the probable state of his/her soul after death by recognizing and displaying a specific "morphology of conversion."[3] According to this morphology, a sinner's successful conversion could be recognized by a series of signs and stages: conviction in sin, fear of God's judgment, desire for redemption, faith-building through prayer and Bible study, realization of justification, manifestation of piety and devotion in thought and action, and vigilance through continual introspection. Although Puritan theologians devised different sequential stages of conversion, they concurred in their basic outline of a teleological process, one that could potentially be identified and rationalized by individual believers and by the outside world as a successful conversion.[4]

For Puritans living in the Atlantic world, the intense and prolonged self-analysis in preparation for salvation needed to be verbalized and

---

[2] The prospects of preparation were, as seen in the previous chapter, at the center of numerous theological debates in Old and New England. For a central study on conversion and preparation in the American colonies, see Norman Pettit, *The Heart Prepared: Grace and Conversion in Puritan Spirit Life* (New Haven: Yale UP, 1966).

[3] Edmund S. Morgan, *Visible Saints: The History of a Puritan Idea* (New York: NYUP, 1963) 66.

[4] The ideal of Puritan conversion is outlined in William Perkins, *A Treatise Tending unto a Declaration, Whether a Man Be in the Estate of Damnation, or in the Estate of Grace* (London: John Porter, 1597) 36-45 and in William Perkins, *The Workes of that Famous and Worthy Minister of Christ in the Universitie of Cambridge, M. William Perkins. The Second Volume* (1631; Early English Books Online, 19653) 13. For a study of intellectual and theological currents underlying the theory of conversion in New England, epitomized especially by Thomas Hooker and Thomas Shepard, see David L. Parker, "Petrus Ramus and the Puritans: The 'Logic' of Preparationist Conversion Doctrine," *Early American Literature* 8.2 (1973): 140-162.

placed in a narrative sequence.[5] While some colonists kept their thoughts and observations private, many sought verification of their conversion experiences by going public, both in speech and in writing. New England congregational churches required candidates to deliver a narrative of conversion before they granted full membership. Due to the ministers who recorded them, these conversion narratives provide unique opportunities for transhistorical eavesdropping. As the first section of this chapter outlines, lay conversion narratives can help understand the personal developments of common colonists and offer rare insights into the spiritual and material concerns and transformations of ordinary men and women. Because the procedure was also applied to the so-called Praying Indians, Native American conversion narratives constitute proto-ethnographic sources that, on the surface, display indigenous attitudes toward Protestantism and illustrate how they sought ways of coping with the trauma brought about by the land-clearing epidemics of the first decades of the seventeenth century.

In most of the texts surveyed in this chapter, physical ailments or infirmities illustrate how conversion crossed the boundaries between mind, body, and semantics. In virtually all personal narratives, illness played an important role in the recognition of sin and in the decision to turn to God after recovery. In some cases, illness served as a means of entering into a covenant with God and with one's community; in others, illness revealed contradictions in the confessor's spiritual estate; in still others, medical experiences and/or discourses assumed a decisively public function. Within this array of spiritual relations, sickness was often depicted as a transformative and preparatory event in the lives of New Englanders, regardless of whether the narrator was identified as English or Indian. While there existed cross-cultural commonalities in the depiction of illness in textual space, a comparison between English and Native conversion relations brings to light significant differences in

---

[5] Geoffrey Harpham divides the conversion process into two parts: a first conversion marked by "an epistemological certainty that heralds a sense of true self-knowledge," and a second conversion that "confirms or actualizes this certainty in a narrative of the self." Geoffrey Galt Harpham, "Conversion and the Language of Autobiography," *Studies in Autobiography*, ed. James Olney (New York: Oxford UP, 1988) 42.

the cultural renderings of medical issues and their narrative representations.

Illness as Covenant: Lay Conversion Narratives

In order to attain full membership in a New England congregational church, which meant eligibility to participate in the Lord's Supper and entailed political influence (only full members could hold office), candidates were asked to deliver an oral report of their conversion experiences. The central purpose of such a public declaration of faith in, and knowledge of, Christ was to ensure the spiritual purity and unity of New England settlements. Those merely feigning conversion were perceived as sources of intellectual and theological subversion that needed to be barred from the church body through the careful examination of the applicant's autobiographical narrative. Colonial churches demanded that potential members organize the narration of their previous spiritual journey around three intimately connected aspects: the confession of sins, the profession of faith, and the declaration about the work of divine grace in the convert's life.[6] To begin the admission procedure, applicants had to submit a report of their spiritual developments, including acts of repentance and familiarity with church doctrines, to the scrutiny of the local minister and the elders. After the interview, the candidate was asked to repeat his/her conversion narrative before the assembled congregation, often followed by a question-and-answer session that could address any uncertain aspect of the conversion narrative. When all possible objections were defused, the

[6] For New England guidelines for conversion (narratives), see Richard Mather, *Church-Government and Church-Covenant Discussed* (1643; Early English Books Online, M1269) 23-24; John Cotton, *The Way of the Churches of Christ in New-England* (1645; Early English Books Online, C6471) 54-55. Francis Higginson, pastor at Salem, published a short pamphlet outlining the main tenets of conversion and church membership in *A Direction for a Publick Profession in the Church Assembly* (1629; Early American Imprints, Series I, no. 100).

candidate would receive the minister's right hand of fellowship as a sign of his/her admission into the congregation.[7]

For many confessors, sharing their innermost spiritual travail, sins, and despair with their neighbors was a difficult and highly emotional undertaking. For some it was even traumatic, depending on the reaction of the ministers and the congregation. Therefore a public conversion narrative constituted a pivotal event and text in the life of many lay colonists. As Kenneth Minkema explains, "[t]he pressure of appearing before an assembly was undoubtedly great, because the conversion relation was more than likely the only formal speech a layman made in his whole life."[8] The confessor was on public display and his or her reputation and spiritual as well as worldly future depended on peer acceptance of the narrative. Yet, the public relation of the conversion experience did not only have consequences for those who gave it. The narration of the self in conversion also allowed the people in the pews to assess their own spiritual estates, and it prescribed patterns and symbols

---

[7] Morgan estimates that the practice of public conversion narratives began in 1634 (66, 74), although it seems more likely that Thomas Shepard introduced it in 1638. Michael G. Ditmore, "Preparation and Confession: Reconsidering Edmund S. Morgan's *Visible Saints*," *New England Quarterly* 67.2 (1994): 298-319. The Cambridge Platform, adopted in 1648, established a series of principles for the Congregational churches of New England, among them the importance of public profession of faith of every prospective member. For a vivid and contemporary summary of a typical New England church admission procedure, see John Fiske, *The Notebook of the Reverend John Fiske, 1644-1675*, ed. Robert G. Pope, *Collections of the Colonial Society of Massachusetts* 47 (Boston: The Society, 1974) 173-174. See also Jim Egan, *Authorizing Experience: Refigurations of the Body Politic in Seventeenth-Century New England Writing* (Princeton: Princeton UP, 1999) 80; D. Bruce Hindmarsh, *The Evangelical Conversion Narrative: Spiritual Autobiography in Early Modern England* (New York: Oxford UP, 2005) 48-49; Daniel B. Shea, Jr., *Spiritual Autobiography in Early America* (Princeton: Princeton UP, 1968) 91.

[8] Kenneth P. Minkema, ed., "The East Windsor Conversion Narratives, 1700-1752," *The Connecticut Historical Society Bulletin* 51 (1986): 12. Some women who applied for full communion failed to withstand the pressure of having to share their conversion experience and, hence, ministers would read aloud a transcript of the relation previously given before the church elders.

of conversion that were to be emulated by other (prospective) church members. By means of private and public expressions of saving faith, conversion narratives hence served to (re)affirm the covenant between the individual and God as well as between the congregation and its minister, which, in turn, constituted New England communities as religious and civil entities. In short, conversion was performed as a ritual so that the community could be established and maintained as a social, cultural, political, and religious body.

The interplays between individual experience and communal validation are central for understanding conversion narratives as an intricate part of New England Congregationalism.[9] The relationship between personal narrative and public recognition of conversion was complicated by the role of the minister. As a mediator between church doctrine and the realities of colonists' lives and experiences, pastors set the guidelines for conversion: how to recognize certain signs, how to deal with doubt, and how to verbalize personal experience so as to make it recognizable to others. Ministers also participated in the production of conversion narratives by recording them in their personal notebooks. It is hence nearly impossible to determine the extent to which lay writings available to us represent the actual relations of common New Englanders.[10]

The act of rationalizing and communicating the experience of conversion entailed a number of difficulties and pitfalls. Lay conversion

---

[9] For the relationship between the individual and the collective with regard to spiritual narratives, see Charles Lloyd Cohen, *God's Caress: The Psychology of Puritan Religious Experience* (New York: Oxford UP, 1986) 21; Shea 111; Murray J. Murphey, "The Psychodynamics of Puritan Conversion," *American Quarterly* 31.1 (1979): 135-147.

[10] Eric Seeman's study offers valuable insights into the ministerial recording process by showing how a mid-eighteenth-century minister from Kingston, Massachusetts revised and rephrased a confessor's relation given in private in order to facilitate a spiritual awakening in his congregants. Seeman's work shows furthermore the deviation of ministerial and lay interpretations of scripture, a fact that counters the notion of a rather homogenous Puritan divinity suggested by an earlier generation of New England scholars. Erik R. Seeman, "Lay Conversion Narratives: Investigating Ministerial Intervention," *New England Quarterly* 71.4 (1998): 629-634.

narratives (like all Puritan life-writings) were energized by an elevated concern with an ego in the process of denying and humbling itself before God because, according to Hartford founder and minister Thomas Hooker's representative dictum, "you cannot be in your selves and in Christ too."[11] Aside from the problem of acceptable self-positioning in narrative space, orators struggled with rationalizing spiritual experiences and estates that were conceived as ultimately inconceivable and inherently incommunicable. The problem of how to verify a confessor's compliance with church doctrines in his/her conversion accounts and thus the validation of probable elect status was of frequent concern for the New England clergy and the laity.[12] Some Puritan ministers held that language concealed rather than revealed truth and hence, words written or spoken could not be trusted as an adequate tool for conveying the inner state of an individual. Other preachers, such as Thomas Shepard, contested this pessimistic assumption, claiming that visible saints (i.e., those who had convinced others of their election) could lift the veil of language, establish a transparent relation between, in modern parlance, signifier and signified and thus allow direct access to their inner estates. As a result of this conviction, the subjective *expression* of advancement in religious instructions and of emotional engagement with the divine was seen as a necessary and adequate proxy for an objectifiable spiritual condition. A proper confession could, according to Shepard, bring to light

> such [things] as may be of special use unto the people of God, such things tend to show, Thus was I humbled, and thus I was called, then thus I have walked, though with many weaknesses since; and such special providences of God I have seen, temptations gone through; and thus the Lord hath delivered me.[13]

[11] Quoted in Jeffrey A. Hammond, *Sinful Self, Saintly Self: The Puritan Experience of Poetry* (Athens: U of Georgia P, 1993) 49.

[12] For a discussion of how colonial New England ministers sought to incorporate empiricism in their quest to discern the validity of conversion narratives, see Sarah Rivett, "Tokenography: Narration and the Science of Dying in Puritan Deathbed Testimonies," *Early American Literature* 42.3 (2007): 471-494.

[13] Thomas Shepard, *The Parable of Ten Virgins* (1660; Early English Books Online, S3114A) 200.

Nevertheless, no early New England conversion narrative on record today includes the words, "I know that I am saved," or "God has elected me for eternal bliss," partly because this was seen as a highly preposterous and dangerous assumption. Time and again, ministers warned their flocks that too much assurance could be a sign of pride, of deception by the devil, or of "a superficially edifying façade of successful piety."[14] In addition, colonists had to be careful to claim a specific moment when God intervened in their lives, since the relation of the immediate working of divine grace upon the sinner's soul could counter the doctrine of *sola scriptura* and thereby pose a dangerous approximation to the free grace position taken by the Antinomians. As one of the consequences of the excommunication and banishment of Anne Hutchinson in 1637/1638, clerical opponents of conversion narratives as church admission requirements argued that, as Patricia Caldwell puts it, "ordinary people cannot be trusted to express themselves on such an abstruse subject as conversion—even their own; and [...] that the evaluation of such expression cannot safely be left up to ordinary people, especially *en masse*."[15] This notion was particularly prominent in England where Protestant church admission procedures initially did not include public relations of sin and faith.

The narrow symbolic and structural corset of conversion narratives further increased the inherent limitations of language for expressing human emotions. Lay relations were marked by recurring

---

[14] Shea 99.

[15] Patricia Caldwell, *The Puritan Conversion Narrative: The Beginnings of American Expression* (Cambridge: Cambridge UP, 1983) 97. In Bunyan's *Pilgrim's Progress*, "Talkative" and "Faith" point out the problem of translating the presence of the divine into recognizable signs, asking "How doth the saving grace of God discover it self, when it is in the heart of man?" John Bunyan, *The Pilgrim's Progress*, ed. Cynthia Wall (1678/1684; New York: Norton, 2009) 64. The most prominent opponent of conversion narratives as mandatory admission tests was John Cotton, who claimed that such relations were futile for individual salvation and only served the self-constitution of the church. Other critics held that the procedure posed an uncalled-for nuisance because migration to America was already a sign that Puritans had likely been elected for salvation (Caldwell 124).

characteristics: a staccato rhythm of the prose, a repeated use of stock phrases, a uniformity of vocabulary, a limited incorporation of the contemporary world, a depiction of the battle between flesh and spirit, the recourse to Scripture, and a structural arrangement that roughly coincided with the morphology of conversion prescribed by the clergy. Lay(wo)men's narratives were further marked by an underlying tension between the abstract stages of conversion and its concrete manifestation in the lives of believers as well as between common features and individual expression. On the one hand, each conversion narrative, in order to be accepted, had to comply with certain patterns of recognizing the reality of conversion. On the other, it had to map an individual passage to Christ.[16] The conversion scheme granted believers a certain latitude of expression, but it was expected that the variations of the narrative remain within the bounds of orthodoxy and avoid the elevation of the self above its station established in Scripture and clerical exegesis. As Tom Webster succinctly puts it: "The disciplines of self-denial and self-examination [were] designed to turn the necessary condition of selfishness to the creation of a self-abnegating selfhood."[17] The intense anxiety about the blurred boundaries between self-examination, self-display, and self-assertion, however, created a tension between adherence to formula and establishment of idiosyncrasy, on which the literary value of lay conversion narratives and, in fact, of all Puritan spiritual self-writing rested and relied.

Patricia Caldwell has shown that New England conversion relations were characterized by an unprecedented complexity in structure, tone, rhythm, and symbols that preclude an easy predictability of the narratives. Indeed, while these texts take recourse to similar narrative elements that concur with an overarching morphology of conversion, the individuality of religious experience outweighs their commonalities and

---

[16] Shea 186.

[17] Tom Webster, "Writing to Redundancy: Approaches to Spiritual Journeys and Early Modern Spirituality," *The Historical Journal* 39 (1996): 43. In a similar vein, Sacvan Bercovitch has argued that "[t]he Puritan's dilemma was that the way from self necessarily led through the self." *The Puritan Origins of the American Self* (New Haven: Yale UP, 1975) 165.

denies a reduction to formula.[18] The epistemological limits of the empirical pursuit of grace inscribed themselves in the lack of closure in most lay conversion narratives. They tend to end anticlimactically, as in the case of Abram Arrington, who ends his public confession with the words: "And hence I was encouraged to seek after himself. Lord let me see my desires were after him and to seek him."[19] The narrator's remaining uncertainty about his spiritual future reflects the belief in the ultimate inscrutability of God's will and signals that the believer has merely embarked on the path to salvation. Arrington's and most other relations were necessarily inconclusive, because conversion was seen not as an arrival at a higher state of spirituality but rather as an indication that one had begun a promising journey toward divine pardon.

Most Puritan quest-for-salvation narratives were prompted by a life crisis that ensued from the death of a loved one or from a severe illness. In mirroring a larger cultural notion according to which bodily infirmities serve as signs of human depravity, of lurking death, and of God's arbitrary and providential intervention in human lives, lay confessants often depicted illness as a pivotal life event during which the seeker assessed and reorganized his/her relationship with God. Although not all prospective church members included illness in their autobiographical narratives before the congregation, those who did tended to interpret their physical afflictions as useful occasions for recognizing their previous thoughts and behavior as sinful and thus as necessities for a higher state of spirituality. In most cases illness appears at the beginning of the conversion process and its narrative representation. One early New England applicant, William Hamlet from

---

[18] Caldwell 26. Aside from certain recurring themes, arrival in America for instance, early New England conversion narratives established a sense of colonial identity and writing by emphasizing ambiguity and open-endedness, where their "Old World" counterparts tended to be geared toward closure. According to Caldwell, conversion narratives constitute a genuine "American" genre because these admission tests preceded similar practices in England (34-35).

[19] Thomas Shepard, "Thomas Shepard's Record of Relations of Religious Experience, 1648-1649," ed. Mary Rhinelander McCarl, *William and Mary Quarterly* 48.3 (1991): 451.

Cambridge, exemplifies this structural placement of illness as a crucial turning point in the formation of the self in Christ. Hamlet's confession, in which bodily afflictions figure as both a sign and a precondition of God's grace, may be taken for numerous other evocations of illness in seventeenth-century conversion narratives. He tells the audience that in his youth,

> the ordinances of God have been unsuitable to me and then I thought the Lord would afflict me and so He did, which was light. And being the first stroke I thought it was light but if I continued in my backslidings He would come out with seven worse plagues and so [I] prayed [to] the Lord that I might be more heavenly in prayer.[20]

For this godly seeker, illness marks the memory of a first knowledge of God's presence, the origin of spirituality. Only few lay relations mention health issues in later stages of the conversion process, even though one may safely assume that diseases played a recurring role in the lives of colonists. For the purpose of relating Puritan conversion, however, illness is primarily understood as fostering the conviction in, and compunction for, sin. An illness renders sin real by transforming certain thoughts and actions into a physical condition, thereby opening them to inspection, interpretation, and judgment. Illness thus becomes a

---

[20] Thomas Shepard, *Thomas Shepard's Confessions*, ed. George Selement and Bruce C. Woolley, *Publications of the Colonial Society of Massachusetts* 58 (Boston: The Society, 1981) 128. Shepard's *Confessions* consists of fifty-one transcripts of lay conversion narratives, recorded between 1638 and 1645. In contrast to Thomas Hooker and other Puritan ministers who received prospective New England church members (only) in private, Shepard required narratives before the whole congregation. For an insightful analysis of the differences and commonalities between pastor Shepard and his congregation, see George Selement, "The Meeting of Elite and Popular Minds at Cambridge, New England, 1638-1645," *William and Mary Quarterly* 41.1 (1984): 32-48. For the specificities of female conversion narratives recorded by Shepard, see Kathleen M. Swaim, "'Come and Hear': Women's Puritan Evidences," *American Women's Autobiography: Fea(s)ts of Memory*, ed. Margo Culley (Madison: U of Wisconsin P, 1992) 32-56.

metonymy that signals a larger shift of conversion from spirit to soma in those searching for Christ.[21]

In many lay relations, including William Hamlet's, the illness-induced realization of previous iniquities causes the believer to enter into a personal covenant with God: if He would only cure the disease, the sufferer would follow His laws, become a devout believer, and thereby forge a new self in Christ. In Hannah Bancroft's confession, for instance, given before the East Windsor congregation in November 1700, illness hinges between compunction and backsliding into previous spiritual and behavioral patterns, another medicine-related characteristic in lay conversion narratives:

> The first awakenings I had was when I [was] dangerously sick about four years ago, and then I made many promises, that if God would spare me I would be better and live another life. And after my recovery I for a while sought to God in the use of means for converting grace, but soon grew weary thereof and left off, and the last sermon I heard from that text, follow peace with all men and holiness without [which] no man shall see the Lord [Heb. 12:14], which was not long after my sickness was awakening to me, and brought to mind my promises which I made to God in my sickness, and now I had broken them so that I betook my self again to the use of means for the good of my soul and in a more diligent manner, than ever before.[22]

The covenant between the individual believer and God, here prompted and sealed by illness, figured prominently on a spiritual level but was also of central importance in Puritans' self-perception as a group. Even though most New England saints realized that "sickbed Promises are usually soon forgotten," as Richard Baxter commented scathingly, the converts relating their experiences stressed how God continued to call the believer and urged to proceed the spiritual

---

[21] In some narratives, illness of a family member functions as a punishment by proxy for the confessor's transgression. See, the conversion narratives of William Adams and Elizabeth Stacey, transcribed in Robert Strong, ed., "Two Seventeenth-Century Conversion Narratives from Ipswich, Massachusetts Bay Colony," *New England Quarterly* 82.1 (2009): 158, 163.

[22] Minkema 27.

pilgrimage in and through covenant-making with God as well as with other members of the congregation.[23]

Hannah Bancroft's spiritual relation also illustrates how most lay conversion narratives echoed the clergy's configuration of illness both as an actual, bodily condition and as a metaphor for a debased spirituality that needed to be remedied by turning to Christ. The covenant made during an illness causes the seeker to shed previous aspects of his/her identity and to reshape the self in accordance with God's laws—through Bible study, prayer, repentance, self-scrutiny, and confessional narration. Once on the path to conversion, the initial commitment to God, the first conversion, is necessarily envisaged as temporary and in need of being confirmed by a second conversion in and through writing. John Bunyan's quintessential Puritan conversion narrative, *Grace Abounding to the Chief of Sinners* (1666), demonstrates aptly the frequent backsliding, temptation, and uncertainty that accompany and constitute the sinner's growth in grace after the journey toward salvation has begun. For English Protestants on both sides of the Atlantic, such deviances from a linear route to Christ were not attributed to flawed theological doctrine or interpretation but were rather seen as essential stages of conversion. Because illness was often accompanied by a promise to reform and then followed by backsliding, it taught the ever-looming danger of false assurance and the necessity of a spiraling and preparatory movement of conversion toward fully accepting Christ; two central lessons to be learned by the applicant and by those listening to or reading the narratives.

Only few extant conversion relations employ illness as anything other than an occasion to recognize and repent previous sins. In a few instances, confessants deviate from the mechanized use of illness as an illustration of how God's sovereign will and power inscribes itself unto the human psyche and body. Cambridge congregant Robert Holmes, for example, admits that, "I was sick to death but took no care for my soul if I died so and sought to buy cattle when well."[24] This is a rather unusual confessional statement because, in contrast to most other illness reports,

---

[23] Richard Baxter, *Reliquiae Baxterianae* (1696; Early English Books Online, B1370) 90.

[24] Shepard, *Confessions* 143.

the state of affliction is not described as a turning point in the spiritual progress of the narrating self. Instead, illness is retrospectively configured as a missed economic opportunity. Rather than viewing the occasion as a sign from God, Holmes misreads and ignores the culturally ascribed meaning of illness and turns toward worldly matters instead. His juxtaposition of spiritual reflection and mundane act (i.e., purchasing cattle) creates a dissonance in his confession that draws attention to the author's insecurity about, or perhaps even his resistance to, accurately reading the cultural script underlying his illness. Instead, the writer's eye and pen are directed toward maintaining and increasing colonial presence in New England (creating order out of "wilderness" disarray), a presence that is fundamentally challenged by disease.

Despite this exemplary deviance from the narrative norm, the theology of illness in lay conversion narratives remained relatively consistent during the seventeenth and well into the eighteenth century. In the Shepard confessions, most prospective members were concerned with how their social and religious expectations about life in the "New World" had been contrasted with a reality marked by material desires and spiritual deadness. By 1700 such early anxieties about the mental and bodily conditions in New England no longer sought expression in conversion narratives. Kenneth Minkema's collection of East Windsor narratives between 1700 and 1752 shows that, while colonial society was shifting toward materialistic issues, the narrative concern with illness tended to follow the paths established by their forefathers. In accordance with its previous cultural configuration, illness functioned as a means of grace along the pilgrim's progress, located between awakening and wearing off.[25] The differences between early and later

---

[25] Minkema 13. Of the fourteen relations written by Timothy Edwards, father of Jonathan Edwards, and edited by cultural historian Kenneth Minkema, ten were recorded between 1700 and 1702, two in 1722 and two in 1725. For the role of conversion in early New England Puritanism and during the First Great Awakening, see Jerald C. Brauer, "Conversion: From Puritanism to Revivalism," *The Journal of Religion* 58.3 (1978): 227-243. It is interesting to note that during and after the Great Awakening (i.e., during the second half of the eighteenth century) references to worldly matters, including health and illness, seem to have disappeared entirely from lay conversion narratives, which are, instead, entirely steeped in religious discourse. Cf. Kenneth P. Minkema, "A

New England lay narratives lies in a deeper entrenchment of certain motifs of conversion and a narrative dramaturgy designed to replicate the advancements and disappointments along the sinner's preparation for saving grace. Early eighteenth-century personal relations also differed from their predecessors in their attempt to counter an awareness of the shortcomings of language by employing more stock phrases that had by then been established as signposts for recognizing a confessant's prospects of salvation.

Relating her autobiographical narrative for the church at East Windsor in the winter of 1701, Anne Fitch, like few others before her, expresses a deep-rooted sense of panic about her spiritual estate while she is suffering from (an unspecified) disease. Her panic translates into a description of overwhelming doubt, guilt, fear, depravity, resistance to Christ, and desire for mercy to a point where the initial physical illness gives way to far more severe crisis of faith:

> And then for several days I expected every hour that I should die and go to hell, and then my sins and God's wrath were so amazing to me that I can't express it, so that though my bodily pain was very great, yet such was the anguish of my spirit that I thought it ten times greater, and so great that no affliction that ever I felt in my life was in any measure like it.[26]

Fitch's inner turbulences are voiced in a stream of short-breathed sentences that aim to capture the abyss of a Puritan soul. The inherent unrepresentability of her spiritual state ("I can't express it") is countervailed by a hyperbolic excess of illness signifiers that function as a foil against which spirituality and assurance can possibly be measured. Representative of the lay conversion genre, Fitch's words anticipate the increasing formalization of personal expression at the turn of the eighteenth century.

---

Great Awakening Conversion: The Relation of Samuel Belcher," *William and Mary Quarterly* 44.1 (1987): 121-126; J. M. Bumsted, "Emotion in Colonial America: Some Relations of Conversion Experience in Freetown, Massachusetts, 1749-1770," *New England Quarterly* 49.1 (1976): 97-108.

[26] Minkema, "East Windsor" 33.

As these examples indicate, private self-scrutiny made public constituted a central topic in a broad array of personal narratives in seventeenth-century New England.[27] For most settlers, life in colonial America, more so than in their mother country, demanded constant vigilance of the self in order to erect and maintain a pious society that could serve as a model for others. When it came to missionizing the local Indian population, the colonists' configuration of illness and medical practice were extended in cultural contacts scenarios. English colonists not only brought their tools, books, plants or animals but also employed disease as a tool of empire, useful not only as pathogens but also as symbols. This discursive colonization, in part facilitated by the increasing dominance of the English rationalization of epidemics, was particularly evident in Native American conversion narratives.

Contagious Conversion: Religion and Medicine in Native American Narratives

As seen in chapter one of this study, disease created a cultural crisis in indigenous communities of hitherto unknown scope and intensity. In the wake of annihilation, loss of traditions, and trauma experienced by disease survivors, many Native people sought the help of their English neighbors. Interpreting the loss of family, knowledge, and way of life since the first major epidemic in 1616 as the result of unfavorable supernatural forces, some Algonquians were particular receptive to the message, meaning, and order which Puritan ministers promised if they converted to the Protestant faith and forsook their previous religious rituals and cultural beliefs. Conversion, in a nutshell, became contagious itself and spread throughout mid-century Native New England villages like a disease.

After a decade of setting up shop, colonists began their concerted missionary efforts among the remaining Algonquians, seeking to bring as many souls to conversion as possible prior to the imminent return of

---

[27] For a study of illness in Puritan spiritual autobiographies and diaries, see my "Making Sense of Morbidity in Early American Autobiography," *The Morbidity of Culture: Melancholy, Trauma, Illness and Dying in Literature and Film*, ed. Stephanie Siewert and Antonia Mehnert (Frankfurt a.M.: Lang, 2012) 69-82.

Jesus Christ. The millenarian impulse for missionizing New England Natives was especially evident in the work and life of John Eliot, preacher at Roxbury, Massachusetts, who devoted much of his energy to spreading the Gospel among the local Natives. Eliot's missionary activities, which began around 1640 and lasted until 1680, were prompted by religious, economic, and political motives. He and other ministers hoped that Native subjects who pronounced their allegiance with the Puritan faith would signify to the world the cultural superiority of English ways and manners, facilitate further trade relations between the two groups, and procure alliances that could prove helpful in the disputes over the boundaries between English and French zones of influence in the Western Hemisphere.[28]

In order to secure funding for their work, Eliot and his colleagues, among them ministers Thomas Mayhew and Henry Whitfield, wrote and published reports in England that attest to the progress of their missionary work. The series of writings, known as the *Eliot Tracts* or *Indian Tracts*, were designed to represent, among other aspects of the

---

[28] English missionary efforts were designed to counter-balance the Spanish "Black Legend" by emphasizing, from the perspective of colonists, peaceful conversion and cooperation with and among the Natives and the newcomers. As colonial late-comers in America, English settlers arrived with preconceived notions about indigenous inhabitants, drawn from reports about Spanish atrocities that had been published by the end of the sixteenth century. In most of these relations, Native Americans were described as friendly and primitive, yet doomed to extinction. Against the background of depictions of the massacres of indigenous Americans, English colonial domination could be justified on the basis of its presumed inferiority to the Spanish model of conquest. For most New Englanders, the colonization of America, it seemed, had hitherto consisted of a struggle among Satan's minions—the heathen Natives and the Catholic *conquistadors*—and now needed to be supplemented by the intervention of God's chosen people. For especially useful overviews of Eliot's missionary activities, see Neal Salisbury, "Red Puritans: The 'Praying Indians' of Massachusetts Bay and John Eliot," *William and Mary Quarterly* 31.1 (1974): 27-54; Dane Morrison, *A Praying People: Massachusetts Acculturation and the Failure of the Puritan Mission, 1600-1690* (New York: Lang, 1995); Richard Cogley, *John Eliot's Mission to the Indians before King Philip's War* (Cambridge, MA: Harvard UP, 1999).

mission, Native conversion in (presumably) their own words, translated by the ministers and thus filtered through an ethnocentric lens. The accounts of Native Americans who recite sermons and Scripture represent a highly fascinating and equally disturbing record of cultural encounters in the "New World." One source of confusion about Indian conversion narratives stems from the meticulousness with which their orators seem to have discarded their former way of living and thinking in favor of a life in Christ. For the majority of indigenous confessants, New England Protestantism appears to have been a means to a practical end: protection from the diseases and their consequences that had appeared with the arrival of the English settlers. Next to medical help, the *Eliot Tracts* detail how Indians, who were most affected by the upheaval brought about by epidemics, sought meaning and personal solace in the words and teachings of the newly arrived preachers.[29]

As a result of English missionary endeavors, the colonies witnessed the temporary formation of a new social and cultural caste: the Praying Indian. Before the outbreak of King Philip's War in the summer of 1675, New England housed approximately 1,000 Indians who prayed to the Puritan God, who had adopted, at least to a certain degree, English manners, and who could no longer live in their traditional habitats. Because English settler communities denied their converting Native neighbors participation in church services, Eliot and his assistants founded fourteen Praying Towns, mostly in the vicinity of Boston, where Natives could learn and live according to English religious and cultural principles and interact with colonists on a regular, though segregated basis. According to the stipulations of the missionaries, Indian conversion meant not only an acceptance of Christ as savior but, also, "the Reformation of their disordered lives," which was considered

---

[29] Eliot, Mayhew, and other New England missionaries versed in Algonquian exercised considerable editorial control over the translation and transcription of oral relations. The exact nature and scope of their interventions remains consigned to history, but one may reasonably assume that the minister-authors wanted to present a successful mission on paper. For this reason, many conclusions about Indian lives drawn from colonial writings, in general, and conversion narratives, in particular, must be viewed with caution because these texts tend to project colonial ideology onto the conquered subject.

to be most feasible in isolated settings that facilitated only selected interactions between the two groups.[30] Nevertheless, the settlements for Praying Indians were from the start cultural contact zones, in which the co-existence of a Puritan-style meetinghouse and wigwams as well as the use of church drums instead of bells epitomized the incomplete acculturation of the Natives. While some Englishmen considered the spiritual and cultural estates of the Praying Indians to be a success on the path to the full dissolution of tribal culture, others, while concurring with the goal of taming the Natives, were appalled by the "freakish" and suspiciously heretic staging of Englishness by the converts.[31]

The primary arenas for such staging were the tribal meetinghouses. There, the Praying Indians hoped to seal their covenant with God and with the belief system of their colonists by relating their conversion experiences before a board of Puritan examiners, notably in their own language, Algonquian.[32] Though not intended as an aesthetic form of

---

[30] John Eliot, *Tears of Repentance: or, A further Narrative of the Progress of the Gospel amongst the Indians in New-England* (1653; Early English Books Online E522) 31 [unpaginated]. Colonists may have considered the building and isolation of Praying Towns as a form of quarantine. It seems hardly a coincidence that plans for founding dwellings for Christian Indians were made shortly after a devastating smallpox epidemic in 1647-1648. By rounding up remaining Natives, offering them a new life and identity in special villages, the English fostered a racial segregation that served to protect the colonists from cultural and biotic contaminations.

[31] This is expressed, for instance, in the narrative of Mary Rowlandson's captivity among the Wampanoag during Metacom's Rebellion (a.k.a. King Philip's War). At one point, she watches an approaching group of Englishmen who turn out to be Indians dressed in European-style clothing. This performative cross-dressing at first puzzles and later appalls the Puritan narrator. Dressing becomes a token for conversion and is then revealed as an appearance that hides an underlying evil reality. Mary White Rowlandson, *The Soveraignty and Goodness of God* (1682; Boston: Fleet for Phillips, 1720) 50.

[32] Puritan efforts to Christianize Native Americans derived from the belief that American indigenes were remnants of the Ten Lost Tribes of Israel who, according to scripture, had to become believers before the Second Coming of Christ. Eliot and his colleagues held that this goal could best be achieved by teaching their missionary subjects in their own language. This decision, which

expression, these ethnic spiritual narratives anticipate a number of features associated with twentieth-century, postmodern performativity. As Joseph Roach has stressed, performance

> make[s] publicly visible through symbolic action both the tangible existence of social boundaries and, at the same time, the contingency of those boundaries on fictions of identity, their shoddy construction out of inchoate otherness, and, consequently, their anxiety-inducing instability.[33]

Applied to the early American colonial scene, Praying Town conversion narratives were not indications of an achieved degree of religiosity but rather demonstrated the impossibility of an Algonquian reciting an authentically Puritan path to conversion. Many colonists, as well as historians and literary scholars today, believed that in their staging of conversion, Native confessors created cultural copies of Englishness in Algonquian that, by the mere fact of language, remained an incomplete surrogate of the Protestant model.

When Praying Indians repeated Englishness with a difference in word and action, they created a hybrid version of the original that threatened personal and collective identities on both sides of the New England cultural and racial divide. On the one hand, converts fostered the demise of traditional tribal cultures; on the other, their performances

---

marked an unusual concession to the colonized in the history of American settlement, was followed by the translation and printing of the Bible and other religious documents in Algonquian, a massive task that Eliot and his Native assistants undertook with zeal and commitment and against the opposition of many New England divines who urged that the funds for the translation would be better spent on Anglicizing the Indians. Michael P. Clark, Introduction, *The Eliot Tracts*, ed. Michael P. Clark (Westport: Praeger, 2003) 24-25.

[33] Joseph R. Roach, *Cities of the Dead: Circum-Atlantic Performance* (New York: Columbia UP, 1996) 39. A Native American conversion narrative constitutes a performance both in the sense of its enacted theatricality and role-playing and in a more philosophical sense as having "no ontological status apart from the various acts which constitute its reality." Judith Butler, *Gender Trouble: Feminism and the Subversion of Identity* (New York: Routledge, 1990) 136.

of religiosity proved deeply disturbing to some colonists, for the enactments of Englishness often charted a refracted image of the colonists' own desires and shortcomings. For most staunch Puritans, the Indian converts' mimicry—resulting from the double-voicedness of the narratives (Algonquian speaker/English translator) and their uncanny stagings of Englishness—posed a danger to New England's cultural, social, and political stability. Native conversion narratives served as a potentially subversive source of agency because the relations rendered the colonial endeavors as immanently incomplete by presenting colonized subjects that were, in Homi Bhabha's famous words, "*almost the same* [as the English], *but not quite*."[34] By mimicking the cultural dominant's means and modes of expressing religious sentiments, some Algonquians used their narratives as a source of empowerment. By employing the inherent ambiguity and open-endedness of the conversion model, some Indians were able to present an ongoing transculturation in narrative space and, thereby, enacted and communicated a sense of cultural resilience vis-à-vis the missionary efforts by Eliot and his colleagues. One of the questions that have directed recent scholarly readings of the *Eliot Tracts* is hence precisely the degree to which Praying Indians were able to deploy conversion in order to re-form tribal communities as distinct social and cultural entities. One can indeed read some confessionals collected and assembled by Eliot and his colleagues as deliberate *ersatz* conversions that imitate an imagined original with an ulterior motive: the recuperation of cultural agency after the disease-induced dissolution of tribal communities.[35]

Indian performances of English Protestantism remained elusive and unstable constructs of identity. Attempting to counter common

---

[34] Homi K. Bhabha, *The Location of Culture* (London: Routledge, 1994) 86.

[35] Because Puritan missionaries recorded all the extant Indian conversion narratives, however, the latitude for conveying Native agency and cultural resistance was certainly limited. One religious practice that lent itself for co-optation by the converting Natives was prayer. Eliot's Indian converts placed a stronger emphasis on the power of prayer than New England church applicants at the time, apparently because the former felt that this novel mode of communication with God could shape their realities and provide protection from illnesses

contemporary suspicions about the verisimilitude of indigenous relations and the potentially threatening consequences for assessing lay conversions, Richard Mather defended the genuineness of Native spiritual experiences based not only on their words but also their emotional displays:

> And though they spake in a language of which many of us understood but little, yet we that were present that day, we saw them, and we heard them perform the duties mentioned, with such grave and sober countenances, with such comely reverence in gesture, and their whol carriage, and with such plenty of tears trickling down the cheeks of some of them, as did argue to us that they spake with much good affection, and holy fear of God, and it much affected our hearts.[36]

According to Mather, the Natives' performance of faith was not to be seen as a fake conversion but rather as a representation of the concurrence between displayed Indian interiority and Protestant requirements for church admission. This advertisement and defense of Native conversion failed to convince the majority of New Englanders, however. Given the suspicion that especially English Protestants housed toward all forms of theatricality, many colonists held that Native conversions revealed the candidate's hypocrisy rather than his/her actual conversion and thus signaled the falsity of the narrative itself as well as of its author.[37] Rather than representations of achieved conversion, many

---

[36] R. Mather quoted in Eliot, *Tears of Repentance* 31 [unpaginated]. Later, Eliot adds: "I have been true & faithful unto their souls, and in writing and reading their Confessions, I have not knowingly, or willingly made them better, than the Lord helped themselves to make them, but am verily perswaded on good grounds, that I have rather rendered them weaker (for the most part) than they delivered them; partly by missing some words of weight in some Sentences, partly by my short and curt touches of what they more fully spake, and partly by reason of the different Idioms of their Language and ours" (*Tears of Repentance* 26-27 [paginated]).

[37] Leibman argues that the hybridity of Native conversion narratives stems from the adaptation of the indigenous story-telling (or *memorate*) tradition to the narrative structure and symbolic reservoir of Christian conversions. The switch from one cultural realm to another may have been less difficult than might be

Native narratives replicate acts of surrogation that point to the theatricality of all conversion narratives, including those by Puritan congregants.

Because Puritans were constantly concerned with the credibility of conversion testimony offered by their peers, their uncertainty about whether the Algonquian converts were hypocrites or true believers reigned prominent in their minds and writings. For many observers, a central dilemma was that Native conversion narratives needed to portray a reformed colonized subject in order to legitimize the American experiment and, at the same time, the Indianness of the convert had to be preserved in order to distinguish the two social and cultural groups and to keep the process of missionizing at pace.

In the struggle over cultural and political hegemony in New England, most colonists were convinced that their spiritual and secular mission was sealed by divine favor that found its expression in disease. This conviction, as seen at the outset of the present study, was firmly entrenched in the thoughts, actions, and writings of the colonists, and the group surrounding Eliot was not exempt from it. In their initial report, *New England's First Fruits* (1643), the missionaries sum up the first decade of colonization and reinvigorate the discourse of medical providentialism:

> Thus farre hath the good hand of God favoured our beginnings: see whether he hath not engaged us to wait still upon his goodnesse for the

assumed because both narrative forms employ similar relations with the supernatural world. "The *memorate* shares some important features with the standard Puritan conversion narrative," Leibman explains, "both can be either told in first person or retold by someone who was not involved in the incident. Just as conversion narratives were often told to gain church membership, *memorates* by *pniesok* (warrior-counselors) and *pawwaws* (shamans) were told as part of the rite of passage to become a spiritual leader, advisor, or practitioner. Unlike conversion narratives or experiences, *memorates* often came in the form of a dream or vision that might be deliberately induced through a 'difficult ordeal' or 'loss of sleep, fasting, and drinking mixtures that may have been hallucinogenic.'" Laura Arnold Leibman, Introduction, *Experience Mayhew's Indian Converts*, ed. Laura Arnold Leibman (Amherst: U of Massachusetts P, 2008) 21-22.

future, by such further remarkable passages of his providence to our Plantation in such things as these: 1. In sweeping away great multitudes of the Natives by the small Pox a little before we went thither, that he might make room for us there.[38]

Here, the author feels compelled to a sense of superiority based on the signs of probable election, in this case conveyed through the ecology of disease that shaped the material and cultural foundation of early New England.

Matters of health, illness, and healing form a repository of recurring tropes throughout the *Eliot Tracts* and appear mainly in two interrelated guises: as part of a cultural battle over Algonquian healing rituals and as signs of Native iniquities. According to the missionaries, the shamanic healer or powwow remained the primary obstacle to Indian conversion. Described as a devilish creature since the early days of New England settlement, the powwow possessed medical skills that the English considered unacceptable and futile, harming rather than curing a patient. Missionaries had to concede, however, that Native healers maintained a revered position in many tribes, despite their obvious inefficacy in light of the avalanche of disease in the early decades of the seventeenth century. Because of his continuous influence and power in tribal affairs, the powwow became a central target of missionary efforts.[39]

As seen in chapter one, most early New Englanders viewed indigenous healing rituals as expressions of the devil. Such an assessment was not only due to the colonists' unfamiliarity with the ceremonies but also because most could not master the language in which the rituals were performed (Algonquian) and thus could not control them. Interestingly enough, the foundation of Praying Towns coincided with a legislation by the Massachusetts Bay Court prohibiting powwow ceremonies. With this measure English settlers set the stage for

---

[38] Anon., *New Englands First Fruits* (1643; Early English Books Online E519) 20.

[39] Eliot's decision to translate the Bible may have inadvertently helped to solidify the position of the powwow in New England tribes because indigenous healers relied on language as a repository of symbols and as a vital link to the past for their curing rituals and ceremonies.

further acculturating the Native population of North America—a process that was to continue well into the twentieth century—by stigmatizing the shaman as "a principal barrier to the eradication of Indian culture."[40] Yet, the powwow was not a fixed person or role in Native New England communities. He (sometimes she) rather reflected a spirituality and way of life that could be enacted by several members. Hence, by merely outlawing the powwow as a recognizable figure in Indian life, colonial agents were unable to eradicate fully a cosmology in which spiritual healing played a central role.

In order to battle and break the cultural power of the powwow, the English continually disseminated accounts that linked the shaman's singing, gesturing, and violent body motions to witchcraft. In the *Eliot Tracts*, Native healing enters the literary stage in the second report, *The Day Breaking* (1647), when the narrator paraphrases indigenous explanations of the powwow's role and then is quick to add his own interpretation:

> Being further askt what doe these Pawwaws, and what use are they of; and they said the principall imployment is to cure the sick by certaine odde gestures and beatings of themselves, and then they pull out the sicknesse by applying their hands to the sick person and so blow it away: so that their Pawwaws are great witches having fellowship with the old Serpent, to whom they pray, and by whose meanes they heale sicke persons.[41]

Aside from providing (erroneous) ethnographic information on Algonquian healing, this section exemplifies how the English narrative voice takes dominance over its Native subject. While the first part of the sentence (before the colon) allows the Indian voice some agency over

---

[40] Virgil J. Vogel, *American Indian Medicine* (1970; Norman: U of Oklahoma P, 1990) 35.

[41] John Wilson, *The Day-Breaking, If not the Sun-rising of the Gospell with the Indians in New-England* (1647; Early English Books Online, S3110) 21. For a similar interpretation of indigenous healing rituals as demonic practice, see Eliot, *Tears of Repentance* 4-6 [paginated]. English colonists also stressed that many Natives feared their shaman because of his perceived ability to inflict illnesses (Morrison 15).

conveying medical information and meaning, the following phrase represents the colonial master in full control of consigning truth and reality about indigenous cultural practices in discursive space. Yet, by attributing the powwow's healing abilities to his allegiance with Satan, the author grants medical efficacy to shamanic healers, implying that their curative powers potentially transcend the boundaries of indigenous communities, affecting the health of Natives and colonists alike.

In order to protect both groups from the perceived black magic employed by Native healers, Puritan missionaries reiterated the necessity of erecting a religious bulwark comprised of prayer, Bible reading, and conversion. Eliot and his colleagues soon realized that the tradition of powwowing could not be ended by a single blow but needed continuous work. Many Algonquians felt that if they gave up powwowing without being fully accepted participants in the Puritan faith, no one would and could cure their illnesses.[42] In order for conversion to work, English missionaries also had to offer deities, symbols, and practices that could connect with the previous beliefs of New England Natives. The demand for mimicry hence involved a politics of surrogation, the exchange or substitution of an indigenous cultural element or practice with one imported from England. For example, Native beliefs in spiritual beings, or *manitowuk*, which suffused the visible and invisible worlds could be merged with, or partly superseded by, a belief in the Christian Holy Spirit.[43]

The outlawing of traditional healers was flanked by an intellectual debate about the efficacy of Indian versus English medical practices. In their cultural battle over the proper social role of the powwow, English colonists repeatedly deployed disease as evidence against heathen practices and in favor of English religion and medicine. John Eliot was quite familiar with rudimentary theories and practices of medicine and used his knowledge to garner support from potential Indian converts and from his sponsors in England. In *The Clear Sun-shine* (1648), for

---

[42] Thomas Shepard, *The Clear Sun-Shine of the Gospel Breaking Forth upon the Indians in New-England*, 1648, *Collections of the Massachusetts Historical Society*, Third Series, vol. 4 (1834): 37-38.

[43] Henry Warner Bowden, *American Indians and Christian Missions: Studies in Cultural Conflict* (Chicago: U of Chicago P, 1985) 122.

instance, Eliot claims that the tribal attachment to powwowing needed to be countervailed not only by religious instruction but also by "secular" medical education. If the prospective Indian proselytes comprehended that Western civilization had produced healing methods superior to traditional rituals and botanical knowledge, then conversion would be a decisive step closer to success. Instruction in medicine and religion implied, therefore, that the missionaries and the missionized were potentially sharing a common intellectual ground. However, with the description of Indians lacking sufficient "skill in physick, though some of them understand the vertues of sundry things, yet the state of mans body, and skill to apply them they have not," Eliot disavows indigenous contributions to medical knowledge.[44] He also stresses the image of Natives as civilizational illiterates who remain in desperate need of teaching in all matters of culture. The English author further argues that for want of better knowledge, Algonquians still have no choice but to seek their powwows in time of sickness.[45] He then turns this circumstance into a reason for asking the London-based Society for the Propagation of the Gospel to fund a medical school in the colonies. This school was to be restricted to English settlers only; Algonquians, while in need of civilizing, were considered too far removed from the gifts of reason necessary to master Western medicine: "Some of the wiser sort I have stirred up to get this skill; I have shewed them the anatomy of mans body, and some generall principles of Physick, which is very acceptable to them, but they are so extremely ignorant, that these things must rather be taught by sight, sense, and experience then by precepts, and rules of art."[46] Eliot deems it enough that Indians recognize the

---

[44] Shepard, *Clear Sun-Shine* 56.

[45] See Eliot's letter printed in Edward Winslow, *The Glorious Progress of the Gospel amongst the Indians in New England* (1649; Early English Books Online, W3036) 15-17.

[46] Shepard, *Clear Sun-Shine* 56. In 1663 Eliot appealed to the College of Physicians in London for support of his medical endeavors among Native Americans, see John Eliot to Richard Baxter, July 6, 1663, reprinted in Michael P. Clark, ed., *The Eliot Tracts* (Westport: Praeger, 2008) 432-433. For Eliot's medical knowledge, see John Eliot to Robert Boyle, 30 September 1670,

possibilities and efficacy of English medicine and receive rudimentary instruction in healing. Once the Natives have been convinced of the efficacy of medical knowledge developed by European civilization(s) and disseminated by New England graduates, they will, Eliot contends, turn their backs on traditional healing and spirituality, ready to accept Christ. Moreover, keeping medical knowledge away from the Natives ensured their dependency on Western healing. By withholding information and assistance, medicine became a tool of colonization, which proved especially powerful in conjunction with the deep religiosity of the colonizers.[47]

For the missionaries, the victory in the discursive battle over medical efficacy, waged in the *Eliot Tracts*, became a central cipher for English cultural superiority. Not only for Eliot, but also for his colleague, Thomas Mayhew, Western medicine (represented by the colonial preacher-physician) and Native healing (represented by the powwow) were engaged in a medical and spiritual contest, with an obvious winner. In *The Glorious Progress* (1649), he cites three examples of tribal members who renounced traditional ways after they had witnessed the medical power of prayer and had realized that Christians remained unaffected by the medical work of the shaman. Mayhew omits all references to English physicians who may have aided in the battle over medical efficacy and cultural superiority and, instead, depicts himself as a medico-religious teacher and practitioner who instructs the heathen about the proper use of prayer for healing purposes. Epitomizing the "angelical conjunction" between preacher and physician, Mayhew was a minister with considerable medical skill, performing a vivisection on one of his Algonquian patients, which (in combination with prayer)

---

reprinted in Martin Moore, *Memoirs of Life and Character of Rev. John Eliot* (Boston: Bedlington, 1822) 123-125.

[47] The usefulness of European medical knowledge for converting New England Natives was first recorded by Edward Winslow, who after his medical visit to Massasoit held "much profitable conference [on religious matters] which would be too tedious to relate, yet was not lesse delightfull to them, then comfortable to us." Edward Winslow, *Good Newes from New England, or A True Relation of Things Very Remarkable at the Plantation of Plimoth in New-England* (1624; Early English Books Online, STC 25856) 34.

yielded his recovery where theretofore the local powwow had failed.[48] These and similar descriptions, despite their ideological biases and reasons for selection, point to the firm conviction of English missionaries that medicine constituted a decisive stepping-stone in their colonial endeavors because it allowed the prospective converts to recognize a cultural practice as superior to their own.

Despite certain successes in their missionary efforts, the repeated English invocations of the advantages of healing as a means of religious and cultural conversion fell short of contributing considerably to the "principal end" of the settlement, fixed in writing in the Massachusetts Bay Charter of 1629: to "wynn and incite the Natives of Country, to the Knowledg and Obedience of the onlie true God and Savior of Mankinde, and the Christian Fayth."[49] The lack of understanding and frustration over the continuation of powwowing is evident throughout the early sections of the *Eliot Tracts* and even though there are no statistics available concerning the actual number of converts and non-converts at the time, the consistent support for traditional healers in tribal communities was both a nuisance and cause for renewed advertising for the missionary work. After staking the intellectual superiority of European medicine, Mayhew complains of the Indians' continuing "bondage to the Pawwawes," explaining at length that members of the Native community continue to resort to old healing practices during an epidemic.[50] Mayhew stresses that, "[t]he Indians having many calamities fallen upon them, they laid the cause of all their wants, sicknesses, and death, upon their departing from their old heathenish ways."[51] It seems, therefore, that the cultural message that "backsliding causes divine wrath" was present in both English and tribal communities. Mayhew fails, however, to counter the revival of powwowing with persuasive religious rhetoric and illustrates, instead, the helplessness of English

---

[48] Winslow, *Glorious Progress* 16.

[49] "The Charter of the Massachusetts Bay Company, 1629," *American Colonial Documents to 1776*, ed. Merrill Jensen (London: Eyre & Spottiswoode, 1955) 82.

[50] Henry Whitfield, *The Light Appearing More and More towards the Perfect Day* (1651; Early English Books Online, W1999) 8.

[51] Whitfield 4.

missionaries in light of continuous Indian adherence to traditional spirituality.

Some readers of this particular tract may have realized the futility of proselytizing the Natives, while others might have felt the urgency of raising more funds for the work of the New England ministers. After having spoken to local Indians, Mayhew concludes that more time and effort is needed in order to propagate the conviction that traditional (healing) ceremonies were inherently sinful. He also insinuates that Western medicine has yet to prove its efficacy to an extent that would convince Algonquians to discard their traditional practices altogether. Instead, Mayhew is forced to acknowledge the failure of extending Western medicine to the colonized subjects. When he reports of an aging man dying of palsy, Mayhew is unable or unwilling to attribute to him any words of probable salvation: "when I spake to him, he fetched many sighs; he is at this day a living and a dead monument of the Lords displeasure, having hurt himself most, and done them most good he hated."[52] Mayhew argues that God manifests his presence in the life of the sick Algonquian, offering little mercy but plenty of punishment. It is obviously too late for the dying man to mend his ways; because he has failed to forsake powwowing, he has reached a point of no return, Mayhew tells his reader. Here, the discursive front drawn by Mayhew in the intellectual battle over medical practice reveals the preoccupation of the ministers with the powwows and, in doing so, demonstrates the power and obstinacy of the indigenous healing figure which emerges out of the act of performative surrogation.[53]

As time progressed and the missionary reports from the New England frontier increased, a noticeable change occurred in the depiction of powwowing. More and more, it seemed, New England Natives abdicated their traditional healing practices. For instance, in *Strength out of Weaknesse* (1652) Mayhew recounts how a shaman had discovered the presumably satanic origin of Native healing. As one of the converts explains to the minister, the celestial powers that energized shamanic healing came in four different shapes:

[52] Whitfield 11.

[53] Joshua David Bellin, "John Eliot's Playing Indian," *Early American Literature* 42.1 (2007): 17.

one was like a man which he saw in the Ayre, and this told him that he did know all things upon the Island, and what was to be done; and this he said had its residence over his whole body. Another was like a Crow, and did looke out sharply to discover mischiefes coming towards him, and had its residence in his head. The third was like to a Pidgeon, and had its place in his breast, and was very cunning about any businesse. The fourth was like a Serpent, very subtile to doe mischiefe, and also to doe great cures.[54]

This passage can be read as a Native shorthand for concepts of the body, illness, and medicine. Illustrated by the animal imagery, nature is seen as the gateway to the healthy indigenous body, where the head (mind) and breast (heart), and health as a state of spiritual and corporeal equilibrium, are presided over by an ambiguous deity, most likely Abbomocho (or Hobbomok). Despite the contextualization of this view as satanic, the Indian narrator manages to inject health-related cultural information into Mayhew's text. This passage is hence a rare indication of how indigenous knowledge and worldview seeps into a colonial narrative. Controlled by the English, the relation of dream figures, taken from the *memorate* tradition, serves to remember a cultural practice by including it in Western modes of representation.

This passage may furthermore be read as an example of early Native American *auto*ethnography, which, according to Mary Louis Pratt's definition, allows people

> to describe themselves in ways that engage with representations others have made of them. [These texts] involve a selective collaboration with and appropriation of idioms of the metropolis or the conqueror. These are merged or infiltrated to varying degrees with indigenous idioms to create self-representations intended to intervene in metropolitan modes of understanding.[55]

---

[54] Henry Whitfield, *Strength out of Weaknesse; or a Glorious Manifestation of the Further Progresse of the Gospel among the Indians of New-England* (1652; Early English Books Online, W2003) 24.

[55] Mary Louise Pratt, "Arts of the Contact Zone," *Profession 91* (1991): 35.

As autoethnographic texts, Algonquian conversion narratives deploy discursive means of resistance as a tactic to undermine the control of Western domination by co-opting and thus disrupting its modes of representation. When the converted powwow relates the tribal interrelation between the human body and cosmos, he introduces an internal break, an insertion of cultural difference that reveals the temporal suspension and deferral of conversion by the confessor. What results, then, is a struggle over negotiating indigenous experiences, especially with regard to medicine, with Christian notions of salvation in and through narrative space. Yet, the rarity of such a performative invocation of agency in Indian conversion narratives renders visible the virtual impossibility of resistance, especially in light of epidemics that eradicated most of the carriers and recipients of Algonquian culture.

In the introductory chapter of *Tears of Repentance* (1653), the author undertakes a crucial narrative shift from third to first person perspective, a change in rhetorical strategy that appears to have been owed to increasing pressures to provide evidence of successful missionary work directly from the mouths of the converts. By the 1650s, the Native testimonials recorded in the *Eliot Tracts* increasingly resembled their English models in structure and content. Now that they are allowed to speak, their speech has become standardized. For instance, many relations place illness during the early phase of the sinner's path to grace. As one man, named Nookau, confesses: "Five years ago, before I prayed I was sick, I thought I should die; at which I was much troubled, and knew not what to do; then I thought, if there be a God above, and he give life again, then I shall beleeve there is a God above, and God did give me life: and after that I took up praying to God."[56] The intensity of spiritual crisis presented here resembles that portrayed in Puritan conversion narratives. However, the confessant expresses a concern over the existence of God that his colonial neighbors would hesitate to reveal. The latter were, as we have seen, much more concerned with the intricacies of following divine law and with the weaknesses of the human heart. By questioning God's presence, Nookau's confession exemplifies a common Native adaptation of English conversion narratives. To the Puritan reader, however, such a confession illustrated

---

[56] Eliot, *Tears of Repentance* 39 [paginated].

the inferior humanity of the Algonquian subject, signaled by its increased susceptibility to illnesses and its lacking religious knowledge.

The approximation of Indian narratives to the English model was in part due to the fact that the first two attempts (1652 and 1654) to persuade a board of colonial examiners of the credibility of Native conversion failed. Only in 1659 did Algonquian oral relations, polished and rehearsed for years, convince Eliot's Roxbury congregation that the Praying Indians should be granted their own church. Toward the end of the collection of Native confessions, powwowing seems to have been fully eradicated from indigenous communities and, indeed, the decreasing descriptions of English missionaries struggling with powwow culture illustrates a similar loss of influence in tribal affairs in reality. Each disease-infected and dying Native further threatened and undermined the influence of the shaman who was increasingly seen as unable to defuse the cultural crisis that shook Algonquian communities. Eliot and Mayhew accordingly inform their readers that shamans have increasingly surrendered their traditional healing ways in favor of accepting Christ.[57] For instance, one promising candidate for salvation named Waban, an aging powwow lately turned Puritan convert, confesses how, during a sickness, he decided to adopt English culture and how he has since become pious. In a later confession, Waban indicates his mastery of contemporary religious medical discourse. He reflects on Matthew 9, in which Christ is described as the physician of the soul: "he healed mens bodies, but he can heale souls also: he is a great Physitian, therefore let all sinners goe to him. Therefore this day know what need we have of Christ, and let us goe to Christ to heale us of our sins, and he can heale us both soul and body."[58] Here, Christ is shown as having been integrated into a tribal social and cultural network of meaning, replacing the shaman as the central healing figure in Native communities. Waban's reference to a theology of healing approximated

---

[57] Eliot, *Tears of Repentance* 8 [unpaginated].

[58] John Eliot, *A further Accompt of the Progresse of the Gospel amongst the Indians in New-England* (1659; Early English Books Online E510) 9. See also Wutasakompavin's meditation on Matthew 8:2-3 (Eliot, *A Further Accompt* 19). Almost all confessions include the following Native transgressions: praying to many gods, not knowing how to pray properly, and misrecognizing sin.

the English original to a degree that would, as Eliot and his colleagues hoped, convince the audience of the possibility and feasibility of true conversion. But the omission of signs of traditional culture in Waban's narrative threatens the authenticity of the report since, according to the Calvinist morphology of conversion, the path to salvation required doubt, wavering, and ambiguity. Hence, the attempt to prove the authenticity of the conversion by including medical issues fails, because it makes the ventriloquism of the narrative all too obvious. When measuring Waban's relation against similar lay Puritan conversion accounts, the overabundance of authentic signs of conversion deconstructs the purpose of the narrative and reveals the lacking mimetic reliability of the text. This is not to deny the Indian convert's sincerity or lack of faith; rather, his performance of religiosity, molded by the words and pens of the missionaries, brings to light the central representational dilemma of all conversion narratives: how to adequately illustrate and communicate a subjective state of being and becoming converted in objective terms.

As Native interpretations of personal illnesses increasingly resembled those established by New England colonists, so did their configurations of collective diseases. If, according to initial English reasoning, God had punished Algonquians as a group because of their alliance with the devil and had saved the English because of their piety, then an increase in Praying Indians must eventually reduce the number of disease-induced Indian deaths. John Eliot, eager to prove to his congregations (in the Praying Towns) that Christianity was in essence a healing faith, and to his English readers that Indian conversions were indeed possible, reports how during the smallpox epidemic of 1649 many converts were spared while English colonists suffered:

> The winter before this last past it pleased God to worke wonderfully for the *Indians,* who call upon God in preserving them from the small Pox, when their prophane Neighbours were cut off by it. This winter it hath pleased God to make lesse difference, for some of ours were also visited with that disease, yet this the Lord hath done for them, that fewer of them have dyed thereof, then of others who call not upon the Lord. Onely three dyed of it, (but five more young and old) of other diseases.[59]

[59] Whitfield, *Strength out of Weaknesse* 1 (emphasis original).

This statement exposes, among other things, the propagandistic quality of early New England medical providentialism, a discourse that configured disease susceptibility along collective, proto-racial lines of division. Twenty years after the arrival of the Winthrop fleet, this master narrative failed to withstand the realities of illness in the colonies. Hence, Eliot postulates a significant revision of the conceptual connections between religion, group membership, and health. In contrast to John Winthrop's interpretation of disease in early New England as divine signs of favor, Eliot's smallpox report stresses the causal links between piety and health, prayer and recovery, rather than between racial-cultural affiliation and disease. In doing so, the author momentarily shifts emphasis away from Native/English health divides toward the commonalities of Indian and English bodies.

* * *

Assurance about one's salvation was the most pressing spiritual concern for pious New England colonists. For some, the knowledge of salvation was revealed directly, whereas others insisted that assurance could only be experienced through Scripture and demanded a formalized narrative but still could never be conclusively confirmed. The attempts to verbalize and perform conversion functioned both as barometers of individual and collective spiritual endeavors and as didactic tools. The description of the emergence of grace through various stages could be discerned as a model of practical divinity, illustrating to every member of the congregation the means and signs through which the recognition of saving faith might become possible.

When colonists attempted to rationalize their spiritual states, illness served to indicate to the believer and to the community that was asked to validate the conversion report that God had indeed intervened and reshaped the internal landscape of the sinner. In most Puritan lay relations, therefore, illness occurred at the outset of the conversion process and its narrative representation; its dominant function was to awake the sinner, making him/her realize as well as repent for the iniquities that have produced states of bodily infirmity. Time and again, church candidates confessed to breaking the promises they had announced to God during illness but had soon forgotten after recovery.

Illness was thus seen as an intricate part of confession: it caused and shaped it, constituted a sign of sinfulness, of human imperfection both physically and spiritually, and delivered the believer into a state of exception in which a turn to Christ followed by continual introspection remained the only viable healing option. It comes as no surprise, therefore, that medicine, as an emerging scientific field and as a means of curing, played a negligible role in practically all Puritan conversion narratives.

The transcultural employment of illness rhetoric in New England conversion narratives illustrates that colonists had devised a system of signs that could represent the inner state of the convert. For the English, these signs were universal. Anyone who convincingly displayed the signs of conversion could be considered among the elect. As part of the conversion endeavor, medical discourse allowed the English to assert the intellectual superiority and practical efficacy of Western knowledge and, at the same time, enabled the representation of partial cultural resilience through the figure of the powwow. As a performative copy or counterfeit that merely approximated an original, Native conversion narratives often present uncanny illustrations of a modernity that becomes contested in the process of transgressing cultural boundaries. Because they showed the impossibility of proving conversion, many Native American conversion narratives threatened the validity and credibility of *all* conversion narratives emanating from a self-examined and god-assured individual. Lay New England conversion narratives, on the other hand, gave voice to the interplays between the crisis of the soul that captivated first-generation colonists and the crisis of representation that public confessions unearthed. That is, these narratives constantly grappled with showing what could not be shown: God's converting grace. It is precisely the contradiction between invisible election and visible conversion that fueled the semiotic engines driving seventeenth-century English and Native American conversion narratives. Their testimony about sin and knowledge of theological doctrine (confession and profession) was itself a ritual designed to achieve spiritual healing and to mend the body personal and the body social. A narrative of conversion, whether kept private or shared with others, whether created by an English settler or an Algonquian survivor, was designed to produce a catharsis of the individual and, if shared, of the community. In other words, similar to other healing rituals such as prayer or communal fasting and thanksgiving, conversion narratives were conceived as paths to personal and public health that not only supplemented medical procedures but that were essentially medical themselves.

# 5. Poetic Responses to Illness

During the early decades of New England's colonization, literature played an ambivalent role. Although English colonists recognized literature's potential for education and edification, they were deeply skeptical of its corruptive function. Many Puritan ministers and teachers criticized the literary culture of "merry England" for presenting false accounts of reality and for providing negative models of behavior for the audience. In a similar vein, many colonists held that literature, when designed to convey beauty and truth, was futile, for all beauty and truth were already revealed in the Bible. John Cotton's dictum that "God's Altar needs not our polishings" encapsulates Puritans' general suspicion about texts that emanate from an inherently imperfect and flawed human mind.[1] As one result, acceptable modes of writing needed to adhere to a plain-style rhetoric. Established as a main principle of New England letters in William Bradford's preface to *Of Plymouth Plantation*, the aim of plain-style rhetoric was to establish a concurrence between language and the world: "I shall endeavour to manifest in a plain style, with singular regard unto the simple truth in all things; at least as near as my slender judgment can attain the same," Bradford writes at the outset of his historical account of early New England settlement.[2] By emphasizing a non-ornamental, reality-directed style of writing, Bradford and other colonists sought to ensure that literature would avoid the trap of representing human vanity and that products of the mind would remain subordinate to the word of God.[3] In any case, for most

---

[1] John Cotton, "Preface," *The Whole Book of Psalms Faithfully Translated into English Metre* (*Bay Psalm Book*) (1640; Early American Imprints, Series 1, no. 4) n.p.

[2] William Bradford, *Of Plymouth Plantation, 1620-1647*, ed. Samuel Eliot Morison (1856; New York: Knopf, 1952) 3.

[3] For a useful introduction to colonial New England conceptions of writing, see N. H. Keeble, "Puritanism and Literature," *The Cambridge Companion to*

seventeenth-century New Englanders the mission to cultivate the land and deal with its Native inhabitants reigned superior to composing words that were designed merely to please or entertain the reader. Hence, many considered engaging in the production and reception of literature to be a sign of idleness and, thus, a sin.

Other colonists, especially beginning in mid-century, argued that the Bible provided a suitable model and illustration for the empowering and enlightening use of metaphors (e.g., in the Song of Solomon or the Psalms). Human beings should, therefore, engage in the production of literature, especially poetry, and use figures and images as an additional means of praising God. As David G. Miller explains, "[m]etaphors for the Puritans, then, were not ornaments of rhetoric but were instead sanctioned, necessary devices for conveying truth to human beings. Christ himself, inspired by the Spirit, used figurative language that should not be confused with statements of literal fact."[4] Most colonial authors considered metaphor to be both useful and dangerous. As a linguistic device it was useful when it revealed the truth of an object or topic through comparison and substitution; it was dangerous, however, when the direction of meaning transfer from one object or topic to another remained opaque or ambivalent. Even though many colonists viewed literature with skepticism and although there was little time to devote to writing, New Englanders produced an impressive number of diaries, spiritual autobiographies, sermons, historical accounts, captivity narratives, poems (especially elegies, promotional verses, and meditations), and other writings that employ metaphor to varying degrees. Such texts were vital for the colonists' monitoring and interpretation of their role and mission in North America as individuals and as a collective.

As shown in the preceding chapters, New England settlers frequently expressed their religious, social, and cultural expectations about, and experiences with, life in America through images of health and illness. One function of medicine-related writings in the formative decades of

*Puritanism*, ed. John Coffey and Paul C. H. Lim (New York: Cambridge UP, 2008) 309-324.

[4] David G. Miller, *The Word Made Flesh Made Word* (London: Associated UP, 1995) 29.

New England was to relieve the collective siege mentality that resulted from contacts with the "wilderness" and from political and doctrinal pressures, especially after the Restoration of Charles II in 1660. Although a broad array of colonial illness writings was energized by these contextual forces, poetry is a particularly insightful and fruitful genre for an analysis of personal and communal responses to life in early America.[5] Michael Wigglesworth, for instance, draws his illness poetry almost exclusively from the realm of Scripture, seeking to elucidate for his Calvinist readers the riddles and lessons of illness. Some of Anne Bradstreet's poems written during her quaternion phase reveal how Puritans sought to uphold Western civilization in an environment that threatened to contaminate human bodies and souls. Many of her meditational poems, moreover, illustrate how human beings, when religion relegates bodily afflictions to an unforeseen, yet ostensibly perfect divine plan, struggle to find a satisfactory interpretation of the pain and grief associated with illness. By contrast, the work of priest-physician-poet Edward Taylor, who took frequent recourse to the medical and alchemical practices of his time, enables us to understand more fully how religion, science, and the occult were not considered as divergent, mutually exclusive epistemologies but, rather, how they worked themselves palimpsestically into early New England literature.

This chapter explores how illness-related passages in the Bible and concepts drawn from Galenic humoralism and Paracelsian iatrochemistry served as a repository of tropes and metaphors for seventeenth-century American poets to advance their aesthetic and religious agendas. The following pages address how early New England

---

[5] For general studies on early New England poetry, see Kenneth B. Murdock, *Literature and Theology in Colonial New England* (Cambridge, MA: Harvard UP, 1949) 137-172; Peter White, ed., *Puritan Poets and Poetics: Seventeenth-Century American Poetry in Theory and Practice* (University Park: Pennsylvania State UP, 1985). A more recent overview of Puritan poetry is provided by Amy M. E. Morris, "Plainness and Paradox: Colonial Tensions in the Early New England Religious Lyric," *A Companion to the Literatures of Colonial America*, eds. Susan Castillo and Ivy Schweitzer (Malden: Blackwell, 2005) 501-516.

poets made sense of suffering and how they sought to reconcile their illness experiences with the aims of religion and the measures of art prescribed by their cultural environment. In a nutshell, the illness poems by Michael Wigglesworth, Anne Bradstreet, and Edward Taylor aim to align private experiences, especially regarding health issues, with New England culture at large.

One of the central questions underlying my reading of early American poetry is the extent to which words were seen or used as medicinal devices, bearing curative and redemptive powers both for the individual patient-poet and the collective readership. As a note of caution, poetry's medicinal efficacy is difficult, if not impossible, to assess because only few extant documents explicitly attest to the healing power of words.[6] The most productive approach to unveil the medicinal potential of language in early New England poetry is, therefore, heuristically, to ask, on the one hand, how colonists conceived of language as tools for the alleviation of suffering, and on the other, how poetry could contribute to the spiritual advancement of the patient. Suffering, as the ensuing analysis of early colonial verse will show, often enters the poem as imagistic, metaphoric, or rhythmic interruption(s). Instances of pain and suffering are projected from the author's interiority to the exteriority of the written page; from the personal experience seeking expression in language that resonates from and within an outside world to the communicative space of the poetic text. Searching for a rhetoric that appropriately expresses pain and suffering and that is able to comfort the sufferer or one of his/her caregivers, seventeenth-century poems offer ample opportunities for healing the illness-induced rupture in the relationship between humanity and God. Since flesh was conceived as inferior to spirit, the healing of the latter would ensure the cure of the former. However, the works by Wigglesworth, Bradstreet, and Taylor, while repeatedly stressing the potentiality of words to transform suffering into edification, at times convey a lingering sense of uncertainty about language's ability to fully extract redemption out of the debilitating state of illness.

---

[6] For a useful overview of the intersections between literature and medicine, see G. S. Rousseau, "Literature and Medicine: Towards a Simultaneity of Theory and Practice," *Literature and Medicine* 5.2 (1986): 152-181.

Michael Wigglesworth, "Physician of the Soul and Body"

Of the three poets discussed in this chapter, Michael Wigglesworth has been the least appreciated colonial author among scholars of early American literature. Following the stigmatization of his work as aesthetically deficient and religiously rigid during the nineteenth century, twentieth-century critics, with few exceptions, have placed Wigglesworth's poetic achievement below that of Anne Bradstreet and Edward Taylor.[7] Wigglesworth was a particularly staunch defender of Puritanism who relentlessly sought to discover evil in his own soul and that of others. Therefore, his poetry was geared toward disseminating doctrine rather than striving for aesthetic innovation. This is particularly evident in his illness poetry. In many of his reflections on sickness as a veiled sign from God, Wigglesworth seeks to give pain a language that can redeem the patient physically and spiritually. Such an endeavor, however, reaches, and must reach, its epistemological and representational limits, for pain and suffering during illness perpetually elude capture in language.

Partly due to his chronic sicknesses that kept him from attending to his ministerial duties at Malden, partly because of his desire to facilitate personal and collective healing, Wigglesworth turned to writing poetry in the mid-1650s. In his works, he casts himself as an idealized Puritan Everyman who is less concerned with conveying beauty or presenting a subject at odds with the world than with expressing his private reflections about God—with the Bible as constant reference and metatext. Written mostly in ballad meter, Wigglesworth's first and most

---

[7] For a review of the criticism of Wigglesworth's poetry, see Ronald A. Bosco, Introduction, *The Poems of Michael Wigglesworth*, ed. Ronald A. Bosco (Lanham: UP of America, 1989) ix-xvii; Allan H. Pope, "Petrus Ramus and Michael Wigglesworth: The Logic of Poetic Structure," *Puritan Poets and Poetics: Seventeenth-Century American Poetry in Theory and Practice*, ed. Peter White (University Park: Pennsylvania State UP, 1985) 210-212. Most references to Wigglesworth's life in section are taken from Richard Crowder, *No Featherbed to Heaven: A Biography of Michael Wigglesworth, 1631-1705* (East Lansing: Michigan State UP, 1962).

popular poem, "The Day of Doom" (1661), unfolds an apocalyptic scenario during which earthly sinners are separated from the regenerate.[8] With unveiled didacticism the speaker urges his reader over a course of 224 stanzas to prepare for an event whose beginnings are already evident in all walks of colonial life: the Day of Judgment and the Second Coming of Christ. Many New Englanders, then and later, considered the year 1661 as a watershed for the colony. It was marked by the end of Puritan reign in England, the contentious debate over the Half-Way Covenant, the steady arrival of settlers of different denominations, new intellectual currents heralding the rise of science (marked by the founding of the Royal Society in London), a variety of natural disasters, appearances of comets, struggles with the Natives, diseases, and witchcraft prosecutions. To the sense that the end of the world as they knew it was near, added the colonists' observation of a seeming increase of immorality and materialism. It is this overall socio-cultural context to which Wigglesworth's poems "The Day of Doom" and "God's Controversy with New-England" (1662) respond.

## Disease and Jeremiad

As a means of rationalizing and assessing the political, cultural, and spiritual turmoil that New Englanders discovered all around them, ministers found (in the Bible) a textual format—the jeremiad—that describes the current state of affairs and compares it to a more glorious past. It also devises a plan of action according to which pious settlers

---

[8] "The Day of Doom" constituted Wigglesworth's first "bestseller" and one of the most widely read literary texts throughout seventeenth-century New England. Scholars of American literature have identified the poem as an exemplar of everything they found appalling about America's Puritan settlers. For instance, John C. Adams argues that "the verses read as if he is speaking with his head barely lifted from a pillow. His neck muscles are straining but concealed, with the sheets pulled up to his chin. He is rasping out the pain-filled rhythms of the *Day of Doom* after reading his Bible for solace in the loneliness of his room—his own analog of hell." John C. Adams, "Alexander Richardson and the Ramist Poetics of Michael Wigglesworth," *Early American Literature* 25.3 (1990): 280. See also, Gerhard T. Alexis, "Wigglesworth's 'Easiest Room,'" *The New England Quarterly* 42.4 (1969): 573-583.

can return to the foundational moral values and standards of the first generation of settlers and, thereby, reaffirm their covenant with God. The purpose of these jeremiads, as Sacvan Bercovitch has shown, was to "direct an imperiled people of God toward the fulfillment of their destiny, to guide them individually toward salvation, and collectively toward the American city of God."[9] As such, the jeremiad marked a ritualized response to a number of signs that the people of Massachusetts Bay Colony interpreted as indications of the declension of the social and religious order.

Wigglesworth employs the jeremiad formula in his first two poems, "The Day of Doom" and "God's Controversy with New-England" and, in doing so, transposes a sermonic theme and structure to verse form. Like all narrative jeremiads, which were sounded from pulpits throughout New England, Wigglesworth's versified history of the region glorifies the arrival of English settlers and reflects on a social formation that is already declining. In sermonic form, jeremiads warn that, if the people of New England fail to fulfill their part in the covenant with God, the downfall of the "city upon a hill" will be imminent. Wigglesworth's poems approach this theme from different intellectual and rhetorical angles. Both works hinge on the Puritan belief in millennialism, the conviction that the apocalyptic destruction of the world is looming and that the Second Coming of Christ and his thousand-year reign, the millennium, is forthcoming.[10] In "The Day of Doom," the sickbed experience is connected to the fate of unrepentant sinners at Judgment

---

[9] Sacvan Bercovitch, *The American Jeremiad* (Madison: U of Wisconsin, P, 1978) 8-9.

[10] The term "millennialism" designates an apocalyptical spirituality according to which the Reformation has set in motion the fall of the Antichrist (Pope) and the ultimate return of Christ to earth. Many Calvinists did not necessarily believe that Christ would re-appear in body, but rather that his influence would increase and that the complete rule of the saints would be established. The millennial promise assured believers that the community they had established acted out a divine plan that would eventually lead towards a positive resolution. See the essays collected in Bernd Engler, Jörg O. Fichte, and Oliver Scheiding, eds., *Millennial Thought in America: Historical and Intellectual Contexts, 1630-1860* (Trier: WVT, 2002).

Day and thus serves as an indication of infinitely more intense suffering in the next life. The unregenerate, in

> pain and grief have no relief,
>      their anguish never endeth.
> There they must ly, and never dy,
>      though dying every day:
> There must they dying every ly,
>      and not consume away.[11]

The use of anaphora and assonance in this stanza illustrates the linkage between illness, death, suffering, and hell, while the rugged rhymes and somber imagery emphasize the overall sense of doom that sickness anticipates and represents.

Wigglesworth's next poem, "God's Controversy with New-England," places the theme of the millennium and the prospects of salvation already staged in "The Day of Doom" in a more immediate context and takes its cue from a recent drought in New England. By directing audience attention toward the spiritual and worldly implications of their previous and current actions, the poem offers a mythologized history of English colonialism. In keeping with the jeremiad formula, Wigglesworth's verse recollects the achievements and righteousness of the early colonists before configuring the Great Migration as a sign of divine election and thus raising the arrival of Protestantism in North America to mythic proportions:

> Until the time drew nigh wherein
>      The glorious Lord of hostes
> Was pleasd to lead his armies forth
>      Into those forrein coastes. (90, l. 37-40)

The New England portrayed by Wigglesworth, complete with the serenity of a small group of Puritan settlers humbly building their

---

[11] Michael Wigglesworth, *The Poems of Michael Wigglesworth*, ed. Ronald A. Bosco (Lanham: UP of America, 1989) 63, l. 1673-1680. In the following, excerpts from the author's poems will be cited parenthetically, with page numbers followed by line numbers.

society of the godly, is reminiscent of Adam and Eve's entrance into Paradise. Indeed, the typological references to Genesis are deliberate attempts at blending earthly and heavenly realms, preparing the reader to accept the historic and cosmic significance of the colonial endeavor. It is by linking "America" with "Eden" that the poem attempts to withstand the current trend of waning spiritualism, designating declension as a typological extension of the Fall that can only be countered by fully engaging in the covenant of grace.

During the 67 stanzas that comprise "God's Controversy with New-England," the poetic voice re-enacts the past as an errand into the wilderness that derived its justification from being part of a cosmic battle between God and Satan. By the time Wigglesworth penned his poetic rendition of the region's history that altogether disavowed its pre-contact past, the narrative of how the colony had been settled in accordance with divine providence was already firmly entrenched in the collective cultural unconscious of New England. Wigglesworth appropriates and versifies this narrative and by emphasizing the rearrangement of Native-English power hierarchies in the wake of diseases, the poem helps to sustain the discourse of medical providentialism. Commenting on how Native Americans reacted to the arrival of epidemics from Europe, he writes,

> Some hid themselves for fear of thee
>> In forests wide & great
> Some to thy people croutching came,
>> For favour to entreat. (91, l. 65-68)

Although the obvious addressee of these lines is God, the poem can easily be re-read to speak to the contemporary New England reader, reminding him/her that there once was a time when God's preference for the English colonists translated into medical signs. In sync with the narrative purported by John Winthrop and other colonists, Wigglesworth's poetic voice casts the events surrounding the arrival of the colonists in historical and biblical terms. Accordingly, New England was cleared by the hand of God, leaving only a handful of Native people who stoop in fear of further diseases and bow in submission to the newly arrived settlers, who seemed to be the likely yet unconfirmed source of disease and, more importantly, the consistently healthier group.

In "God's Controversy with New-England," the past with its
providential medical occurrences is contrasted with a present that
appears strikingly different because the colonists have failed to build the
intended heaven-directed society. From the poem's subtitle, "New
England planted, prospered, declining, threatened, punished," the reader
already infers that the colony's spiritual decline is inevitable. The poem
firmly erects a vision of a colony whose purpose is still justified and
intact, and who only needs to maintain the path laid out by Christ. The
turning point occurs in verse 16 when the speaker deplores the passing
of "thy first, / [...] thy best estate" (93, l. 141-142). Here, the titular
controversy unfolds as Wigglesworth's speaker recedes into the
background and gives way to God's voice between stanzas 18 and 48.
Set off from the previous section in theme, tone, orthography, and
supported by a shift from ballad meter to a more complex verse structure
(five decasyllabic lines and a concluding hexameter), the second voice
in the dramatic staging is introduced by an interrogating refrain: "Are
these the men that [...]" (94-95). This accusatory anaphora underlines
the overall reprimand for New England's backsliding that guides the
poem's rhetorical maneuvering as a whole. Wigglesworth's
impersonation of God's voice conveys a wrathful deity that is appalled
by how the colonists have departed from the foundational vision of
utopian brotherhood on the American strand:

> How is it, that Security, and Sloth,
> Amongst the best are Common to be found?
> That grosser sins, in stead of Graces growth,
> Amongst the many more and more abound?
> I hate dissembling shews of Holiness.
> Or practise as you talk, or never more profess. (96, l. 229-234)

Through the "dissembling shews of Holiness," the authorial staging
of a disappointed Creator presents a warning against hypocrisy and
conversion accounts that avoid the truth about the confessants' inner
estates. The author's hermeneutics of suspicion about New Englanders'
prospects for individual and collective salvation extends to the
relationship between the poetic voice and the audience: on the one hand,
the reader is the object of education; on the other hand, the depravity of
the sinning colonial subject must remain intact for the poem's *raison
d'être* to prevail.

As Jeffrey Hammond has observed, the persuasive success of the poem, as well as of other doomsday writings, depends on "the rhetorical split between the reading self and the saintly metaself."[12] In Wigglesworth's poem, the reading self is directed towards realizing its deviance from the ideals of its saintly metaself, an idealistic persona constructed by the poem's speaker to describe the contours of a devout and pious Puritan destined for eternal bliss. By outlining the discrepancy between the actual and ideal selves, Wigglesworth urges his reader to take responsibility for the current fall of New England. Since the author considers himself as a buffer between the wrath of God and the sins of His people, he can attempt to direct the actions of his fellow wo/men by offering words designed as an antidote to the spiritual sickness that presumably afflicts the colony as a whole. In order to facilitate collective recovery, the reader is asked to align his inner self with the Puritan metaself, an act of healing purported to alleviate the current crisis of the New England way.

After the original poetic voice returns to the foreground, the attention shifts to how the warnings about God's punishment for unappreciative New Englanders are already becoming manifest outside the poem's internal chronotope. Following the New England sermonic tradition, Wigglesworth's explication outlined in the previous sections of the poem and the application of Calvinist doctrine centers around two divine signs: epidemics and droughts. The former are introduced in the last third of "God's Controversy with New-England":

> Our healthfull dayes are at an end,
>     And sicknesses come on
> From yeer to yeer, becaus our hearts
>     Away from God are gone.
> New-England, where for many years
>     You scarcely heard a cough,
> And where Physicians had no work,
>     Now finds them work enough. (99, l. 359-366)

---

[12] Jeffrey A. Hammond, *Sinful Self, Saintly Self: The Puritan Experience of Poetry* (Athens: U of Georgia P, 1993) 52.

As the poetic voice laments the arrival of illness as a sign and consequence of declension, it supports the discourse of medical providentialism while, at the same time, turning the original narrative of New England's foundation on its head. The explanation for the decline of colonial health is, according to the poem, solely rooted in the loss of immunity granted by the divine. Epidemics and providence are not divergent in the poem because as much as Native Americans died "for a purpose," so this time the collective illnesses of colonists are justified by the previous backsliding of the community. Here, however, divine providence as a hermeneutic model is turning against itself. By positioning the colonists as the afflicted, the narrative of biological determinism established by the first generation of New Englanders is revised and reversed:

> Now colds and coughs, Rhewms, and sore-throats,
> > Do more and more abound:
> Now Agues sore & Feavers strong
> > In every place are found.
> How many houses have we seen
> > Last Autumn, and this spring,
> Wherein the healthful were too few
> > To help the languishing. (100, l. 367-374)

Wigglesworth's speaker subtly shifts from the individual to the multitude: the first illnesses represented in the stanza—"colds and coughs, Rhewms, and sore-throats" (367)—represent the author's own afflictions.[13] Then, the poetic self discovers that illness has become de-personalized, as it were, spreading throughout the settler community. Sickness no longer signifies a disturbed relationship between the individual sinner and God but signals the metaphorical contamination of the New England covenant by the settlers. The last two lines of the stanza echo Bradford's depiction of Algonquian smallpox survivors who are unable to help their dying peers, as seen in chapter one. The original New England disease scenario, during which suffering and dying Native

---

[13] Cf. Michael Wigglesworth, *The Diary of Michael Wigglesworth, 1653-1657. The Conscience of a Puritan*, ed. Edmund S. Morgan (1946; New York: Harper, 1965) 88.

Americans evoked pity and sympathy in English observers, is repeated in Wigglesworth's poem, albeit with a significant difference. This time, illness, as a tool and sign of divine will and power, no longer follows a person's religious affiliation, social status or physiological features; instead, the causes and consequences of illness are portrayed as universal. As the colonists are humbled by disease, their weakness is exacerbated by more epidemics (and droughts), all of which are posited as divine means reminding English colonists of their initial mission:

> One wave another followeth,
>> And one disease begins
> Before another cease, becaus
>> We turn not from our sins.
> We stopp our ear against reproof,
>> And hearken not to God:
> God stops his ear against our prayer,
>> And takes not off his rod. (100, l. 375-382)

The repetition of to "stop [an] ear" establishes a reciprocity between the elect's renunciation of God's providential plan and the deity's similar, yet infinitely more causative aversion from His chosen few. Hence, the continuation of punishment ("And takes not off his rod" [l. 382]) is portrayed as utterly justified and deserved. The speaker's own position is that of observer, commentator, and fellow sinner, whose alliance with the reader is established by the pronoun "we." As part of the community, the speaker casts himself as an individual who is, to some extent, responsible for the events that are unfolding. Similar to the question recorded in Wigglesworth's diary, "Sicknesses, death of godly ones, wants, divisions have not my sins a hand in these miserys?," the relationship between personal sin and communal suffering is here also apparent: the speaker continually oscillates between being an observer and being among the observed.[14] Since most colonists believed that due to their covenant with God, individual transgressions entailed far-reaching consequences for the community as a whole, the sin of one member reflected that of all.

---

[14] Wigglesworth, *Diary* 82.

One of Wigglesworth's main remedies for the sicknesses of New England, then, is a personal and communal re-alignment with the laws of Scripture rather than turning towards science.[15] The statement, "Unless thou quickly change" (101, l. 426), opens up a window of opportunity for action on the part of the colonists and thus counters the notion that illness, as part and parcel of divine providence, must be humbly endured. In anticipating later, more full-fledged jeremiads, Wigglesworth's poem claims that the signs of the time signal the declension of New England; however, the fate of the colony rests, in part at least, in the hands of the settlers, whose thoughts and actions are envisioned as potentially pleasing to God and as still being able to avert His punishing rod. This is especially evident in the final stanza of the poem, when the reader is led to the conclusion that there remains time and opportunity to act:

> Cheer on, sweet souls, my heart is with you all,
> And shall be with you, maugre Sathan's might:
> And whereso'ere this body be a Thrall,
> Still in New-England shall be my delight. (102, l. 443-446)

Wigglesworth's message seems clear at this point: if spiritual deadness, stasis, and distance from God is New England's disease, then prayer, repentance, obedience, and piety is the cure. What the poem fails to mention, though, is that illness will prevail no matter how close the collective approximates divine will and adheres to His laws, because sin according to Christian logic is inevitable. For the author, any scientific explanatory approach or remedy for the current state of New England needs to be disavowed and suppressed because it would question the assumption that underlies the colonial project as a whole: that there was

---

[15] We know from various elegies that Wigglesworth was a respected physician and more than likely supplemented his meager income by offering his medical knowledge to ill colonists. Wigglesworth owned a copy of Harvey's 1628 treatise on blood circulation, a few alchemical books, Culpeper's *English Physician*, and other medical standards of his age. See the library list in Adams 130.

a healthier time in New England due entirely to God's blessing and that this state can be recovered by religious means. In sound jeremiad fashion, the only way to turn the affliction of the colonists into something positive is to view it as an affirmation of the Puritans' special status as covenanted believers.

## Meat Out of the Eater, Or How to Become a True Christian Sufferer

In "Meat Out of the Eater" (1670), Michael Wigglesworth turns from epidemics as divine punishment to the spiritual significance of diverse kinds of afflictions, among them illnesses. The main theme in "Meat Out of the Eater" is how to draw blessings out of tribulations, a theme which rests on the premise that to be worthy of Christ, one must suffer through illness.[16] The title of the poem paraphrases Samson's riddle in Judges 14:14—"Out of the eater came forth meat, and out of the strong came forth sweetness"—and recasts a central Christian dilemma that is addressed throughout the ensuing meditations and songs that comprise the work: why does God allow those who follow His word to suffer on earth? "Meat Out of the Eater" is organized along a number of riddles whose poeticized solutions are geared toward possible answers to this pivotal question. By offering the reader various poetic musings on an ensemble of enigmas and paradoxes that a believer may encounter during the search for salvific evidence in his/her life, Wigglesworth designs a poetic manual for dealing with a broad array of human afflictions: sickness, physical weakness, poverty, confinement, solitude, sorrow, and death. For the reader, a first clue to the riddle of how to gain spiritual advancement from afflictions may be derived from merging the two nouns of the poem's title ("meat" and "eater") into the word "meter." Seen this way, poetry, particularly his own, is presented as Wigglesworth's guide to discovering a potential solvent for bodily and spiritual illnesses, one that is explicitly designed to supplement, rather than to substitute, biblical means of coping with affliction.

---

[16] For a more general reading of Wigglesworth's poem, see Walter Hughes, "'Meat Out of the Eater': Panic and Desire in American Puritan Poetry," *Engendering Men: The Question of Male Feminist Criticism*, ed. Joseph Allen Boone and Michael Cadden (New York: Routledge, 1990) 102-121.

In the first section of "Meat Out of the Eater," entitled "Light in Darkness," the minister-poet-physician offers a synopsis of the major afflictions and their treatment in the poem. Illness is closely linked to the patient's spiritual constitution when Wigglesworth's speaker relates:

> While Physick is at work,
> Ill Humours are disturb'd:
> So while Chastisement are at work,
> Corruptions may be stirr'd.
> They do but shew what was
> Within the heart before:
> They may discover hidden Lusts,
> They do not make them more. (156, l. 33-40)

Here, the speaker connects the rearrangement of bodily humors underlying sickness to divine punishment intervening in the sinner's life. Illness disrupts what Jacques Derrida, following Jean-Jacques Rousseau, would later call a "continual present" in and through God by introducing a temporality, a before, during, and after.[17] This temporal discontinuity shapes not only the patient's disease experience but also its representation in poetic space. For the reader, engaging with the poem entails viewing the illness as an occasion for dealing with the relatively mild effects of sin *now* (through introspection and repentance at regular intervals) rather than bearing the full brunt of God's wrath *later*, at the Day of Judgment.

Wigglesworth's attempt to render his denomination's medico-religious doctrine of divine affliction acceptable among colonists from all walks of life is further evinced in the next stanza.

> Gods Physick is at work
> To purge Corruption out:
> And this in time he will effect,
> Believe and do not doubt.
> He first discovereth sin,
> Shews thee what wanting is,

---

[17] Jacques Derrida, *Of Grammatology*, trans. Gayatri C. Spivak (Baltimore: Johns Hopkins UP, 1976) 249.

Makes thee to feel thy need of help,
        And mourn for what's amiss. (157, l. 57-64)

In other words, for an ideal colonist, affliction means more than
mere punishment or trial: it includes the potential for redemption. With
this conceptual approach, Wigglesworth's poetics of illness ties in with
and amplifies "the discourse of afflicted specialness," which New
Englanders repeatedly employed to justify and drive their colonizing
endeavors.[18] According to this discourse, God punished the English with
disease (and other calamities) not merely as a sign of His wrath but also
as an indication of His continued interest in, and favor for, the
establishment of pious and devoted settlements.

After a general introduction of the notion of afflicted specialness,
Wigglesworth groups a series of meditations on the spiritual advantages
of illness under the title "Sick Mens Health." Again, the author's
wordplay gives ample room for interpretation since "Sick Mens Health"
can be read as "the health of sick men" or as "sick means health." With
this religious riddle, Wigglesworth anticipates a solution to the enigma
of illness and other kinds of human suffering that he addresses at the
outset of "Meat Out of the Eater." Illness occurs, he claims, to humble
the sufferer and to make him/her stronger through faith, "the substance
of things hoped for, the evidence of things not seen" (Hebrew 11:1).

Among the difficulties that the author faced in his poetic theodicy
was that his rather abstract approach to Christian paradoxes needed to
resonate with the reader's daily experiences. To achieve this end,
Wigglesworth clothed the joys and pains of God's intimate presence in
an imitable narrative so that readers could appropriate the poem's
prescriptions. Jeffrey Hammond argues that "Wigglesworth introduces
readers to themselves, inviting them to overhear a debate between doubt
and faith presented not as theological abstractions but as conflicting
halves of the reading self."[19] For the Malden poet, the key to solving
Christian enigmas and paradoxes lies in accepting that even the elect
suffer from illness (and other afflictions) and that this actually indicates

---

[18] Theresa Toulouse, "'My Own Credit': Strategies of (E)valuation in Mary
Rowlandson's Captivity Narrative," *American Literature* 64.4 (1992): 662.

[19] Hammond 74.

that God (still) cared. As a means of grace, illness could be brought to a productive end when the sufferer realizes that sin can be interpreted as a useful intervention from the invisible world and that humility marks a central pillar of salvific experience. Salvation, in this view, results from the imitation of Christ—the ultimate example of humanity—whose own controversy with God at the cross signaled the necessity of human acceptance of divine righteousness and promise of redemption. In short, affliction can bring about edification and/or signify election. As John C. Adams explains:

> Whether one is healthy or chronically ill, one must be prepared to let go of this world gracefully, with assurance, if one is going to experience one's own death, or its anticipation as an inevitability, in peace. Wigglesworth's personal suffering is a reminder that old age, chronic suffering, and infirmity are not necessarily signs of God's abandonment, but may be parts of a natural teleological progression that moves toward a positive good.[20]

Wigglesworth is clearly writing from his own experience when he outlines possible approaches to investing illness with meaning. Any chronic illness, especially if it lasted almost thirty years as in the case of Michael Wigglesworth, must have gnawed in the devout Puritan's mind.[21] While a recovery from a relatively short sickness can be deemed a sign of successful repentance, a chronic disease may signal that the sufferer has not yet fully (re)turned to Christ, a thought which must have seemed particularly baffling and worrisome for a man of learning, piety, and devotion such as Wigglesworth.

---

[20] Adams 283.

[21] Due to a lingering illness, Michael Wigglesworth was unable to attend to his ministerial duties at the church of Malden from 1657 to 1685. His illness had begun around 1652 while still a tutor at Harvard, and we know from Cotton Mather's funeral sermon for Wigglesworth that he had to give up preaching in public shortly after his ordination. Wigglesworth perhaps suffered from asthma, perhaps from a psychosomatic disorder. John Ward Dean, *Memoir of Rev. Michael Wigglesworth, Author of The Day of Doom*, 2nd ed. (Albany: Munsell, 1871) 57, 61-62.

Furthermore, Wigglesworth adds to colonial conceptualizations of illness by addressing all stages of life and not merely as an initial realization of sin as it is proposed in many lay conversion narratives. At the outset of the section "Sick mens Health," for instance, the speaker positions himself as an observer who is outside the medical marketplace of New England but dependent on it. His medicinal prescriptions are not geared at alleviating bodily conditions but to mend their underlying spiritual causes:

> I shall not intermeddle
> With the Physicians Art:
> Nor Medicines prescribe, which may
> Relieve thy Body's smart.
> But what may help thee bear
> Thine outward Misery
> With Patience, as becomes a Saint,
> And to get good thereby. (177, l. 17-24)

For Wigglesworth, the value of affliction such as illness lies in both its temporal and its spiritual dimension. Only by being relieved again after a time of intense uncertainty and suffering can the sinner reaffirm his/her faith. Illness thus becomes part and parcel of preparing for salvation; instead of merely accepting illness passively, the affliction presents an occasion to work toward one's salvation. Illness thereby retains its inherent ambiguity: it is a sign of God's hand acting on those who believe in Him, and this is actually good news.

Throughout the poem, Wigglesworth constructs his solution of the Christian paradox—the enigma of illness as source of pain and spiritual advancement—around a specific typology, namely the suffering of Job. Resounding the biblical directions on dealing with illness in the Book of Job, the speaker in "Meat Out of the Eater" claims that suffering is sent to test the moral stamina of those professing to be His people. The mystery that illness poses must be answered by a continued and renewed adherence to the New England way. Although such reflections on illness were tied to a specific time and place, Wigglesworth's speaker addresses a *universal* aspect of illness: it forces any patient to concentrate on a certain body part and triggers a thought process that aims to invest his/her suffering with meaning. In such a situation it seems necessary, even justified, to muse upon the cause behind, course of, and chances for recovery. At the same time, however, Wigglesworth's poetic responses to illness highlight many ways of conceptualizing and textualizing illness that are specifically Puritan. Like Job, Wigglesworth's speaker learns that there is still a world of wonders behind affliction and that seemingly undeserved suffering may constitute a sign of election and the covenantal relation between God and the elect:

> Diseases bodily
> May help thee to do well:
> But Soul diseases, if not cur'd,
> Will carry thee to Hell.
> Our Bodies may sometimes
> Need Physick, more then Food.
> So may our Souls need Sicknesses
> And Pain, to do them good. (183, l. 33-40)

In order to bring his overall argument to full fruition, the speaker needs to retrace repeatedly the problem of how the wicked who prosper and the holy who suffer fit into the larger godly design of the course of events on earth. In Wigglesworth's poetic interpretation of this design, the soul literally requires illness and pain for its approximation of Christ. Illness can only be re-inscribed affirmatively by configuring the relationship between soul and body as negatively reciprocal (what is good for the body is dangerous for the soul and vice versa) because "Our Bodies Sicknesses / Are Physick for the Soul" (l. 41-42). For the poet, illness becomes a source of strength when it functions as a test of righteousness rather than a mere punishment for sin. In other words, the question why New England Protestants suffer can only be answered in a meaningful way when sickness is considered in terms of the spiritual benefits it entails for the patient. In this sense, Job and the poem can speak of the curative purpose of sickness, sent to remind the sinner of the heavenly rewards that God grants His chosen people.

In "Sick mens Health," Wigglesworth's speaker uses the image of bloodletting as part of God's divine curative panoply, for "he purgeth out / Bad Humours, namely Pride, / Self-love, Impatience, Worldliness" (184, l. 57-60). The release of "corrupted" blood in poetic space becomes a cathartic act similar to the drinking of holy wine during the

Lord's Supper and is positioned as a means of cleansing impurities of the body and the soul.[22] The author's choice of words seeks to produce an edifying effect in the reader. In the closing stanzas of the poem, Faith and Fear are employed as allegorized companions to those Puritans subjected to a serious illness and stage a debate whose resolution resounds Wigglesworth's central message that illness should be considered as a source of, and opportunity for, spiritual advancement. Once again, the patient is asked to both endure in humility all the negative bodily sensations and spiritual battles, including pain, fear of wrath, looming death, and to withstand the Jobean temptation to renounce God as the sovereign and righteous mover of all things on earth. If successful, the suffering Puritan will not only regain his health but will emerge from the illness as a more refined and pious believer.

In sum, Wigglesworth's work aims to rationalize diseases as highly significant spiritual experiences through poetic compression of Calvinist discourse on matters of health and illness. Largely devoid of elaborate metaphor or symbolism, the plain-style rhetoric of the Malden poet strives to capture the theological essence of illness by approaching the poetic arts with the firm notion that language means what it states. Expressing the author's belief in the essence of language and Christian presence, his poems repeatedly address a paradox between the bodily experience of pain, agony, and suffering and the affirmative spiritual meaning these corporeal sensations can potentially generate. For Wigglesworth, poetry may heal by providing access to biblical directions on how to transform illness into salvific occasions. One should not, therefore, dismiss Wigglesworth's poetry for being trite or simplistic all too readily. He was certainly a gloomy poet whose doggerel verse reflecting humanity's spiritual condition lacks the artistic merit that most twenty-first-century readers look for in a good poem.

---

[22] As Patricia Watson explains, "[a]lthough the practice of blood letting dates back to the time of Hippocrates, with the rise of Christianity, phlebotomy may have taken on a religious aura: as Christ 'gave his blood' to redeem mankind of his sins, so man's blood becomes 'corrupt' in many illnesses, and he must 'give blood' like Christ did in order to purify the body and restore the balance of the four humours." Patricia Ann Watson, *The Angelical Conjunction: The Preacher-Physicians of Colonial New England* (Knoxville: U of Tennessee P, 1991) 87.

However, his plain-style rhetoric and general denial of metaphor create a predictability that offsets the tumultuous pangs of the soul addressed in the poems' contents. In this sense, Wigglesworth's poetry was almost ideally suited for Puritan edification and education. The poetic structure offers a sense of serenity, calmness, and predictability that anchors the seeking and doubting believer in Christ. Although most verses leave the reader anxious about the consequences of evoking God's wrath, the predictable verse structure and thematic resolutions aim to offer solace and a soothing anticipation of salvation for the devout recipient. The difficulty of having to explain the axiom "Christians suffer" lies in accounting for why and how God blesses humanity through chastisement, especially illness. Using language that is accessible and comprehensible for his seventeenth-century audience, Wigglesworth explains the paradox of illness while, at the same time, warning that the desire for health should never exceed the desire for holiness. Sickness temporarily separates the believer from God, the poet claims, but if faith is maintained, the reunion with the divine will be all the more rewarding.

Meditations on illness as poeticized by Michael Wigglesworth were central for the Calvinists' emphasis on practical divinity, because they addressed tangible occasions for transforming doubt and uncertainty into assurance. When seeking knowledge of salvation with Puritan zeal, however, the ubiquity of disease in colonial America posed continual and often life-long challenges for devout New England colonists. While writing about how to cope with illness in the rather abstract and sermonic mode of the jeremiad, Wigglesworth's private experience with illness rarely controls the direction of his verse. By contrast, Anne Bradstreet takes her illnesses as self-referential moments that induce intimate meditations and seek expression in verse.

Rebellion Reconsidered: Anne Bradstreet's Medical Verses

Writing poetry throughout her life, Anne Bradstreet aimed at serving practical rather than theoretical ends. "Many can speak well, but few can do well," she begins the second entry of her meditations, arguing that "[w]e are better scholars in the theory than the practic [sic] part, but he is a true Christian that is a proficient in both."[23] This fundamental intellectual trajectory can be traced in most of Bradstreet's artistic works and distinguishes her, among other things, from Michael Wigglesworth. Her illness poems, especially, are concerned with the doctrinal as well as practical implications of bodily distempers. Similar to most other colonial writings at the time, the recourse to biblical models marks a constant undercurrent of her illness poetry; however, her reflections on sickness often transgress the boundaries of mere doctrinal affirmation. Bradstreet's illness poems attempt to translate her intellectual approach to theory and practice into a poetic principle by emphasizing deeds over words. On several occasions in her writing, Bradstreet highlights the notion that words randomly assembled can only insufficiently grant God full gratitude for his manifold gifts to humanity. True thanksgiving requires "speech acts" and hence the transformation of words into poetic offerings is considered as one possibility of action in return for deliverance. According to Bradstreet's artistic agenda, by versifying and abstracting base human experiences, poetic language can take on a material quality and as such constitutes a deed, both as a renewal of the covenant in the legal sense, and as an act or performance by a devout, intelligent, and responsible agent in a practical sense. While poetry is thus conceptualized and employed as a useful response to poor health, illness itself becomes an impetus for practicality, for it prompts the colonist to take up her pen and write a poem of gratitude, reflection, and education.

Much of the twentieth-century debate about Bradstreet's work has revolved around the question whether her verse presents a speaking voice that accords with, or deviates from, Puritan orthodoxy. Ann Stanford, for instance, has detected a division in Bradstreet's poetics between dogmatism and rebellion. She argues that, "in her determination to write and in her defense of the capability of women to reason, to contemplate, and to read widely, she showed herself capable of taking a stand against the more conservative and dogmatic of her

---

[23] Anne Bradstreet, *The Works of Anne Bradstreet*, ed. Jeannine Hensley (Cambridge, MA: Belknap P of Harvard UP, 1967) 272. In the following, Bradstreet's words will be cited parenthetically; poems will be quoted with line number following page numbers.

contemporaries."[24] In more recent considerations of Bradstreet's religious and poetic stance, scholars have unraveled many of the complexities involved in her affirmation or contestation of Puritan orthodoxy. They have shown her rebellion to be either sparked by gender issues (Harvey) or by her anti-Puritan sentiments (Stanford) and her compliance with doctrine (Daly).[25] I concur with Jeffrey Hammond's New Historicist assessment that once we view Bradstreet's poetry in the context of colonial New England religious culture, her occasional rebellion against God emerges as part of the morphology of conversion and was thus largely in keeping with seventeenth-century religious dogma.[26] Hammond's context-specific approach to reading Bradstreet's work seems especially useful for an analysis of her medical verses. Similar to her grief and love poems, Bradstreet's illness poetry emphasizes that suffering should be seen as a pedagogical tool of the divine, urging the believer not to attach him/herself too strongly to the material world. Her poems attempt to "make sense" of illness by illuminating the constant circling back and forth between doubt and assurance. Bradstreet's illness poetry hence serves a crucial salvific function in presenting a self who has embarked on a pilgrimage to salvation during which the traveler frequently deviates from her path toward Christ, especially during times of poor health.[27]

[24] Ann Stanford, "Anne Bradstreet: Dogmatist and Rebel," *New England Quarterly* 39.3 (1966): 378.

[25] Tamara Harvey, "'Now Sisters ... Impart Your Usefulnesse, And Force': Anne Bradstreet's Feminist Functionalism in *The Tenth Muse* (1650)," *Early American Literature* 35.1 (2000): 5-28; Robert Daly, *God's Altar: The World and the Flesh in Puritan Poetry* (Berkeley: U of California P, 1972) 82-127; Stanford 380-382.

[26] Hammond 84-85.

[27] For a more concise version of the following sections, see my "'Too Many My Diseases to Cite': Anne Bradstreet's Illness Poetry," *The Writing Cure: Literature and Medicine in Context*, ed. Alexandra Lembert and Jarmila Mildorf (Münster: LIT, 2013) 115-134.

Galenic Poetry: "Of the Four Humours in Man's Constitution"

Since the 1960s scholars have tended to divide Bradstreet's work into two phases: her early (public) poems, which display the poet's reverence for Renaissance learning, and her later (private) writings, which are often conceived of as more liberated and personalized works of self-reflection.[28] In the more recent past, this division into a public/imitative and a private/original phase and voice in Bradstreet's poetry, particularly when each is valued according to artistic standards from a twentieth-century perspective, has been challenged in the secondary literature. Robert Daly suggests, for instance, that readers should recognize the multiple sense of voice and presence expressed in Bradstreet's poems, especially when they enact dialogues between several speakers.[29] This is the case throughout her work, especially in "The Flesh and the Spirit," "A Dialogue between Old England and New," and in the quaternions.[30] The latter comprised the bulk of

[28] Kenneth Requa, "Anne Bradstreet's Poetic Voices," *Early American Literature* 9.1 (1974): 3-18.

[29] Robert Daly, "Powers of Humility and the Presence of Readers in Anne Bradstreet and Phillis Wheatley," *Puritanism in America: The Seventeenth through the Nineteenth Centuries*, ed. Michael Schuldiner, Studies in Puritan American Spirituality, vol. 4 (Lewiston: Mellen, 1993) 9-10. Cf. Rosamond Rosenmeier, *Anne Bradstreet Revisited* (Boston: Twayne, 1991) 114, who considers the alleged private/public split in Bradstreet's poetry as overly schematic. For a similar argument, see Eileen Margerum, "Anne Bradstreet's Public Poetry and the Tradition of Humility," *Early American Literature* 17.2 (1982): 152-160. The multivocality in Bradstreet's work is analyzed in Kimberly Cole Winebrenner, "Bradstreet's Emblematic Marriage," *Puritanism in America: The Seventeenth through the Nineteenth Centuries*, ed. Michael Schuldiner, Studies in Puritan American Spirituality, vol. 4 (Lewiston: Mellen, 1993) 45-70.

[30] Since Adrienne Rich's foreword to *The Works of Anne Bradstreet* (1967), the quaternions have often been read as inferior to the poet's later poems and have only recently received attention that looks beyond their ostensibly "pedestrian, abstract, mechanical" characteristics. Adrienne Rich, "Anne Bradstreet and Her Poetry," *The Works of Anne Bradstreet*, ed. Jeannine Hensley (Cambridge, MA: Belknap P of Harvard UP, 1967) xii. For an important revisionary study of

Bradstreet's first publication, *The Tenth Muse Lately Sprung up in America* (1650), a collection of poems that after its publication in England was celebrated as emblems of colonial American writing and for upholding European values and advancements in the "wilderness." The poems' echoes of learnedness from the shores of America seek to convince their readers of Western civilization's ability to prosper in different regions of the globe. They display the female author's familiarity with world knowledge in steps of four: the elements, humors, life-stages, and seasons. These "apprentice poems" make almost no reference to religious doctrine but rather rejoice in the visible world, human capacities, and the ability of the poet to mold academic knowledge into rhyme and meter.[31] With this approach, the quaternions function as performative statements through which the poetic self asserts itself in and through Renaissance learning rather than through Christ proper.[32]

The second of the four quaternions, "Of the Four Humours in Man's Constitution," follows Protestant poetic guidelines, echoed in Sir Philip Sidney's dictum (drawn from Horace) that verse should "teach and delight," and reflects the author's intent to write pedagogical texts for local students.[33] The poem is orchestrated as an allegorical dialogue

---

Bradstreet's quaternions, see Carrie Galloway Blackstock, "Anne Bradstreet and Performativity: Self-Cultivation, Self-Deployment," *Early American Literature* 32.3 (1997): 222-248.

[31] Jane Donahue Eberwein, "The 'Unrefined Ore' of Anne Bradstreet's Quaternions," *Early American Literature* 9.1 (1974): 19.

[32] This is not to say, however, that Bradstreet's quaternions can easily be enlisted to support the argument that her work counters Puritan orthodoxy. Rather, the realm of acceptable knowledge in seventeenth-century New England evoked and even demanded expressions of worldly learning.

[33] Sir Philip Sidney, *Defence of Poesie* (1581), trans. Richard Bear, University of Oregon, 1992 <http://poetry.eserver.org/defense-of-poesie.txt> 3 March 2011. Elizabeth Ferszt has pointed out that the quaternions were in all likelihood written in response to the 1642 Massachusetts law that required parents to instruct their children in reading and writing. She considers Bradstreet's early poems as easily adaptable for classroom use, teaching history, medicine, husbandry, and the human condition in general. Elizabeth Ferszt, *Rejecting a*

between choler (or yellow bile), blood, phlegm, and melancholy (or black bile). Rather than conveying specific medical treatment methods, Bradstreet's medical quaternion, which consists of 611 lines, uses Galenic humoralism to devise a corporeal and mental lesson for the reader. In the course of the poem, Bradstreet lets each of the four humors, which are depicted as daughters of the four elements, enter the stage of the poem successively. Each then voices her special benefits and exposes the threats other humors pose to human health and constitution. For instance, the first allegorical figure, Choler, who resides in the heart, develops her poetic monologue around a defense of her territory in the body against the remaining three humors and, by doing so, sets the tone and diction for the contest over preeminence in the human body. The anatomical instruction of the reader continues when Choler grants Phlegm supremacy over the brain and Melancholy dominance over the spleen. The appearance of Blood in the second section of the poem allows the poetic voice to contest Choler's claim of superiority by highlighting the negative aspects of the other humors (e.g., Blood states that Choler is responsible for anger and pride and causes jaundice). In doing so, the poem extends the physiological lesson, outlining the location and function of each humor in the body, to the realm of the mind. Because the four voices allegorize and enact human character traits, they also teach the reader how to understand and deal with different personalities.

When Melancholy takes issue with the statements of her previous two contenders, her strategy of asserting her exceptional role in the body refrains from rhetorical attacks on Choler and Blood—"But rather I with silence veil her [Choler's] shame / Than cause her blush, while I relate the same" (46, l. 473-474). Melancholy thus introduces a different strategy of interaction and conflict-resolution when, toward the end of her monologue, she states her role in causing mental illnesses. Rather than highlighting her own advantages and the disadvantages of her siblings in an attempt to declare her preeminence in the body, Melancholy prepares the reader for the resolution of the poem in which peaceful coexistence is stressed over a confrontation about hierarchies.

*New English Aesthetic: The Early Poems of Anne Bradstreet*, Diss. Wayne State U, 2006, 5-6.

Before Melancholy can fully unfold her message, however, Phlegm
takes the stage and changes the terms of contest and debate by
portraying herself as lacking the rhetorical and physiological weapons of
her predecessors. Phlegm claims her place and value in the human body,
not by boasting about her own abilities or denigrating those of her
sisters, but by arguing that, because she is located in the brain, she
connects all four humors and thereby formulates the central idea and
theme of the poem: unity. Having reached the final lines of the
quaternion, Bradstreet uses Phlegm to express her conviction that "thou
and I must make a mixture here" (50, l. 589) to the reader.

As a text for students to learn vocabulary, grammar, and rhetoric, the
quaternion   outlines   the   theoretical   background   necessary   for
understanding the human body and mind.[34] However, the poem does
more than merely teach physiology. The poem's pivotal theme and
lesson is unity, suggesting that coexistence among the battling humors
and a balance of their individual strengths and weaknesses is vital for
human health. This application also stresses balance as a necessity for
the psychosocial unity of the community of colonial readers who, as
individuals, are forced to recognize their own character traits in the
figures staged in the poem. In other words, when read as an allegory of
the body social, the assertion of individuality of each member of the
Puritan community is less important than the realization of mutual
dependence, integration, and equilibrium.[35] While unity was crucial for

---

[34] Helen McMahon has shown how the employment of contemporary
physiological terms and references to ancient knowledge in the poem was
influenced by Dr. Helkia Crooke's *Mikrokosmographia: A Description of the
Body of Man* (1615), while the debate structure, imagery, and diction was
largely borrowed from Joshua Sylvester's 1614 translation of "Panaretus" by
Jean Bertault. Helen McMahon, "Anne Bradstreet, Jean Bertault, and Dr.
Crooke," *Early American Literature* 3.2 (1968): 118-123.

[35] Seen this way, "The Four Humors" implicitly echoes the Pauline conception
of corporal unity in Christ (1 Corinthians 12-31), which is also the central theme
in John Winthrop's seminal sermon "A Modell of Christian Charity," delivered
on the eve of the Great Migration and probably attended by Bradstreet, who was
a passenger aboard the *Arabella*. See Donald P. Wharton, "Anne Bradstreet and
the *Arabella*," *Critical Essays on Anne Bradstreet*, eds. Pattie Cowell and Ann
Stanford (Boston: G. K. Hall, 1983) 262-269.

the political and economic survival of the Bay Colony, Bradstreet disavows the importance of hierarchy for building a plantation in the "wilderness" and omits some of the negative religious implications that the notion of unity inheres. For some Puritan divines, Bradstreet's celebration of mixture would have constituted a cause for concern, since one of the fundamental aims of the settlers was to maintain and defend the purity of the English Protestant movement in America and to avoid a blend of regenerate and unregenerate colonists in New England meeting houses as much as possible.

The lacuna of theocratic abstraction in Bradstreet's academic poem is further evinced by the absence of Calvinist concepts and of references to the mechanisms of divine healing. Although the ending proclaims unity as a desirable personal and collective state, "Of the Four Humours in Man's Constitution" highlights the actual absence of unity because the humors are engaged in an interlocking battle with each other throughout much of the poem. Health, therefore, as determined by the contention between the four humors, can only be a temporary epiphenomenon, while illness, disunity, and imbalance constitute states of normalcy for the body personal and the body politic.

Upon Several Recoveries from Illness

Anne Bradstreet's ten personal illness poems have not yet received sustained scholarly attention. Most critics have treated her verses on sickness as mere affirmation of the author's firm grounding in Puritan dogma. This may be owing to Adrienne Rich's early dismissal of Bradstreet's poetic reflection on medical issues as "in fact curiously impersonal as poetry; their four-foot-three-foot hymn-book metres, their sedulous meekness, their Biblical allusions, are the pure fruit of convention."[36] Since they ostensibly lack the rebellious potential evident in some of her grief and love poetry, the illness poems have appeared as curious side notes in scholarly discussions of Bradstreet's work.[37]

---

[36] Rich xviii.

[37] Rosenmeier (2-3), for instance, does not include illness poems in the list of exceptional Bradstreet poems. See also, Ann Stanford, *Anne Bradstreet: The Worldly Puritan* (New York: Burt Franklin & Co., 1974) 3. Even four decades

However, it is precisely the alleged simplicity and predictability of Bradstreet's illness poems that calls for further scrutiny. Although her reflections on poor health generally follow acceptable spiritual guidelines—they read bodily signs for their otherworldly significance—a number of Bradstreet's poems are more than mere "fruits of conventions" (Rich), as I hope to show in the following. Her employment of artful language and an aesthetic of gratitude as a means of alleviating personal suffering actually compare to few other colonial American texts. Hammond's remark that the "movement from pain to doctrine reflects the speaker's attempt to overcome human words with the redemptive antidote of God's Word," applies to most of Bradstreet's illness poems.[38] It is indeed noteworthy that the metaphors and intellectual strategies she uses to cope with her illnesses indicate her conviction that this mode of textualizing health matters is not merely a trite religious exercise but an act of spiritual healing and advancement.

This conviction is outlined in further detail in Bradstreet's prose writings. Among the lessons of life conveyed in her autobiographical letter, "To My Dear Children," Bradstreet offers sound advice on how to deal with illness. In her early teens, she suffered under "a long fit of sickness which I had on my bed," and "often communed with my heart and made my supplication to the most High who set me free from that affliction" (241). Many of her journal entries consist of similar narrative meditations on illness, followed by short poems. In May of 1657, after suffering from "a sore sickness," Bradstreet's retrospective assessment of this time in her life touches on practical and spiritual consequences of her illness-induced absence from the household of the family (255). Illness has rendered Bradstreet unable to perform the regular duties of a colonial housewife and mother. It has made impossible Bradstreet's calling in life and has, in doing so, denied her the main source of identity. Forcing the New England subject to radically examine itself in

---

after Rich's dismissal, an introductory entry on Bradstreet claims that "her impulse toward rebellion is evident throughout the body of her writings," but remains silent about her illness poems. Ronald A. Bosco and Jillmary Murphy, "New England Poetry," *The Oxford Handbook of Early American Literature*, ed. Kevin J. Hayes (New York: Oxford UP, 2008) 121.

[38] Hammond 133.

the sickroom, illness hence creates a state of exception from seventeenth-century gender and cultural norms. This state of exception ought to be reconfigured as a time of renewed self-fashioning, Bradstreet asserts. Precisely at the moment when human agency is threatened by a bodily distemper, the believer can turn to God and receive redemption and an opportunity to re-create her self in and through Christ. The key for Bradstreet is to accept that the decaying body actually signals its opposite: the flourishing of the soul. In September 1657, the author has to concede that God had chosen her for a series of confining and debilitating illnesses. Again, the only productive outcome from her affliction is the lesson it teaches her and—through her—Bradstreet's children and grandchildren. This time, she realizes that one ought to consider illness as an opportunity for continual praise and reform and not simply as a momentary occasion for self-improvement. Similar to Wigglesworth's approach to coping with disease, punishment through illness is for Bradstreet a desirable state of being and consciousness—"I can no more live without correction than without food" (257)—essential as eating and breathing.

In another prose meditation, titled "May 11, 1661," after four years of relative health, Bradstreet's tone and mood are less optimistic than on previous occasions. Rather than integrating the illness into the evolving fabric of the Christian self, the poet now grapples with the insufficiency of (her) words. There is also a sense that the speaker finds her illness to be a cause for self-scrutiny but that the rules for behaving as a devout believer are increasingly difficult to follow and accept. She hence asserts that if she were only able to use language properly, the praise for God would finally be real. While being ill discontinues the existence of an economic agent producing material goods, it also enables the creation of a more spiritual self that produces mental and artistic values. These values are generated in the process of voicing human gratitude for regaining health in meaningful statements.

In this meditation on illness, Bradstreet not only reflects on bodily dysfunctions but also draws from them the rudiments of an aesthetic program. After recovery, she writes:

> I cannot render unto the Lord according to all His loving kindness, nor take the cup of salvation with thanksgiving as I ought to do. Lord, Thou that knowest all things know'st that I desire to testify my thankfulness

not only in word, but in deed, that my conversation may speak that Thy vows are upon me (259).

The speaker, in a self-reflexive instance, recognizes that (her) words are not enough to express the full scope of gratitude for deliverance. The self-scrutiny during the preceding illness has granted insight into more proper and devotional behavior for the Christian pilgrim, and now the problem is how to re-present this to God and the world. The final sentence outlines an aesthetic of gratitude based on the principle that writing constitutes a branch of human creativity spurred by the divine that can turn word into deed. In short, Bradstreet considers a poem on the page as a deed, a material offering and sacrifice written in gratitude and humility after recovery from illness. In keeping with the dictum that theory and practice need to coincide in order to constitute pious and useful Christian behavior, she illustrates what she means by "not only in word, but in deed" when she adds short and rather simple poems that express her gratitude for recovery from illness to her prose meditations. Included under the meditation dated "May 11, 1661," Bradstreet's verse is conceived as an illustration of the insight received during illness and as a testimonial offering to God and to the world:

> An humble, faithful life, O Lord,
> Forever let me walk;
> Let my obedience testify
> My praise lies not in talk.
>
> Accept, O Lord, my simple mite,
> For more I cannot give.
> What Thou bestow'st I shall restore,
> For of thine alms I live. (259-260, l. 13-20)

This poem constitutes a deed in the sense that it enacts words that express sincere devotion to God in a formalized and controlled manner. Such a poem can be read as an attempt to keep and confirm sickbed promises and thus to reinvigorate the covenant with God. In order not to forget illness and the spiritual lessons it teaches, Bradstreet's illness poems seek to remind the patient/sinner of his/her duty to acknowledge the power and mercy of God. Despite her attempt to downplay the value of her work, calling her poem "my simple mite" (260, l. 17), Bradstreet is convinced that being able to transform sickness into a poem of praise and thanksgiving—an aesthetic of gratitude—would be recognized, by herself as well as the reader, as a sign of probable salvation.

These conclusions result from years of coping with bodily distempers. In fact, illnesses were such an ubiquitous part of Bradstreet's life that they provided her with the initial impetus to write poetry. Her first (published) attempt at verse, titled "Upon a Fit of Sickness, Anno 1632 *Aetatis Suae*, 19," presents an early New England subject who is exploring internal worlds rather than the unfamiliar landscape of the American "wilderness." What concerns the speaker most is how her corporeal condition resonates with her prospects of salvation and not how the natural environment shapes her sense of self, her relation to God and the community. Reflecting on a previous, unspecified distemper, the young author begins "Upon a Fit of Sickness" by evoking illness as a crossroads between life and death:

> Twice ten years old not fully told
> > since nature gave me breath,
> My race is run, my thread is spun,
> > lo, here is fatal death. (222, l. 1-5)

As the poem unfolds, the speaker attempts to pinpoint the significance of illness in a person's spiritual pilgrimage on earth. In doing so, she abstains from versifying internal tensions between doubt and affirmation that characterizes much of Bradstreet's later writings; rather, illness has caused the poetic voice to forsake the material world without explicitly siding with God. "Her point is not," Robert Richardson observes, "that tribulation or suffering compels her to turn to Christianity; it is rather an expression of contempt for this life in the medieval tradition."[39] After the first eight lines, the speaker switches from meditating on impending death to an almost grudging and defiant affirmation of life. She records her spiritual progress, and by

---

[39] Robert D. Richardson, Jr. "The Puritan Poetry of Anne Bradstreet," *Texas Studies in Language and Literature* 9 (1967): 317-331. Rpt. in *The American Puritan Imagination: Essays in Revaluation*, ed. Sacvan Bercovitch (London: Cambridge UP, 1974) 108-109.

implication, her seasoning to life in New England, as a series of successes and setbacks. After yet another eight lines of subdued jubilation about the prospects of salvation, the speaker retreats to reflect about the end of life that illness has foreshadowed: "O bubble blast, how long can'st last? / that always art a breaking" (222, l. 17-18). In contrast to many of her later personal poems, which end with a clear (and at times seemingly formulaic) evocation of godliness, Bradstreet's first poem culminates in a short dialogue with the devil:

> The race is run, the field is won,
> the victory's mine I see;
> Forever known, thou envious foe,
> the foil belongs to thee. (222, l. 29-32)

Especially when placed concomitantly with the homely images of the beginning of the poem and to the image of salvific assurance at the end, the repetition of winning a symbolic and typological race (taken from 2 Timothy 4:7) seems problematic. Here, the quest for righteousness does not conclude in the hands of the heavenly Father. As Rosamond Rosenmeier explains, "[t]he poem does not end on a note of conventional piety. It ends with the use of a figure that renders ambiguous life's apparent finality: it appears to give death the victory, while at the same time suggesting in the implied planting metaphor that 'envious' death acts in the service of life."[40] Whereas Rosenmeier reads "thou envious foe" as a metaphor of death, I would suggest that Bradstreet is actually referring to the devil in the poem's concluding couplet. Seen this way, claiming that the Fallen Angel receives nothing but defeat and disgrace from the redeemed patient/sinner, the speaker configures illness as a satanic tool of temptation and not primarily as a trial or judgment of God. By giving the devil a presence in the final two lines, Bradstreet misses the chance to end the poem according to convention, that is, with praise or thanks to her Lord. Regardless of whether the conclusion is seen as a sign of her poetic immaturity or as a deliberate display of Puritan devotion, the poem's closing couplet renders visible a culturally constructed role of the devil in the illness

---

[40] Rosenmeier 77.

theatre on earth that is lacking in other colonial New England illness writings.

Bradstreet repudiates this rather unusual poetic resolution in her second poem on illness, entitled "Upon Some Distemper of Body," which is one of the most aesthetically sophisticated representations of illness in the texts surveyed for this study. The preposition "upon" in the title of the first and second illness poems in Bradstreet's work situates the speaker in an elevated, albeit attached position with regard to the object of poetic contemplation. The word "upon" signals not only the belatedness of human reflection but also claims a territory that has been mastered intellectually. The speaker of the poem is quite literally attempting to draw agency away from illness after a time of painful suffering and uncertainty about her life's course. The energy necessary to compose words about pain and suffering in an artistic manner is itself already an indication that the author has survived and recovered from illness, or is at least healthy enough to engage in contemplative work about her previous experience. To do so, the nature of the illness itself is no longer relevant and hence the actual disease is never referenced.

> In anguish of my heart replete with woes,
> And wasting pains, which best my body knows,
> In tossing slumbers on my wakeful bed,
> Bedrenched with tears that flowed from mournful head,
> Till nature had exhausted all her store,
> Then eyes lay dry, disabled to weep more;
> And looking up unto his throne on high,
> Who sendeth help to those in misery;
> He chased away those clouds and let me see
> My anchor cast i' th' vale with safety.
> He eased my soul of woe, my flesh of pain,
> and brought me to the shore from troubled main. (223, l. 2-13)

The speaker employs a number of aquatic images (bedrenched, tears, clouds, anchor, vale, shore, main) that might refer to dropsy or a related illness. But more important than the disease itself is the way in which Bradstreet hides the specificity of her illness experience behind a metaphoric veil. While the water imagery echoes thematically the reflections on moisture in "Of the Four Humours in Man's Constitution," the act of distancing the speaker from her actual illness through metaphor in "Upon Some Distemper of Body" serves to illustrate her contemporaneous approximation of God which is facilitated by a deeper understanding of her bodily and spiritual condition.

In Bradstreet's first two illness poems, religious doubt and rebellion, the ostensible hallmark of her poetry according to many scholars, play a negligible role. This changes in "For Deliverance from a Fever," which is composed in ballad form and cast as a dialogue between the poetic voice and God. The poem revolves around the patient's physical agonies on the sickbed, her lack of agency, the fear of divine punishment, and her inability to attribute meaning to divine signs. The turning point occurs in the fourth quatrain when the focus shifts from the immediate illness experience to the poet's relation to God:

> "Hide not Thy face from me!" I cried,
> "From burnings keep my soul.
> Thou know'st my heart, and hast me tried;
> I on Thy mercies roll." (247, l. 14-17)

Bradstreet's statement, "Hide not Thy face from me," can be read either as a lamenting plea that mirrors psalmic diction and imagery or as an exhortation with which the speaker oversteps the boundaries of piety and devotion. As Robert C. Wess has pointed out, this poem embodies and illustrates a tension between simple faith and religious doubt that is evident especially in Bradstreet's grief poems but lacking in her more straightforwardly orthodox poems such as "The Vanity of All Worldly Things" or "As Weary Pilgrim."[41] However, while Bradstreet's statement can be seen as a subtle act of rebellion against God, who dares to avert His gaze and favor from a devout believer, it remains in line with dogma, according to which moments of separation from God are integral and even necessary components in the salvific dialectic of doubt and affirmation. As Beth Doriani explains in her analysis of the influence of David's lamentations on Bradstreet's poetry, the interrogating statement "Hide not Thy Face" illustrates the poet's desire

---

[41] Robert C. Wess, "Religious Tension in the Poetry of Anne Bradstreet," *Christianity and Literature* 25.2 (1976): 30-36.

for close acquaintance with God and echoes Psalm 6, in which David calls God to alleviate human suffering in similar terms (cf. also Psalms 27, 69, 102, 143).[42] Much as God's turning away from Bradstreet's speaker during times of distress signals her temporary separation from the deity, the ultimate recovery from illness, which is already evident from the word "Deliverance" in the title, marks the reunification with God, "Who hath redeemed my soul from pit" (247, l. 28). This poem, therefore, introduces a recurrent theme in Bradstreet's illness meditations: sealing the speaker's unity with the divine and the unity of body and mind after recovery. At the same time that Bradstreet configures illness as an emblem of death (cf. "Upon a Fit of Sickness"), she interprets recovery as an emblem of her salvation and thus as a reason to praise and give thanks to God.

The notion that writing verses of praise and gratitude also constitutes a religious *duty* is evinced in "Upon My Daughter Hannah Wiggin, Her Recovery from a Dangerous Fever," a poem comprised of only two quatrains:

> Blest be Thy name who didst restore
>     To health my daughter dear,
> When death did seem ev'n to approach,
>     And life was ended near.
>
> Grant she remember what Thou'st done
>     And celebrate Thy praise
> And let her conversation say
>     She loves Thee all Thy days. (262, l. 4-11)

Again, this poem can be seen as a deed, a performative act, whose artifactuality of gratitude constitutes the gratitude itself. This short poem, however, can hardly conceal the speaker's short breath and hesitation to write at all. Its brevity suggests that the author felt compelled to compose words designed to form and order her meditation on affliction that would otherwise be lost in the mind of the individual.

---

[42] Beth M. Doriani, "'Then Have I ... Said With David': Anne Bradstreet's Andover Manuscript Poems and the Influence of the Psalm Tradition," *Early American Literature* 24.1 (1989): 57.

Furthermore, the leap from thought to verse, and from word to deed, manifests a Puritan anxiety about relying exclusively on works as signs of salvation. The intensity with which the poetic voice desires her daughter's proximity to God is emphasized by the gap between the two stanzas when Bradstreet turns to express her wishes for the future.

The theme of thanksgiving resonates also in "From Another Sore Fit" and "Deliverance from a Fit of Fainting." In both poems, Bradstreet's speaker is primarily concerned with how to repay adequately God's decision to facilitate the patient's recovery; they revolve around the question: "What shall I render to my God / For all His bounty showed to me? (248, l. 14-15). While "From Another Sore Fit" finds solace and resolve in "My heart I wholly give to Thee" (l. 18), "Deliverance from a Fit of Fainting" illustrates some of the problems associated with expressing gratitude in ways that are meaningful to the speaker's saintly metaself. In both poems, complete dependence on God is poetically exercised through the use of hyperbole: "From Another Sore Fit" uses words such as "wasted flesh" (l. 10) and "how in sweat I seemed to melt" (l. 8). "Deliverance from a Fit of Fainting" employs the conceit of a "spider's web cut off" (l. 6) to represent the patient's illness-induced state of corporeal depravity. In contrast to the former poem, the latter problematizes the feasibility of praising God as a justified and necessary reward for redemption from illness: "Worthy art Thou, O Lord, of praise, / But ah! It's not in me" (249, l. 2-3). Already established in the opening lines of the poem, the notion that the speaker is unable to express her gratitude properly suffuses all four stanzas and is supported by a dominance of cold vowels. Although God has helped the sufferer to overcome her sense of uncertainty that has accompanied the fit of fainting (from which Bradstreet suffered repeatedly in her life), the spiritual recovery after the return of health remains a cause for concern for the speaker. "Deliverance from a Fit of Fainting" hence subtly expresses the difficulties of a New England poet to reconcile her illness experiences with the cultural script of divine healing, according to which personal afflictions aid the speaker's spiritual advancement. This argument is supported by the ending of the poem—"O Lord, no longer be my days / Than I may fruitful be" (l. 15-16)—which deviates from Bradstreet's previous insight that illness brings the patient sufferer closer to God. Instead, this particular poem stands out by voicing a sense of resignation that corporeal demise is not only inevitable but perhaps may be inseparable from spiritual uncertainty and even declension.

Overall, Bradstreet's poetics of illness is consistently geared toward investing illness with spiritual meaning. The distribution of the illness topos throughout her verse renders visible not a simple shift from public to private phases, as suggested in earlier readings of Bradstreet's work, but rather a transformation of language, voice, and vantage point. The colonial poet expresses her concurrence with the Puritan belief that illness, as all forms of suffering, is a currency of exchange between the believer and her Savior. While all her illness poems underline and insist on the affirmation of doctrine, Bradstreet's poetic deeds serve as a means of "artfully distancing and transforming physical suffering."[43] By retroactively and metaphorically distancing herself from the realities of illness, Bradstreet aims to seal the therapeutic process.

To reiterate a central point of my argument concerning Bradstreet's illness poetry: the rebellious stance that can be detected in her love and grief poems remains largely absent in her reflections on illness. Only rarely do doubt and anger break through the surface of her gratitude for having recently regained her health. Bradstreet's poetic responses to illness therefore contest the notion that bodily afflictions or overwhelming losses must threaten the faith of the elect, especially if the believer is a woman. Jean Marie Lutes has argued that Bradstreet's spiritual configurations of illness "circumvents medical assertions of female weakness," because they consistently portray a speaker who appropriates Michael Wigglesworth's advice to convert the humbling experience of illness into spiritual edification and elevation.[44] Rather

---

[43] Raymond A. Anselment, *The Realms of Apollo: Literature and Healing in Seventeenth-Century England* (Newark: U of Delaware P, 1995) 18.

[44] Jean Marie Lutes, "Negotiating Theology and Gynecology: Anne Bradstreet's Representations of the Female Body," *Signs: Journal of Women in Culture and Society* 22.2 (1997): 312. See also, Ivy Schweitzer, "Anne Bradstreet Wrestles With the Renaissance," *Early American Literature* 23.3 (1988): 293. While I agree with Lutes' overall line of argument, I would challenge her assumption that the poetic configurations of illness by Wigglesworth and Bradstreet are essentially the same (320). Although Bradstreet adheres to the notion that illnesses provide opportunities to derive strength out of weakness, Lutes' comparison overlooks the role of gender and Bradstreet's emphasis on practice

than pieces of rebellion against Puritan orthodoxy, her illness poems function as anchors of memory for the author and for the reader. The mnemonic poems write against forgetting the lesson that each illness has taught the author: maintaining an intimate relation with God. Occasionally, the poems also express the author's difficulty in fully internalizing this lesson. Apparently, Bradstreet needed repeated confirmation that her several illness experiences had made her a better Christian. At first sight, it may seem surprising that she returns repeatedly to the topic of illness with such vigor and effort. Does her devotional and recurring poetic treatment of illness suggest that she needed to convince herself time and again of the lessons that illness teaches about humanity's physical and spiritual condition? One might argue that if she had been fully able to accept illness as demanded by colonial culture at large (i.e., illness as punishment and/or test of faith), she would have abandoned the topic at some point in her life. A second glimpse at Bradstreet's work shows that rather than viewing her poetic return to illness as a sign of her trembling faith or overwhelming doubt, the loss of health functions as a religious catalyst that energizes devotional practice in poetic form. One of the reasons that there are a number of thematically similar reflections on illness was that Bradstreet thus showed to herself and her reader that she is indeed blessed by affliction and that she had been tested enough to warrant her election. Hence, the continued reflection on illness is caused by Bradstreet's uncertainty about its inherent message and concurred with the Puritan dictum of continual spiritual renewal throughout the sinner's path to salvation.

When considered as a group of connected poems, Bradstreet's meditations on illness reveal a frequent shifting between devotional, confessional, and didactic voices. These voices urge the audience in various ways to consider illnesses as part of a larger spiritual journey rather than as merely distressing moments whose larger significance for salvation cannot yet be grasped. In her later work, the frequent invocations of illness experiences and interpretations illustrate the pilgrim's continuous need and desire for divine correction. Conversion,

and deeds that clearly put her reflections on illness in a different tonal and conceptual register than Wigglesworth's illness poetics.

the apex of the pilgrim's inner life, is thus facilitated by illness; the cause of illness lies, in typical Calvinist fashion, in human action and God's displeasure. The poetic expression of suffering hence becomes a crucial part of the early New England confessional mode because the speaker repeatedly implies that illness is self-inflicted through sin. Dealing with illness becomes as compulsive a behavior as the examination of the soul. In fact, for Bradstreet the two are coterminous: illness can be nothing but an occasion for soul-searching, reflection, and meditation. As a result, sickness takes up a central position in the experience and representation of conversion and salvation, a point that connects Bradstreet's work to that of Edward Taylor, one of the many readers and admirers of her poetry in colonial New England.

Illness Matters: Edward Taylor

Like Wigglesworth, Edward Taylor was a revered preacher, who provided medical treatment for his congregation and wrote an extensive body of poetry.[45] Rather than basing his healing practice on Galenic premises alone, Taylor sought to facilitate recovery from illness through prayer, introspection, and reform and, moreover, by adhering to Paracelsian principles. Taylor left no medical records or account books that would allow historians to retrace his healing practice, but he kept a collection of recipes and treatment methods copied mainly from Culpeper and Paracelsus. Taylor "distilled" the medical books he had read in order to assemble a portable *material medica* that would be of practical use when traveling to remote settlements to attend sick congregants. His "Dispensatory" is comprised of two volumes, which include directions for the application of numerous minerals, metals, plants, as well as animal and human parts for medicinal purposes.[46] In

---

[45] His journey across the Atlantic, his entry into Harvard, and the call from the newly-founded settlement of Westfield to serve as minister are recorded in Edward Taylor's diary, transcribed and published in *Proceedings of the Massachusetts Historical Society* 18 (1880-1881): 5-18.

[46] Taylor's knowledge of the healing theories and practices of his day can be evinced from the ten medical books contained in his personal library, listed in Thomas H. Johnson, "Taylor's Library," *The Poetical Works of Edward Taylor*,

the first section of the "Dispensatory" the Westfield minister-physician lists medicinal applications of earth, water, stones, gems and minerals, before he shifts attention to the curative use of metals. Typical of Taylor's adherence to Paracelsian medical theory, he then describes the correspondences (or sympathies) of certain metals to planets (e.g., silver/moon, gold/sun), reflects on the Philosopher's Stone, and records remedies whose recourse to magic is at times indistinguishable from medical practices that were considered as signs of witchcraft in other New England settlements.[47]

As Kenneth Murdock has explained, Taylor's poetry deviates from the doctrine of plain-style rhetoric championed by most first-generation Puritan writers. This deviation constitutes "a rebellion dictated by a

ed. Thomas H. Johnson (Princeton: Princeton UP, 1966) 201-220. For Taylor's scientific influences, see William J. Scheick, "Edward Taylor's Herbalism in Preparatory Meditations," *American Poetry* 1.3 (1983): 64-71; Lawrence Lan Sluder, "God in the Background: Edward Taylor as Naturalist," *Early American Literature* 7.3 (1973): 265-271. For an analysis of Taylor's medicinal use of human body parts, see Karen Gordon-Grube, "Evidence of Medicinal Cannibalism in Puritan New England: 'Mummy' and Related Remedies in Edward Taylor's 'Dispensatory,'" *Early American Literature* 28 (1993): 185-221.

[47] Edward Taylor, "Dispensatory," n.d., Beinecke Rare Book and Manuscript Library, Yale University, ms. 36-39. For Taylor's fascination with Paracelsian medicine, see Catherine Rainwater, "This Brazen Serpent is a Doctors Shop": Edward Taylor's Medical Vision," *American Literature and Science*, ed. Robert J. Scholnick (Lexington: U of Kentucky P, 1992) 18-38. Taylor took a deep interest in alchemy, involving all practical and theoretical aspects. For studies on this topic, see Karen Gordon-Grube, *The Alchemical 'Golden Tree' and Associated Imagery in the Poems of Edward Taylor*, Diss. Free U Berlin, 1990; Reiner Smolinski and Kathleen B. Freels, "'Chymical Wedding': Rosicrucian Alchemy and Eucharistic Conversion Process in Edward Taylor's Preparatory Meditations and in Early Seventeenth-Century German Tracts," *Transatlantic Encounters: Studies in European-American Relations: Presented to Winfried Herget*, ed. Udo J. Hebel and Karl Ortseifen (Trier: WVT, 1995) 40-61; Joan Del Fattore, "John Webster's *Metallographia*: A Source for Alchemical Imagery in the Preparatory Meditations," *Early American Literature* 18.3 (1983): 233-241. Cf. Cheryl Z. Orevicz, "Edward Taylor and the Alchemy of Grace," *Seventeenth-Century News* 34 (1976): 33-34.

feeling that the fundamental spiritual verities were too mysterious for logical or prosaic exposition and demanded instead all the rich emotional and intellectual suggestiveness of complex 'metaphysical' poetry."[48] Considered by many critics as one of the last proponents of the English Metaphysicals, Taylor artistically sided with John Donne, George Herbert, and Henry Vaughan, whose devotional and introspective poetry he appropriated to project his own spiritual meditations. The following pages seek to elucidate Taylor's appropriation of Metaphysical poetry with a specific focus on the author's employment of alchemical and medical references. These show, once again, how the attempt to arrest pain and suffering in poetic language remained a futile and unattainable undertaking for New England colonists.

Whereas Anne Bradstreet consistently aims to personalize in poetic space the pain and suffering that accompany her poor health, Edward Taylor's poetic meditations often create a distance between the experience of illness and the writing self through an extensive employment of metaphor and conceit.[49] The disjointing between authorial voice and the lived realities of illness is primarily facilitated by staging surprising connections between an object and its assigned (meta)physical referent in various sections of his two major works *Preparatory Meditations* (1682-1725) and *God's Determinations Touching His Elect* (c. 1680). For instance, in "Meditation II.67[A]," Taylor's poetic voice states:

> The Spirits and the Vial both are sick.
> The Lump Consisting of them both so trim
> Is out of trim, sore wounded to the quick
> Distemperd by ill Humours bred therein.
> Some poyson's in the golden Cup of wine,
> The treason works against the king Divine. (193, l. 19-24)[50]

---

[48] Murdock 170.

[49] For a study of Taylor's meditional poetry, placed in larger Puritan traditions, see Ursula Brumm, "The Art of Puritan Meditation in New England," *Studies in New England Puritanism*, ed. Winfried Herget (Frankfurt: Lang, 1983) 139-167.

[50] Edward Taylor, *The Poems of Edward Taylor*, ed. Donald E. Stanford (New Haven: Yale UP, 1960) 78. In the following, excerpts from Taylor's poetry will

Symbolized by the vial, disease has transcended the outer boundaries of the human body and reached the core of the sinner/speaker, whose chances for recovery rely significantly on gaining a deeper, more transparent realization of Christ. The edifying passage begins in the fourth line of the stanza when the speaker addresses internal corruptions, paradoxes within the soul, and the perpetual temptations sown by the devil to lure the believer away from the path of Christian virtue. Later in the poem, the Sun of Righteousness, "With healing in his Wings Physicianswise" (193, l. 34), materializes the light of Christ which grants not only wisdom, healing, and grace but also courage. "The fear is bad: in them diseases grow" (l. 36), Taylor continues and thus claims that illness is a self-perpetuating bodily state that depends as much on external remedies (herbs, chemicals) as it does on the mental and spiritual estate of the believer. Taylor meditates further on the notion of "healing in his wings" in the following poem, "Meditation II.68[A]," which again is inspired by the biblical description of Christ as the sun of righteousness, who frees a sin-sick world from its spiritual and physical diseases (cf. Malachi 4:2). As David G. Miller has suggested,

> Taylor's pun on sun/son highlights his belief in the sufficiency of the light of Christ to transcend and to redeem the metaphorical language. The possible confusion of the homonym pair seems divinely ordained to express the full truth that Taylor wants to convey. Christ's relationship to God is filial but also revelatory.[51]

And, I would add, it is precisely the extension of this relationship to the interaction between humanity and the divine that will produce true healing and salvation, according to Taylor. Here, healing is used as a metaphor for salvation in and through Christ. This is not a shift in a different connotative direction of the term "healing," but rather a logical extension of the theology of disease brought from Europe and developed during the first decades of New England settlement.

---

be cited from this edition, with page numbers in parentheses, followed by line numbers.

[51] Miller 91.

As the poem continues, the motif of the soul's longing for God's medicinal word is encapsulated by linking the speaker's spiritual condition to scurvy and by portraying the "sweet medicating rayes" (197, l. 12) of Christ as divine curative occurrences. But before healing can proceed, the patient has to avert "The Fiery Darts of Satan" (l. 19), which Taylor envisions as diseases that attack the body. To portray the magnitude of this invasion from the realm of evil, disease names "infect" the poem in stanza 5 which consists of an enumeration of illnesses plaguing humanity:

> Yea, Lythargy, the Apoplectick Stroke:
> The Catochee, Soul Blindness, Surdity,
> Ill Tongue, Mouth Ulcers, Frog, the Quinsie Throate
> The Palate Fallen, Wheezings, Pleurisy.
> Heart Ach, the Syncopee, bad stomach tricks
> Gaul Tumors, Liver grown; spleen evills Cricks. (197, l. 25-30)

For Jeffrey Jeske this "intrusion of sheer physicality" challenges the complex thematic and structural balance between the otherwise shady allures of the physical realm and the rewards of heaven.[52] It is by listing and linking disease signifiers that Taylor's speaker ironically elevates the significance of "the Chilly World" (196, l. 8), mentioned in the second stanza of "Meditation II.67[B]," which he then seeks to leave behind while searching for otherworldly treasures. Taylor's list of illness signifiers that spill into the following stanza can also be read as an illustration of the contaminating potential of scientific language for New England culture at large and thus represents the declension of Puritan religiosity at the outset of the eighteenth-century. Or, it can be seen as the remaining threat of the destructive power of Satan, designed to humble writer and audience. In addition, Taylor's poetic voice prepares his reader for words of divine healing that redeem the patient:

> The Kidny toucht, The Iliak, Colick Griefe

[52] Jeffrey Jeske, "Edward Taylor and the Traditions of Puritan Nature Philosophy," *Essays on the Poetry of Edward Taylor in Honor of Thomas M. and Virginia L. Davis*, ed. Michael Schuldiner (Newark: U of Delaware P, 1997) 58.

The Ricats, Dropsy, Gout, the Scurvy, Sore
The Miserere Mei. O Reliefe
        I want and would, and beg it at thy doore.
        O! Sun of Righteousness Thy Beams bright, Hot
        Rafter a Doctors, and a Surgeons Shop. (197, l. 31-36)

More than mere blessings of healer's shops, medicine must be suffused by religiosity because true relief can only come from Scripture and an active engagement with Christ. In the closing stanzas of the poem, the list of painful and debilitating diseases that have threatened human beings in verses 5 and 6 is contrasted with an enumeration of healing images. This time, Taylor's conceits come from medical practice, specifically the utensils used in healing procedures:

And ply my wounds with Pledgets dipt therein.
        And wash therewith my Scabs and Boils so sore,
And all my Stobs, and Arrow wounds come, bring
        And syrrindge with the Same. It will them Cure.
        With tents made of these Beams well tent them all.
        They Fistula'es and Gangrenes Conquer shall. (198, l. 61-66)

Here, the poetic voice, which again presents itself as that of a Puritan Everyman, prays to God to relieve him of a major illness. Toward the end of his meditations on sickness (II.67[A]-68[B]), Taylor creates an analogy between Christ and "the Heavenly Alkahest" (199, l. 19) and thus illustrates his versatility, similar to John Winthrop Jr., in Puritan and alchemical language and concepts. The power to bring about healing is granted solely by the divine but can be discovered, in part at least, by human beings knowledgeable in the old and new sciences. At the same time, however, Taylor's rare inclusion of discursive fragments from the realm of science and his insistence on the supremacy of religious interpretations of the world evidences the limitations of a mere rational approach to understanding and governing diseases and the world at large.

Taylor concurs with Bradstreet and Wigglesworth in his fundamental conceptualization of illness and its role for the elect. Like most New England colonists, Taylor believed in, and witnessed incessantly, the utter depravity of the body—"I'm but a Flesh and Blood bag," he writes in "Meditation I.30" (49, l. 27)—and similarly subscribed to the notion that illness constitutes a divine punishment for human iniquities. However, the Westfield minister-physician poeticizes the terrors that illness and death brought to his own family to a degree that is lacking in other early colonial poetry: "But oh! the tortures, Vomit, screeching, groans, / And six weeks Fever would pierce hearts like stone," Taylor laments in "Upon Wedlock, and Death of Children" (345, l. 19-24). In this poem, the interdependence between illness and spirituality is rendered visible by linking fever and heart which, like all metaphors, symbols, and conceits in Taylor's poetry, strive to culminate in spiritually elevating verse. Edification is arguably one of the primary aims of his meditative and declarative poetry and is best achieved when the state of the sinner/speaker is portrayed as utterly humbled and debased. And Taylor can do so most forcefully when he poeticizes the spiritual depravity that illness brings about. Patricia Watson remarks that "[s]ince ancient Greek times, philosophers had relied upon medical metaphor to symbolize the grievances and turmoil of the soul as bodily disease, and this pattern of expression proliferated throughout the rise of Christianity."[53] As heir to this tradition, Taylor assumes the role of a poet who seeks to transform the distress of illness into meaningful statements about the self and its relation to the divine.

"Meditation II.14" begins with an image of decay and another seventeenth-century version of a Deleuzian "body without organs" that is "Half Dead: and rotten at the Coare: my Lord! / I am Consumptive: and my Wasted lungs" (104, l. 1-2).[54] The rottenness at the core is what concerns the speaker throughout his poetic tracing of a journey through illness. He is desperately seeking the wisdom (a word that is repeated seven times throughout the poem, more than any other) that he finds in Christ and that allows him to locate the significance of his disease in the healing of his soul. The metaphoric intertwinement of sin and sickness is not described as an outgrowth of human depravity, however. Rather, the intimate link between sin and sickness occurs at the level of curing, that is, of curing both sin and sickness so as to bring about health and salvation. In stanza 4, Taylor's divine knowledge is associated with

---

[53] Watson 86.

[54] Gilles Deleuze and Felix Guatarri, *Thousand Plateaus*, trans. Brian Massumi (1980; London: Continuum, 2004) 40.

"Chrystall Cupping Glasses" (105, l. 21) that allow for the extraction of ill or abundant humors from inflicted sections of the body. More than a mere reference to a specific medical practice, the cupping glass is a material artifact that symbolizes the advancement and refinement of Western medicine in the "wilderness" and, at the same time, points to a curative technique (sucking illness from the body) that was also practiced by New England Natives. Aside from its cross-cultural overtones, the cupping glass is also symbolic of religious edification and salvation. Taylor's linkage of health and salvation, healing and holy, is one of the major strains of abstraction in his illness poetry and the "Chrystall Cupping Glasses" one of the most vivid conceits.

Taylor's symbolic repository also includes objects or occurrences that his colonial reader would be thoroughly familiar with. In fact, the metaphysical conceit calls for an expansion of symbolic connections and thus creates a larger set of poetic material that finds its inspiration in the realm of the everyday. Whether spinning wheels, gardens or spiders, Taylor constantly contemplates, dissects, and analyzes the material world in order to find analogies with, or references to, a higher, metaphysical truth. The mining of natural objects for conceit poetry culminates in a peculiar list of medical plants in "Meditation II.62," when Taylor enumerates plants placed on earth by God that have curative powers because they are closely intertwined with spiritual powers (184, l. 16). Hence, "[f]or Taylor, both the chemical practitioner and the alembic itself represent God, the great transformer of man's soul; and the medicines chemically prepared in the alembic symbolize God's saving grace."[55] Moreover, "Meditation II.62" pays tribute to the rich repertoire of medical herbs that are imbued with spiritual and medical healing potential. In contrast to this clear reference to Galenic medicine, "Meditation II.67B," which continues the previous reflection on Malachi 4:2, relies again on iatrochemical procedures which are integrated into a larger religious set of references. By evoking pantheistic visions of plants and placing them vis-à-vis allusions to Paracelsian medicine, Taylor balances old and new medical knowledge and approaches in his poetic enactment of the world. "It is here, if anywhere," Jeffrey Jeske observes, "that we see Taylor moving—if only

---

[55] Watson 103.

preliminarily—along the path leading to modern, secular science."[56] Jeske's note of caution concerning the preliminary nature of Taylor's recourse to secular science is important. It provides a central caveat that is missing in Catherine Rainwater's claim that medical discourse shaped Taylor's overall hermeneutic system.[57]

Shifting from the realm of the private to the realm of the public, Taylor's occasional poem "Upon the Sweeping Flood Aug: 13.14. 1683" directs attention from personal salvation to that of the community. In the opening lines, the speaker employs the image of fire before turning to its elemental opposite when "those liquid drops [...] Came" (347, l. 3) and destroyed the speaker's habitat. In the second stanza, the poetic voice uses a metaphor of illness to attribute meaning to the destructive force of the flood:

> Were th'Heavens sick? must wee their Doctors bee
>    And physick them with pills, our sin?
>    To make them purg and Vomit, see,
>       And Excrements out fling?
> We've griev'd them by such Physick that they shed
> Their Excrements upon our lofty heads. (347, l. 7-12)

Similar to Wigglesworth's configuration of disease in "God's Controversy with New-England," Taylor's employment of nature images hints at the omnipotence and inscrutability of God's providence. He alone can unleash sweeping floods and epidemics, and the exact time and reason for doing so remain hidden from human knowledge, is what Taylor's speaker claims in agreement with the Puritan belief in providence. Unlike Wigglesworth, however, Taylor offers an ironic reversal of the doctor-patient relationship that serves as a metaphor for the relation between Christ and humanity, in the second stanza of the poem: "Where th'Heavens sick? Must wee their Doctors bee / And physick them with pills, our sin?" (l. 7-8). The poetic speaker has already realized the healing potential of sin, which is here portrayed as the actual remedy to cure the sickness of the heavens (which is,

---

[56] Jeske 55.

[57] Rainwater 22-23.

implicitly, at this point of the poem, responsible for divine punishment through natural disasters). The flood is similarly envisaged as a cleansing process that transports excess out of the body social just as medicine "make[s] them purg and Vomit, see" (l. 9). The repeated reference to the shedding of "Excrements" is an indication that the healing process has already set in because the searching and self-examining subject has begun to learn the lesson of illness remission. Nevertheless, true resolution of the conflict between the speaker's community, Taylor's "we," and God can only, and must, occur outside of the world of the poem. A closer look at "Upon the Sweeping Flood" shows that underlying its surface intent of illustrating the inscrutability of God's design lingers the problem of human desire for agency. Although God continues to be the revered guide and operator of the universe, the poem emphasizes how human actions are both the cause for the flood and the epidemic (presumably, in Taylor's view, brought about through sin) and the remedy for abating these natural conditions (supposedly through repentance and prayer). In this sense, Taylor attributes power to human beings that according to the Calvinist cultural script rested solely with God.

While "Upon the Sweeping Flood" attempts to reserve a crucial sense of agency for humankind, thus potentially intruding in God's sphere of responsibility, Taylor's last poem on illness returns to the harbor of Puritan orthodoxy by relegating all decisions to the divine. "Upon My Recovery out of a Threatening Sickness," written in December 1720, could hardly differ more from a Bradstreet poem bearing a similar title because in Taylor's version, illness is almost entirely displaced from the body of the poem. The way to celebrate regained health is to enact the absence of illness from the work of art, by relegating the affliction to a distant past. That is, the speaker never references illness conditions or experiences but places himself wholly in the present "beams of grace," a recurrent salvific motif in Taylor's *oeuvre*. This poem thus supports Hammond's observation that the minister-physician-poet constantly sought "to translate the past into current redemptive experience."[58] Through this translation, and through the distancing of illness via metaphor and conceit, the poetic self, shortly

[58] Hammond 152.

before the death of the author, attempts to reach a peaceful coexistence with his bodily afflictions. Halfway into the poem, the speaker shifts emphasis away from a self that has recovered from illness without having gained assurance, as is evinced in the opening lines of the poem: "What, is the golden Gate of Paradise / Lockt up 'gain that yet I may not enter?"[59] The focus of the following stanzas lies on images of weaving to describe the relation between speaker/sinner and Christ. Yet, illness can no longer be contained in the past. Against all efforts by the poet and his language to arrest it, sickness inevitably returns towards the end of life. As a final realization of the significance of illness, Taylor has to admit that only if he considers bodily afflictions as uncertain signs of future election, is he able to battle his corporeal infirmities.

Towards the end of his life, Taylor came to realize that the epistemological conflict between religion and medicine had become increasingly unmanageable and, perhaps, even unbridgeable. One of the central questions for Taylor and other colonial New England writers was whether the body (microcosm) was still connected with the universe (macrocosm) or whether it was beginning to unravel itself from both (meta)physical and ideological boundaries. It is especially Taylor's employment of alchemical, religious, and natural images that illustrates the poet's overall concern with the uncertainties that accompany the transformation of the body's cultural position at the advent of medicine as a science.

* * *

In times of illness, as Wigglesworth, Bradstreet, and Taylor concur, human beings are faced with a unique opportunity to come into contact with the divine, to experience God by being subjected to His wrath and, possibly, His mercy. In early New England poetry, illness often serves as a reminder of approaching death and of Christ's suffering at the cross for the benefit of the elect. The fear and, at times, panic to fail God's expectations marks a lingering undercurrent in the works surveyed for this chapter and often entails a positioning of health and sickness as

---

[59] Edward Taylor, *Edward Taylor's Minor Poetry*, eds. Thomas M. and Virginia L. Davis (Boston: Twayne, 1981) 218, l. 1-2.

adverse contraries. The conflict between the two can only be remedied by placing illness on a higher level of spiritual reflection. To do so, poetry is but one means, albeit a highly useful one, as the three colonial poets consistently insinuate. By configuring disease as an opportunity to approximate God and as a sign that salvation may be imminent, Wigglesworth, Bradstreet, and Taylor employ the specificities of poetic language—metaphor, rhyme, and meter—to edify their readers for whom illness was a common corporeal occurrence and often a threatening spiritual experience. In comparison, Taylor surpasses his contemporaries in his awareness of language and his ability to mold complex spiritual concerns raised by illness into meter and rhyme. The three poets agree in their conviction that by healing various bodily afflictions, God is also curing illness-induced doubts and anxieties about the patient's relation to the divine. For Bradstreet, Wigglesworth, and Taylor, poetry offers a unique textual format for bodily and spiritual healing because through the meditative and creative process it forces the writer to extract spiritual solace from the illness experience.

The works of the early New England writers studied here also indicate that poetic diction is not always or necessarily conducive to healing. One must take into consideration that the repeated treatment of illness especially in Bradstreet and Wigglesworth's works might suggest that poetry's "formal language does not always communicate the depth of an illness or the extent of the grief; its predetermined forms and prescribed resolutions do not always console."[60] Hence, Bradstreet and Wigglesworth's recurring treatment of distemper and the predictability of its poetic mapping and significance actually signal the impossibility of words and metaphors to fully master the experience of disease. In addition, on a larger historical level, the versified treatment of illness in the works of Wigglesworth, Bradstreet, and Taylor can be seen as jeopardizing official versions of colonial subjectivity, causing a collapse of comforting constructions of identity and the integrity of the body that a number of promotional tracts and historical narratives tended to present to the reader. By charging illness with meaning, the three colonial poets address medical questions from the locus of the self and

---

[60] Anselment 18.

illustrate its relation to, and at times its detachment from, a more encompassing, culture-shaping theology of disease.

For the three colonial poets pain is a *rite de passage* necessary to arrive at a stage of redemption and deliverance in a physical and spiritual sense. According to common reasoning in the colonial era, pain was a part of life, a punishment from God, and something whose endurance strengthened people. For Wigglesworth, Bradstreet, and Taylor poetic language constitutes a suitable medium through which the translation from pain into spiritual gain can be achieved, not least because poetry provides an arena in which the consummation of the individual's relation with God can be multiplied through audience reception. Making sense and poetry out of illness, therefore, is considered as a curative or at least soothing undertaking for the writers and is designed to instruct the colonial reader through example. As Harold Schweitzer has claimed, "[i]f suffering [...] cannot be authorized or mastered, it can yet be told—told as one tells stories, sings songs, paints pictures, or recites poetry."[61] This "telling," according to many literary critics and medical humanists, contains cathartic power by ordering, approximating, or distancing the experience of illness. The validity of this assumption is generally confirmed in the illness poems surveyed here. Yet, in some instances, the healing power of poetry is implicitly denied or at least configured as questionable. Since all poets record their illness meditations in retrospect, the possibility of employing writing as an assertion of voice tends to be portrayed as something that had been lost in or to illness and had to be regained subsequently. Illness, especially when accompanied by severe pain, induces speechlessness and silence, and hence poetry can only represent the belatedness of interpreting and expressing illness experience. Therefore, "[e]ven when it is understood," as Theodor Adorno has claimed in observing the role of art in a post-traumatic world, "suffering remains mute and inconsequential."[62] It is the muteness of suffering from illness, the inability to bridge the gap between body and meaning,

---

[61] Harold Schweizer, "To Give Suffering a Language," *Literature and Medicine* 14.2 (1995): 218.

[62] Theodor W. Adorno, *Aesthetic Theory*, trans. C. Lenhardt (1970; London: Routledge, 1984) 27.

that early American poetry seeks to overcome but cannot avoid amplifying.

A similar rendering of illness experience is evident in Cotton Mather's works. In contrast to poetry, the famous Boston minister chose narrative formats (sermon, treatise, essay, and handbook) to grapple with the challenges posed by new scientific discoveries and by the persistence of folk and Native therapeutics in colonial New England. As the following chapter will show, medical interventions from outside of the official theology of disease repeatedly threatened the tenets of New England Puritanism, whose authoritative power over interpreting the body was increasingly waning at the turn of the eighteenth century.

# 6. Thresholds of Modernity: Cotton Mather's Medical Writings

By 1663, the year of Cotton Mather's birth, the religious and communal vision that the first-generation New England Puritans had held seemed no longer realizable. This increased the pressure on the young Cotton Mather to continue the legacy of civil and ecclesiastical leadership of his grandfathers and Puritan teachers, John Cotton and Richard Mather. After intense preparation in learning by his father, Increase Mather, who served as pastor at the Second Congregational Church in Boston and as president of Harvard University, Cotton Mather entered college at the age of eleven. Due to his stammer, which many scholars regard as a sign of the anxieties caused by the expectations his name inevitably raised, he feared that his ostensible destiny, following his father and grandfathers to the pulpit, could not be fulfilled. In search of an alternative career, Mather turned to the study of science and became particularly interested in the emerging field of medicine. The curriculum at Harvard at the time was still geared toward a solid theological education, but it also offered students a relatively broad liberal background, including mandatory studies in logic, mathematics, Aristotelian philosophy, and metaphysics.[1]

After Mather had overcome his stammer, apparently due to intense religious devotion, and had taken his master's degree, he was ordained

---

[1] Winton U. Solberg, Introduction. Cotton Mather, *The Christian Philosopher*, 1721, ed. Winton U. Solberg (Chicago: U of Illinois P, 1994) xxiv-xxvii. Physics became part of the Harvard curriculum in 1687, when Charles Morton's *Compendium Physicae* was catalogued in the university. Morton's book, which was revered by Mather and other colonists, introduced new scientific concepts and knowledge about findings by Copernicus, Galileo, Descartes, and Boyle to the British colonies. It also included a section on the alchemical transmutation of metals. William R. Newman, *Gehennical Fire: The Lives of George Starkey, an American Alchemist in the Scientific Revolution* (Cambridge, MA: Harvard UP, 1994) 35-36.

as a minister in 1685 and assisted his father in Boston. Despite his religious duties, which required the preparation of several sermons per week and the involvement in the affairs of the congregation, Mather continued to nourish his interest in medicine and science. After leaving college he maintained a particular fascination with the healing arts and acquired a substantial medical knowledge by studying the European masters, from the Ancients to medical experts of his own time. As is evinced by the list of books in his personal library, Mather was deeply immersed in the on-going discussions about medicine (and science in general) of his time without becoming an active medical practitioner himself.[2]

This chapter seeks to trace how Mather's medical writings concurred and grappled with a salient transition in Western civilization which no longer viewed God's manifestation on earth solely in terms of providential interventions, but increasingly held that His presence was discernible in natural laws. According to many eighteenth-century intellectuals, it was humanity's right and duty to discover these laws and actively shape the course of worldly events, including illness. Mather's writings on various health issues can hence be divided into two main phases: between 1698 and 1712 Mather conceptualized illness and healing almost exclusively in accordance with the doctrine of theological pathogenesis; from 1712 until shortly before his death in 1728 his writings were increasingly influenced by contemporary advances in science and also by curative knowledge acquired from sources beyond New England's and Europe's ecclesiastical and medical elites, especially from the laity, Native Americans, and Africans. Throughout his life as a medical amateur and theological professional, Mather engaged with various theories and practices of medicine as well as with the cosmologies that underwrote them and which, by and large, threatened to "contaminate" his Calvinist views on medicine and its underlying cultural substratum.

---

[2] By the end of his life in 1728, Mather's library, in which he took great pride, contained almost 4,000 books and thereby constituted the largest private collection of knowledge in colonial America at the time. In addition, Mather frequently consulted the Harvard library, especially its growing collection of scientific books. Solberg, Introduction xxvii.

Theology and Disease, Redux

Like all members of the New England clergy, Mather conceptualized illness in the ways that his profession prescribed. Time and again, the Boston minister claimed that diseases belong to the "many *Grievous Things* that are the *unavoidable Portion* of Mankind. [...] there is no Avoiding, there is no Preventing, there is no Escaping of it."[3] His first publication on medical matters, *Mens sana in corpore sano* (1698), is entirely in sync with how Puritans conceived of illness as the result of human iniquities. Regardless of whether God inflicts illness directly or through mediators, especially through Satan's army of demons and/or through natural causes, Mather places a corresponding relationship between virtue and health, sin and illness, at the center of his conceptualization of disease. In addition, he posits a crucial correlation between mind and body, as is evinced by the title of his 1698 sermon, "A healthy mind in a healthy body," in which the body is considered as a plane onto which God projects His disapproval of human actions.

Socialized in colonial New England and having become one of its most rigorous supporters, Mather locates the *vera causa* of disease in original sin. "First, Remember," he warns his audience with the typical grim and fatalistic tone of Puritan sermons, "That the *Sin* of our *First Parents*, was the *First Parent* of all our *Sickness*."[4] Not only can all illnesses be accounted for by Adam and Eve's transgression from the law of God; inherent in Mather's statement is also the idea, held by many medical proponents at the time, that all illnesses are essentially one, albeit with different manifestations. Illness, in whatever shape or form, is hence regarded as a corporeal representation of humanity's original and continuing transgression of divine law and should, as a result, induce utter humility before God. To achieve full recovery, the

---

[3] Cotton Mather, *Insanabilia: An Essay upon Incurables* (1714; Early American Imprints, Series 1, no. 1691) 18 (emphasis original).

[4] Cotton Mather, *Mens Sana in Corpore Sano: A Discourse upon Recovery from Sickness* (1698; Early American Imprints, Series 1, no. 829) 22 (emphasis original).

afflicted is called upon to muse on his/her sins and the depravity of humankind following Adam and Eve's fall from divine grace.

Based on the assumption that sin is "the *Natural* as well as the *Moral* Cause of Sickness," Mather reminds his audience that God also forgives transgressions of His law.[5] For all intents and purposes, the Boston minister, similar to Michael Wigglesworth's poetic voice in "Meat Out of the Eater" (1670), claims illness as a medicine for the soul. In order to grasp the reasons for God's wrath, to realize the prospects of redemption through Christ, "the Physician of the *Sin-sick* Soul," and thus to retain and maintain health, Mather at length advises the patient to engage in self-examination, prayer, repentance, and Bible study.[6] By exchanging his life at the cross for humanity's exoneration from sin, Christ has also offered a special medical treatment that the faithful must apply in order to treat illness at its very root. After his/her recovery from sickness, the believer ought to contemplate the undeserved mercy of God through which health has been restored. In sound Puritan fashion, the faithful should use the illness as an opportunity for spiritual growth, for leading a pious life without special sins in the future, and as a constant reminder of the sovereignty and righteousness of God. Thus, illness, like all human afflictions, is to be regarded as a positive sign and event, one that indicates that God is willing to aid the improvement and progress of believers through a healing of sinful ways.[7] If the believer fails to reform, Mather warns, "God has *Reserves* of *Arrows* in his *Quiver*," and will inflict even greater bodily calamities on those who continue to stray from His word.[8] In a nutshell, Mather, in keeping with Puritan ideology established by the first generation of New England colonists, and echoed

[5] Cotton Mather, *A Perfect Recovery: The Voice of the Glorious God, unto Persons, Whom His Mercy Has Recovered from Sickness* (1714; Early American Imprints, Series 1, no. 1696) 11 (emphasis original).

[6] Cotton Mather, *The Great Physician, Inviting them that are Sensible of their Internal Maladies, to Repair unto Him for His Heavenly Remedies* (1700; Early American Imprints, Series 1, no. 926) 11 (emphasis original).

[7] Mather stresses this point at length in *Mare Pacificum: A Short Essay upon those Noble Principles of Christianity* (1705; Early American Imprints, Series 1, no. 1216).

[8] Mather, *A Perfect Recovery* 39.

in many writings on illness, conceived God's punishment through disease as both vindictive and corrective. The close connection between punishment and blessing, all occurring under the guise of divine providence and wisdom, marks one of the fundamental pillars of Mather's rationalization and textualization of illness throughout his writing career. Virtually all of his medical texts contain a deep structure that is intimately connected to this dialectic: as a sign of God's providence, illness induces a consistent morphology of "humiliation followed by deliverance."[9]

According to the theory of theological pathogenesis, sin is the most important, albeit not the only cause of illness. Mather and other colonists insist that "there is no man that sinneth not" (1 Kings 8:46) and hence every human being is potentially prone to illness. An additional answer to the question why God inflicts illness was grounded in the belief that it constitutes a divine test of patience and faith. In his 1714 lecture *A Perfect Recovery*, Mather advises his audience "to use a due *Caution*, in passing a Judgment on the Sick," because illnesses may also be employed by God to make His hand manifest to the afflicted as well as to others.[10]

Until 1712, Mather's essays and sermons position illness exclusively within a religious framework; natural remedies are by and large omitted from his publications on medicine. Mather's turn toward scientific explanations and natural healing measures become evident when in a guide on treating measles, published 1713, he avoids suggesting patient, silent, and humble endurance and, instead, offers considerable practical advice on how to ease illness symptoms, among them to keep warm, eat lightly, induce gentle vomits, and use herbal concoctions. Along with this advice, Mather also recommends that patients abstain from common

---

[9] Parker H. Johnson, "Humiliation Followed by Deliverance: Metaphor and Plot in Cotton Mather's *Magnalia*," *Early American Literature* 15 (1980/81): 237-246.

[10] Mather, *A Perfect Recovery* 12 (emphasis original). Mather advocated that a sick member of a given family demanded spiritual contemplation, prayers, repentance, and thanksgiving by *all* members. Cf. Cotton Mather, *Wholesome Words: A Visit of Advice, Given unto Families that are Visited with Sickness* (1713; Early American Imprints, Series 1, no. 1630).

treatment methods of the time (e.g., bloodletting) and warns that the sequel of measles is much more threatening, and thus worthy of particular medical care, than the actual disease. In addition, Mather is careful not to infringe on the realm of physicians, advising that in severe cases, a doctor should be consulted.[11]

## "Curiosa Americana:" Letters to the Royal Society

By 1714 Mather had recognized that placing illness and healing exclusively under the auspices of theology contested with early Enlightenment ideas that had already reached New England in various books, pamphlets, and letters in the closing decades of the seventeenth century. The emphasis on reason, many contemporary philosophers and medical experts insisted, demanded a different approach to illness than a mere theological one. In this respect, one of the most radical critiques of conventional epistemology and disease etiology was voiced by Benedict (Baruch) Spinoza (1632-1677), who asserts in *Ethics*:

> Among so many conveniences of nature they [i.e., theologians; M.P.] were bound to find some inconveniences—storms, earthquakes, and diseases, etc.—and they said these happened by reason of the anger of the Gods aroused against men through some misdeed or some omission in worship; and although experience daily belied this, and showed with infinite examples that conveniences and their contraries happen promiscuously to the pious and impious, yet not even then did they turn from their inveterate prejudice. For it was easier for them to place this among other unknown things whose use they did not know, and thus retain their present and innate condition of ignorance, than to destroy the whole fabric of their philosophy and reconstruct it. So it came to pass that they stated with the greatest certainty that the judgments of God far

---

[11] Cotton Mather, *A Letter, about a Good Management under the Distemper of the Measles, at This Time Spreading in the Country* (1713; Early American Imprints, Series 1, no. 4376). John Duffy, *The Healers: A History of American Medicine* (Urbana: U of Illinois P, 1976) 35. See also the striking similarities between Mather's medical advice, Thomas Sydenham's *Methodus curandi febres* (1668), and Thomas Thacher's 1677/78 broadside on smallpox and measles.

surpassed human comprehension: and this by itself was enough to keep truth hidden from the human race through all eternity, had not mathematics [...] offered to men another standard of truth.[12]

Spinoza's call for a reason-based skepticism of previous and current authorities in all fields of knowledge, including medicine, was echoed and modified in numerous writings throughout Europe and did not escape Mather's attention. Influenced by the turn toward rationalism and empiricism in the field of ideas and of the sciences, but also sparked by his preexisting interest in natural philosophy, Mather's writings underwent a lasting shift from a medicine based on religion to one that included, often to a startling degree, scientific discoveries and theories. This is not to claim that Mather discarded his theological approach to medicine; rather, he endeavored to integrate religion and science, while maintaining the interpretive authority of the former.

Mather's shift is especially evinced by his decision to send a series of letters to the Royal Society in London—the major clearing house for new knowledge from around the world at the time—in which he reported strange occurrences that he had heard of or witnessed in his country. Aside from pleasing his aptitude for science, Mather thereby sought to advance his reputation beyond the confines of New England, where he had increasingly become an object of mockery and dislike, especially after his involvement in the Salem witchcraft trials of 1692 and its aftermath. As the forty-four letters sent between 1712 and 1724 indicate, Mather was not a true Newtonian scientist, who would conduct experiments that affirm or falsify a hypothesis and that could be repeated by others. Rather, he presented himself as a man of learning who possessed the skills and the confidence necessary to observe the world around him and to interpret it within a religious cosmology,

---

[12] Quoted in Stuart Hampshire, ed., *The Age of Reason: The 17th Century Philosophers* (New York: New American Library, 1956) 124-125. Mather at length answered Spinoza's (and Hobbesean) criticism of traditional Bible exegesis, especially with regard to the Mosaic authorship of the Pentateuch, in his "Biblia Americana." Reiner Smolinski, "Authority and Interpretation: Cotton Mather's Response to the European Spinozists," *Shaping the Stuart World, 1603-1714: The Atlantic Connection*, ed. Arthur Williamson and Allan MacInnes (Leyden: Brill, 2006) 175-203.

supplemented by advances in the sciences.[13] This supplement, however, became increasingly difficult to apply and to justify, as Mather's correspondence with the Royal Society demonstrates.

Mather's claim to fame in the Royal Society—he became a member in 1713, after his first series of observational letters had met with interest and approval—lay in his ability to report natural peculiarities that were endemic to the "New World" and that would, so he hoped, meet with the broad scope of scientific interests represented in the Royal Society, including natural history, botany, biology, medicine, astronomy, mathematics, climatology, engineering, and husbandry. While Mather reports about both universal and site-specific natural curiosities, the letters "contain an embryonic element of nationalism," because the Boston minister writes as an *American* and about occurrences in America.[14] Most letters convey both a sense of the author's pride and embarrassment in living in and writing from America, a region which he admitted to be lacking philosophers and scientists comparable to those in Europe, while at the same time hosting a unique natural and cultural habitat that was worth being related to the rest of the world.[15]

---

[13] By 1713, Mather had become what might be called "a naive Newtonian," meaning that the Boston minister often sided with an idealized version of Newton. Had Mather read Newton's comments directly, he would probably have been shocked by Newton's deep skepticism toward the "correct" form of Protestant worship.

[14] Kenneth Silverman, *The Life and Times of Cotton Mather* (New York: Harper, 1984) 245.

[15] Even though English scholars devoted to the emerging natural sciences of the time greeted Mather's letters enthusiastically, none of the reports seem to have been significant enough to deserve publication, with the exception of a summary that contained short excerpts taken from the first series. Cf. "An Extract of Several Letters from Cotton Mather, D. D. to John Woodward, M. D. and Richard Waller," *Philosophical Transactions* 29 (1714-1716): 62-71. One of the reasons that the reports were not published was that Mather's language failed to conform to new standards in scientific writing and thinking that attempted, unsuccessfully, to depart from, metaphors and puns. A convincing critique of Mather's letters to the Royal Society is offered by Susan Scott Parrish, who contends that their diction and contents were hopelessly behind the new standard

Of the first thirteen letters, which Mather composed between 17 November and 29 November 1712, the early "Curiosa Americana," six deal with medical topics: New England plants used for medicinal purposes (no. 2), the influence of the imagination on illness and healing (no. 4), birth deformities ("monsters") and abnormal tissue in the uterus (no. 5), remedies revealed in dreams (no. 6), wounds that should have killed the afflicted but which were healed (no. 7), and a Native American antidote against rattlesnake bites (no. 11).[16] The tone of the medical letters (as well as of those on other topics) is that of a writer who humbles himself for his scientific backwardness. At the same time, he displays his broad knowledge of the Ancients and of the most state-of-the-art healing methods, anatomical discoveries, and medical theories. Except for occasional references to the Bible, the letters contain only few religious interpretations of illness; instead, the author attempts to represent natural curiosities as detached and as objective as possible.

What is especially interesting in the first series of letters to the Royal Society is how Mather simultaneously fortifies and crosses the cultural dividing line between Algonquians and English settlers. In the first letter, the author discards indigenous knowledge, stating that "there is very little in any Tradition of our Salvages, to be rely'd upon," only to

in representing natural occurrences. Susan Scott Parrish, "Scientific Discourse," *The Oxford Handbook of Early American Literature*, ed. Kevin J. Hayes (Oxford: Oxford UP, 2008) 292.

[16] As of today, the letters comprising the "Curiosa Americana" have only been published in fragments. George Lyman Kittredge catalogued the letters in "Cotton Mather's Scientific Communications to the Royal Society," *Proceedings of the American Antiquarian Society* 26 (1916): 18-57. Short excerpts of some of the letters can be found in Cotton Mather, *Selected Letters of Cotton Mather*, ed. Kenneth Silverman (Baton Rouge: Louisiana State UP, 1971). For scholarly analyses of the letters, see David Levin, "Giants in the Earth: Science and the Occult in Cotton Mather's Letters to the Royal Society," *William and Mary Quarterly* 45 (1988): 751-770; Michael P. Winship, *Seers of God: Puritan Providentialism in the Restoration and Early Enlightenment* (Baltimore: Johns Hopkins UP, 2000) 93-110; Otho T. Beall, Jr., "Cotton Mather's Early 'Curiosa Americana' and the Boston Philosophical Society of 1683," *William and Mary Quarterly* 18 (1961): 360-372.

praise and advertise the efficacy of medical remedies that originated from an ostensibly unreliable cultural tradition in the second and eleventh letters.[17] In his observations on indigenous healing from 18 November 1712, the real and imagined boundaries between Native people and colonists are cast aside for the time being, and Indians are posited as credible purveyors of curative knowledge, especially in the field of botany. Mather lists a number of Algonquian remedies for dropsy, jaundice, gangrene, sore throat, scurvy, syphilis, ulcers, and scrofula (the King's Evil), which colonists have learned from their Native neighbors and have applied successfully.[18] Four years later, he relates a recipe that "was first communicated to [him], by an Indian, who did very strange cures upon cancers, by a decoction of it inwardly taken, and a cataplasm of the boiled plant at the same time laid unto the place afflicted. [...] the secret was obtained from him."[19] The final clause indicates that the acquisition of indigenous healing knowledge was not always an easy task. Furthermore, Mather explains that colonists transferred Native cures to other diseases: in this case, the plant was also used for diseases whose symptoms resemble leprosy and against fever and fatigue.

Of particular interest for the New England correspondent are Native remedies against snake poisoning, to which alone he devotes two letters. On 27 November 1712, Mather reports: "Would you have expected, Syr, to have mett with a Rich Medicine, & a very noble cordial, in the *Gall of the Rattlesnake*?"[20] He then describes how colonists use a Native New England cure by drying the liquid from the rattlesnake's gallbladder as an antidote against venomous bites. Rather than speculating on this curiosity by, for instance, evoking the medical doctrine of similars, Mather closes the letter with a two-page rendition of the serpent in

---

[17] "Cotton Mather to John Woodward, 17 November 1712," Royal Society, London, EL/M2/21.

[18] "Cotton Mather to John Woodward, 18 November 1712," Royal Society, London, EL/M2/22.

[19] "Cotton Mather to John Woodward, 13 July 1716," British Library, Sloane Ms. 3340, folio 297.

[20] "Cotton Mather to Richard Waller, 27 November 1712," Royal Society, London, EL/M2/31 (emphasis original).

religious history. Apparently, Mather's report about an antidote from the poison agent drew the interest of the Royal Society because the second series of letters, sent between 2 July and 24 July 1716, includes another letter on a Native remedy against snakebites. This time, however, the Boston minister neglects the expected duties as a scientific observer and devotes the bulk of his correspondence to the role of the serpent in Antiquity and in Scripture.[21] One can safely assume that this failed to please the members of the Royal Society, because Mather's final letter on snake poisoning is almost devoid of historical and religious references. Written on 4 June 1723, Mather states that he will not continue a discussion of the allegorical significance of serpents depicted in the Bible. Instead, he informs his interlocutor of a plant that his Algonquian neighbors call "poor Robin's Plantain." According to Mather, the name of the plant was derived from a Native American who had observed how a bird (a Robin) treated its snakebite with a specific plant and who then applied it successfully after a rattlesnake had released its venom into his body.[22]

With his repeated inclusion of indigenous medical remedies, Cotton Mather momentarily suspends the commonly held view that the original inhabitants of America were "a satanic parody of the Puritans" and as, on the whole, culturally inferior to their English neighbors.[23] At the same time, Mather's appropriation of Native medicinal knowledge assures that its exotic otherness is retained and thus serves to advance the reputation of the colonists that Mather represents for his European audience. As will be emphasized again at a later point in this chapter, once certain aspects of indigenous cultures have been incorporated to achieve this end, the author returns to suppressing indigenous medicinal knowledge.[24] In the letters to the Royal Society, the Boston minister can

---

[21] "Cotton Mather to John Woodward, 11 July 1716," British Library, Sloane Ms. 3340, folio 291-293.

[22] "Cotton Mather to James Jurin, 4 June 1723," Royal Society, London, EL/M2/38.

[23] Silverman 239.

[24] I am hence contesting Vogel's claim that "Mather showed an uncommon openmindedness, for his time, in his willingness to credit the remedies of the 'tawney serpents.'" Virgil J. Vogel, *American Indian Medicine* (1970; Norman:

still safely include Algonquian medical knowledge, but only because it constitutes a curiosity, a novel and strange occurrence that exceeds ordinary experiences or perceptions of reality.

Against the background of a comparatively scant understanding of causation in the field of medicine at the time, Mather's letters also delineate a number of unusual corporeal conditions and symptoms of colonial New Englanders, *curiosa* that include a dead body without intestines, various malformed births, a woman who became hydropical and voided twelve gallons (!) of water, and people who vomited foreign objects (e.g., pins or small animals).[25] Such accounts, Mather hoped, would heighten his scientific reputation within the growing European and transatlantic network of knowledge exchange, and inject his religious opinions on medical topics into contemporary discourse. This is especially evident when he reports and comments on several sick New England colonists who had cures communicated to them in their dreams. Among them was Lydia Ingram of Boston, who suffered from pain and swelling in her side and stomach, accompanied by a suppression of urine. After local physicians had declared her ailment incurable, a man appeared to her in her dreams and offered her a remedy with directions, which she failed to remember accurately the next morning. After the dream healer had returned and specified the recipe, her physician consented to the application. When the remedy finally matched the dreamed prescription, the patient recovered. In order to avoid an interpretation that would attribute the cure to magic or demonic interventions, Mather stresses the religious piety and devotion of Lydia

---

U of Oklahoma P, 1990) 45. In *Magnalia Christi Americana*, Mather has nothing but disdain for Native medical practices, which he identifies as merely consisting of sweat baths and healing rituals: "Their *physick* is, excepting a few odd specificks, which some of them encounter certain cases with, nothing hardly but an hot-house or a powaw [...]." Cotton Mather, *Magnalia Christi Americana; or, The Ecclesiastical History of New England*, Vol. I (1702; Hartford: Andrus, 1855) 558.

[25] "Cotton Mather to John Woodward, 24 November 1712," Royal Society, London, EL/M2/27; "Cotton Mather to John Woodward, 3 July 1716," British Library, Sloane Ms. 3340, folio 280-282; "Cotton Mather to James Jurin, 22 September 1724," Royal Society, London, EL/M2/48.

Ingram, who stated upon remission that, "[a]ll things are possible with God. [...] give God all the glory; give God all the glory." Towards the end of his medical report, Mather attempts to synchronize religion and the emerging sciences by citing Robert Boyle's (one of the founders of modern chemistry) claim that "celestial spirits" in the shape of angels may indeed appear in the dreams of sick persons, offering efficacious remedies.[26]

Mather's overall attitude of scientific connoisseurship, displayed throughout his letters to the Royal Society, allowed him to venture into topics of inquiry and cultural territory that many devout Christians at the time would have regarded as belonging exclusively to the realm of either divine providence or the devil. In contrast to his father's attempts to prove God's intervention in earthly affairs, assembled in *An Essay for the Recording of Illustrious Providences* (1684), Cotton Mather approaches natural curiosities through a scientific-theological double lens. This affords him the opportunity to engage in scientific discourse and knowledge production, while, at the same time, insinuating that many strange occurrences actually lie outside of the explanatory purview of the budding natural sciences and, hence, reveal the presence and power of God. One such occasion of divine revelation was the outbreak of smallpox in 1721, which threatened the lives of thousands of Bostonians. Miraculously, for Mather, the minister had previously read scientific reports, supplemented by pagan sources, on a new and hardly-tested inoculation procedure, and was ready to engage in an intellectual debate about the pros and cons of preventive medicine.

Medicine and Power: The Boston Smallpox Inoculation Controversy

In the early modern Atlantic world, smallpox was one of only a few clearly identifiable diseases: it had a clinical basis, could be studied according to a mechanistic model of transmission, and produced specific and thus recognizable symptoms. European physicians had long attempted, with little success, to treat smallpox patients. At the beginning of the eighteenth century, the Royal Society published a

[26] "Cotton Mather to John Woodward, 22 November 1712," Royal Society, London, EL/M2/26.

report from Turkey that outlined a novel method designed to prevent the painful and often lethal outbreak of smallpox. The news of inoculation or variolation, as the procedure of artificial immunization was also called, soon reached the New England colonies where the reactions to the new method were divided: either overly enthusiastic or deeply skeptical. Between 1721 and 1722, as smallpox was spreading throughout Boston, ministers and physicians engaged in a heated debate about the efficacy and ethics of inoculation that was to have a lasting effect on the political balance of power established in the founding years of Massachusetts Bay Colony. Even though the ministers who favored the new method, among them Cotton Mather, were on the right side of medical truth, the inoculation controversy heralded a significant shift in the interpretive authority over disease treatment from the preacher-physician to the lay practitioner in the course of the eighteenth century.

Smallpox had repeatedly threatened and ravaged Boston since its foundation in 1630. The first reported outbreak dates back to 1633, when Dutch ships brought the disease to the shores of New England from the West Indies. In the following years, Bostonians and other colonists faced annual visitations but also inexplicable absences of the scourge, despite growing trade activities with the Caribbean and Europe during the seventeenth century. Major outbreaks of this unpredictable disease in Boston, which the English called the speckled monster and which caused a mortality rate between ten and thirty-five percent, occurred in 1677-1678, 1689-1690, and again in 1702. After a respite of almost twenty years, *variola major* returned with a vengeance to the commercial and intellectual center of New England when the HMS Seashore arrived from the West Indies in April 1721. Despite efforts by the town leaders to quarantine ships arriving in Boston Harbor, the population at large was again virtually defenseless against the disease because a whole generation of young Bostonians was disease-prone (i.e., lacking sufficient antibodies) and memories of the horrors of previous outbreaks had by and large disappeared. As a consequence, between September and November 1721, the Boston funeral bells were ringing almost incessantly, and on every street red flags with the emblazoned words "God have mercy on this house" were flying over infected houses. When the epidemic abated in the spring of 1722, about 6,000

Bostonians—roughly half of the city's population—had been infected, of whom 844 died and 288 were saved by inoculation.[27]

Cotton Mather, who had contracted the disease in his teens, understood that when a person survived a smallpox infection, s/he would not fall prey to the disease again. In contrast to most New England physicians at the time, he was also aware of an artificial immunization technique practiced in other parts of the world, especially the eastern Mediterranean and in Africa.[28] In 1716, he wrote a letter to the Royal Society in which he corroborates the success of the procedure based on a similar account related to him by his African slave, Onesimus:

> I am willing to confirm you, in a favorable opinion, of Dr. Timonius's Communication; and therefore, I do assure you, that many months before I mett with any Intimations of treating the Small-Pox with the Method of Inoculation, I had from a Servant of my own, an Account of

---

[27] For a more elaborate account of the history of smallpox in Boston, see Ola Elizabeth Winslow, *A Destroying Angel: The Conquest of Smallpox in Colonial Boston* (Boston: Houghton, 1974) 24-29. Cf. Henry R. Viets, *A Brief History of Medicine in Massachusetts* (Boston: Houghton, 1930) 56; Gerald N. Grob, *The Deadly Truth: A History of Disease in America* (Cambridge, MA: Harvard UP, 2002) 78. For mortality rates and population numbers, see Otho T. Beall, Jr. and Richard H. Shryock, "Cotton Mather: First Significant Figure in American Medicine," *Proceedings of the American Antiquarian Society* 63.1 (1953): 147; John B. Blake *Public Health in the Town of Boston, 1630-1822* (Cambridge, MA: Harvard UP, 1959) 247-249.

[28] The first news of inoculation was published in the *Philosophical Transactions* in 1714 by Emanuele Timoni (Timonius), a Greek physician, educated at Padua and Oxford. The second report, which Mather also read, appeared three years later in the same publication and was composed by Giacomo Pilarino (Jacobus Pylarinus), another Greek physician. Babette M. Levy, *Cotton Mather* (Boston: Twayne, 1979) 165n15. In 1717, Lady Mary Wortley Montagu, wife of the British ambassador in Turkey, learned a similar inoculation technique and published her findings in London, which were rejected by the medical establishment. In 1721, she publicly inoculated her three-year old daughter and thus popularized the method among the aristocracy. Soon thereafter, English newspapers reported on the religious and medical ramifications of the procedure and provided Bostonians with argumentative fodder for the controversy over inoculation. Winslow, *Destroying Angel* 59-65.

its being practiced in *Africa*. Enquiring of my Negro-Man *Onesimus*, who is a pretty Intelligent Fellow, Whether he ever had the Small-Pox, he answered *Yes* and *No*; and then told me that he had undergone an Operation, which had given him something of the Small-Pox, and would forever preserve him from it, adding, That it was often used among the *Guaramantese*, and whoever had the Courage to use it, was forever free from the Fear of the Contagion. He described the Operation to me, and showed me in his Arm the Scar, and his description of it made it the same that afterwards I found related unto you by your Timonius.[29]

In this passage Mather's servant is cited as a cultural authority on early preventive medicine. Considering the widespread attitudes towards Africans as intellectually inferior, it seems remarkable that the minister even deploys such testament. Margot Minardi, who carves out salient notions of race underlying the Boston smallpox epidemic and its ensuing controversy between the religious and secular elite, explains that "because inferiority had not yet been *indelibly* written onto the bodies of Africans, their intellectual and spiritual worth seemed plausible enough for Cotton Mather to take seriously Onesimus's explanation of inoculation."[30] Interestingly enough, in his retrospective account of the smallpox epidemic in *The Angel of Bethesda* (completed in 1724), Mather also relates how he learned about artificial immunization from other African slaves in Boston. Here, however, his narrative voice, which consistently represents a learned theologian and scientific observer, changes for one paragraph:

I have since mett with a Considerable Number of these *Africans*, who all agree in one Story; That in their Countrey *grandy-many* dy of the *Small-Pox*: But now they Learn This Way: People take Juice of *Small-Pox*; and cutty-skin, and putt in a Drop; then by'nd by a little *sicky, sicky*: then very few little things like *Small-Pox*; and no body dy of it; and no body have *Small-Pox* any more. Thus in *Africa*, where the poor Creatures dy

[29] Cotton Mather to John Woodward, 12 July 1716, British Library, Sloane Ms. 3340, folio 294-296 (emphasis original).

[30] Margot Minardi, "The Boston Inoculation Controversy of 1721-1722: An Incident in the History of Race," *William and Mary Quarterly* 61.1 (2004): 50 (emphasis added).

of the *Small-Pox* like Rotten Sheep, a Merciful God has taught them an *Infallible Praeservative.*[31]

It is worth speculating why Mather chose such a shift in narrative voice. One might read this passage as an early version of literary *local color* and thus as a way of adding authenticity and verisimilitude to the reported inoculation procedure. In fact, some twentieth-century commentators praise Mather's willingness and ability to listen to and incorporate what African slaves had to say on matters of life and death.[32] The shift in narrative voice can also be seen as proof of the author's condescending view of Africans, who are portrayed as collectively lacking the ability to speak Standard English. The use of vernacular in his authoritative prose, therefore, solidifies the Africans' ostensible cultural inferiority and social status and thereby precludes full participation in colonial society. As Kathryn Koo has pointed out, "[w]ith their childlike diction and unquestioning faith in a medical procedure that was surely beyond their comprehension, the Africans that Mather 'ventriloquized' on the printed page only reaffirm the notion of a simple-minded people who would helplessly perish 'like Rotten Sheep' without the good graces of their Maker."[33] Mather's use of ethnic ventriloquism at once complicates the power/knowledge hierarchy between Africans and Puritans—suggesting a brief instance of role reversal between teacher and student—while at the same time keeping this hierarchy and status quo firmly in place. Although it seems that the African slaves are independent agents speaking *through* the Puritan

[31] Cotton Mather, *The Angel of Bethesda*, ed. Gordon W. Jones (Barre: American Antiquarian Society and Barre, 1972) 107. For the sake of readability, further quotations from Mather's medical book will be cited parenthetically throughout this chapter and all emphases are original, unless stated otherwise.

[32] Levy 125.

[33] Kathryn S. Koo, "Strangers in the House of God: Cotton Mather, Onesimus, and an Experiment in Christian Slaveholding," *Proceedings of the American Antiquarian Society* 117.1 (2007): 145. See also, Minardi 63. For the notion of "ethnic ventriloquism," see also Mita Banerjee, *Ethnic Ventriloquism: Literary Minstrelsy in Nineteenth-Century American Literature* (Heidelberg: Winter, 2008).

minister, he is actually speaking *for* them, thus asserting his position of cultural power and superiority, as well as that of the colonists Mather is representing. His remark that "a Merciful God has taught them an *Infallible Praeservative*" represents a crucial argument in the ensuing public controversy over variolation because it qualifies the procedure introduced by the cultural Other as a sign of divine grace and providence rather than as (merely) a pagan ritual. This particular reference to God becomes an act of containment, one which aims to bring a foreign and heathen medical practice into the domain of Christianity. However, Mather's performative act of containment ultimately lacked the persuasive strength intended by the author: one of the reasons the majority of Bostonians rejected inoculation was precisely because it had been introduced by Africans.[34]

As a result of his acquaintance with the preventive medical measure, Cotton Mather attempted in 1716 to convince local physicians to inoculate all citizens of Boston as soon as the next outbreak of smallpox was evident. Unfortunately, his attempt was not successful. During the 1721 epidemic, Mather was able to put to the test the method he had learned from various non-European sources after encouraging Zabdiel Boylston, a Boston physician, to undertake the following procedure: take the pus from pustules of a person infected with *variola major* and inject the inoculants into the bloodstream of a person that has not yet contracted the illness. Within a few days the patient will develop minor

---

[34] Mather defended the credibility of his African slave throughout the public inoculation controversy. In 1721, for instance, he wrote: "And I don't know why 'tis more unlawful to learn of *Africans*, how to help against the *Poison* of the *Small Pox*, than it is to learn of our Indians, how to help the *Poison* of a *Rattle-Snake*." Zabdiel Boylston, *Some Account of What is Said of Inoculating or Transplanting the Small Pox* (Boston: Gerrish, 1721) 9. Even though this essay was published by Zabdiel Boylston, the diction of the text, as well as the preface, indicate that most sections were written by Mather. Apparently, the two had considered it wise for Boylston to bear the brunt of the controversy and, also, to take credit for introducing inoculation to the British colonies. Cf. Mather's letter to the Royal Society in which he praises Boylston: "*This* is the gentleman who first brought the way of saving Lives, by the *Inoculation of Small-pox*, into the *American* world." "Cotton Mather to James Jurin, 15 December 1724," Royal Society, London, EL/M2/57 (all emphases original).

symptoms related to smallpox, but the illness will not be lethal. After about two weeks s/he will be healthy and immunized. Boylston first confirmed this procedure after inoculating his son and his African servants in the summer of 1721. In the following weeks and months, Boylston treated 247 Bostonians and undertook the first American clinical test of a medical procedure by meticulously recording the names, age, and race of the patients, the dates of incision, and a brief description of the course of disease, followed by a concluding interpretation of the statistical evidence.[35]

Although the method proved successful from a medical point of view, Cotton Mather's local reputation suffered as a consequence of Boylston's experiment, because the majority of Bostonians as well as the medical establishment (with few exceptions) rejected artificial immunization. Between 1721 and 1722, Boston became the American battleground of a culture war that had been waged vociferously in Europe between ecclesiastical and civil camps since the advent of the Age of Reason. One of the most striking aspects of the controversy in New England was that the clergy rather than university-educated doctors were suggesting a progressive medical procedure. "Here was a strange spectacle indeed," Otho Beall and Richard Shryock write in their investigation of Mather's place in the history of American medicine, "[o]n the one side, it was the physicians who opposed the advent of preventive medicine without even deigning to observe the results, and opposed this on religious as well as on scientific grounds. On the other, it was the clergy who not only aided Boylston, but who also defended a liberal theology against the doctors and the populace at large."[36] As the epidemic peaked and then subsided, the proponents and opponents of

---

[35] Zabdiel Boylston, *Historical Account of the Small-Pox Inoculated in New-England* (1726; Boston: Gerrish, 1730).

[36] Beall and Shryock 146. The full chronology and summary of the controversy cannot be provided here. For an account of the unfolding of the smallpox inoculation debate, see Silverman 336-352; Winslow 44-86. A critical evaluation of Cotton Mather's role during the inoculation controversy can be found in Perry Miller, *The New England Mind: From Colony to Province* (Cambridge, MA: Harvard UP, 1953) 345-366; for a more generous treatment of the Boston minister, see Beall and Shryock 138-161.

variolation engaged in a rancorous pamphlet war that became increasingly personal and vindictive. Whereas the *Boston Gazette* served as the main mouthpiece of those in favor of the preventive measure, the *New England Courant* and the *Boston News-Letter* voiced the opinions of the opponents, particularly that of Boston's one of ten medical doctors, William Douglass.[37] Douglass' motivation for opposing inoculation were in part monetary—attending to the sick was, after all, his main source of income—and stemmed in part from personal dislike of an overly ambitious and annoying minister (Cotton Mather) meddling in his profession. His official rejection of the technique rested on the assumption that the reports on inoculation in the *Philosophical Transactions* were unscientific and that the applicability of the prescribed technique was highly questionable since it meant infecting people with a deadly disease.[38] For a medical profession attempting to establish itself in the colonies, the fear of being perceived by the public as practicing iatrogenesis (i.e., doctors causing illness instead of curing it), proved a powerful factor in rejecting inoculation in 1721-1722. Douglass and other Boston physicians furthermore refused inoculation as a viable public health measure because they saw it as an irresponsible and unlawful clinical trial of questionable medical modality, undertaken by men who lacked the necessary training.

As the controversy intensified, the initial concerns about saving human lives took a backseat to issues of moral and socio-political power. Smallpox, one of the most lethal communicable diseases at the time, produced what Paula Treichler has called with regard to

---

[37] The most salient newspaper articles during the inoculation controversy are assembled and reprinted in David E. Copeland, ed., *Debating the Issues in Colonial Newspapers: Primary Documents on Events of the Period* (Westport: Greenwood, 2000) 13-25.

[38] William Douglass, *The Abuses and Scandals of Some Late Pamphlets in Favour of Inoculation of the Small Pox* (Boston: Franklin, 1722), esp. 2, 9-11. Indeed, certain aspects of the procedure were still worthy of improvement, for instance, the physical separation of the inoculated from healthy persons in order to contain the spreading of the epidemic (Duffy 37).

HIV/AIDS in the twentieth century an "epidemic of signification."[39] In early 1722, the medical debate turned into a turf war between clerical and civic leaders that centered on the question who was authorized to make statements of truth concerning the body and to initiate actions accordingly. Anti-inoculators joined forces with secular Bostonians and unleashed a wave of anti-clerical sentiments. Many residents had not forgotten Cotton Mather's justification of the executions at Salem in 1692 and now claimed that the minister was once again siding with murderers who proposed a treatment based on a different kind of spectral evidence. Some opponents held that in order to maintain their power and influence over social affairs, the Boston ministers were "deliberately wreaking their vengeance upon a society they could not dominate by infecting it with smallpox."[40]

Other anti-inoculators argued that the Boston Africans who, with the help of Satan, had contrived a devious plan to kill their masters through inoculation had deceived Mather and other proponents of variolation. Still others pointed to the Sixth Commandment ("Thou shalt not kill") and Job 2:7, citing how the devil "went forth from the presence of the Lord and smote Job with sore boils from the sole of his foot unto his crown" and that, therefore, the Boston epidemic had to be humbly endured. In essence, the opponents of inoculation asserted that the clergymen were contradicting their own teachings that natural disasters, including individual and collective illnesses, were signs of divine providence and sovereignty. Whereas Scripture allows and encourages the use of medical remedies *after* God had inflicted his punishment or test of faith through illness, they argued, it leaves no room for preventive measures, such as inoculation, with which a person seeks to anticipate and ultimately elude divine judgment and correction *in advance*.[41] By advocating artificial immunization, opponents claimed,

---

[39] Paula A. Treichler, *How to Have Theory in an Epidemic: Cultural Chronicles of AIDS* (Durham: Duke UP, 1999) 1.

[40] Miller 348.

[41] Samuel Grainger, *The Imposition of Inoculation as a Duty Religiously Considered* (Boston: Nicholas Boone, 1721) 4-15; John Williams, *Several Arguments, Proving, That Inoculating the Small Pox Is Not Contained in the Law of Physick, either Natural or Divine, and Therefore Unlawful* (Boston:

Mather and his colleagues not only proved to be medical amateurs but were recasting the foundational covenant between God and the New England colonists. Instead of prescribing quasi-medical practices derived from dark-skinned pagans and suggesting deliberate self-infliction of a potentially lethal illness, the clergy's sole answer to the epidemic should have consisted of utter repentance and reform as well as prayer and fasting.[42]

The nature of the prescribed intervention—injecting pathogens in order to remain healthy—appeared so innovative and self-contradictory that it required justification on both medical and theological grounds. Stung by this trenchant criticism, Mather and other Boston preachers (with few exceptions) responded that it was their moral duty to help the population of Boston stay healthy so that God could be served in the first place. It was no longer sufficient to postulate illness-as-medicine in a metaphorical and spiritual sense; the literal, bodily implementations of this apparent paradox had to be placed under the auspices of religious necessity and interpretive authority. In 1721, the minister William Cooper attempted to answer the religious concerns of his fellow Bostonians, claiming that divine providence had provided inoculation to preserve those who believe in Him from imminent danger and had, therefore, to be accepted with gratitude. Cooper affirmed that smallpox constituted a just punishment for human transgression, yet "at the very same time [...] God [showed] us a way to escape the *Extremity* and Destruction."[43] To refuse such a way to escape divine wrath would

Franklin, 1721) 2. In addition to risks to the individual and the community, Douglass was opposed to the procedure on religious grounds, asking "how the trusting more the extra groundless *Machinations of Men* than to our preserver in the ordinary course of Nature, may be consistent with the Devotion and Subjection we owe to the *all-wise Providence* of GOD Almighty." William Douglass, *Boston News-Letter*, 24 July 1721, reprinted in Copeland 17 (emphasis original).

[42] Silverman 353.

[43] William Cooper, *A Letter to a Friend in the Country, Attempting a Solution of the Scruples and Objections of Conscientious or Religious Nature, Commonly Made Against the New Way of Receiving the Small-Pox* (1721; Early American Imprints, Series 1, no. 2247) 7. See also, Boylston, *Some Account* 18-21.

constitute a breach of the New England covenant. Because God was not only wrathful but also compassionate, supporters of artificial induction of immunity reminded the Boston population, He "furnishes every country with the particular remedies for all the distempers with which it may be affected."[44] As a consequence, the method suggested by Mather and practiced by Boylston marked in the eyes of the clergy no more or less an intervention in God's providence than venesection or other medical procedures.

Another reason for the support of variolation by the clergy was related to the fate of the local Native Americans in the seventeenth century. Time and again, ministers and officials had announced in speech and in writing that the virtual eradication of Algonquian communities was caused and sanctioned by god-sent diseases. Increase Mather and others had observed that the speckled monster was one of the most lethal illnesses Algonquians had to face as an increasing number of English colonists settled the land. A mere acceptance of the smallpox epidemic in Boston despite a tested counter-measure hence contradicted the belief in a divine providence that favored the elect over the Natives. For if the Anglo population, and among them many who could be expected to be on the side of the elect, would die in great numbers from the same illness that had helped to clear the way for settlement, then this had to be yet another sign that God was withdrawing his special treatment from the people of New England. Such a line of argument echoed the central message contained in the many jeremiads preached and published during the second half of the seventeenth century, in which ministers incessantly pointed to

---

[44] Solberg, Introduction lxxxiv. Mather makes this point in *The Christian Philosopher* (1721), when he modifies Paracelsus' "*Ubi Virus, ibi Virtus*" into a site-specific medical dictum, commonly held at the time: "Where there is a disease, there is a remedy." Paraphrasing John Ray and Johan van Beverwyck, Mather claims: "It is very remarkable, that our compassionate God has furnish'd all Regions with *Plants* peculiarly adapted for the relief of the *Diseases* that are most common in those Regions" (145). One aspect of Mather's theodicy is his description of venomous animals which were put on earth by God for the benefit of humanity. Similarly, he argues, there are plants that can be both poisonous and medicinal. Hence, in his view everything in nature is of use; nothing wasted, nothing placed without a divine purpose (142).

ubiquitous signs that God was revoking the covenant and removing his providential support of the New England way. However, bemoaning the religious backsliding that caused God's withdrawal was only part of the jeremiad's structure and rhetoric; preachers also consistently urged their audiences that it was not too late to reform and to regain His favor. According to this logic, the Boston clergy could interpret smallpox as a barometer of sinfulness and inoculation as a tool revealed by God to one of his special children, Cotton Mather, to save the elect from a pestilence originally designed to wipe out the Natives. It was thus a sign that God was still siding with the visible Massachusetts saints.[45]

The responses of the Boston clergymen to the reproaches put forth by the anti-inoculation camp highlighted seminal changes in colonial society and religion of the time. As Roy Porter points out, eighteenth-century Christian theologians began to "cast aside certain vestiges of medieval mortification and unconcern for the welfare of the flesh," replacing them with a more benign view on issues concerning human corporeality.[46] By prescribing new advances in medicine, the Boston ministers modified the doctrine of theological pathogenesis in an attempt to maintain the old order according to which it was the clergy's duty and privilege to interpret illnesses and their cures. Yet, the contradiction of simultaneously upholding tradition and embracing innovations was unresolvable and, as a consequence, the clergy continued to lose influence over secular affairs in eighteenth-century New England. Perry Miller sums up the aftermath of the controversy, stating that:

> The conflict was a crisis within the culture, of which the ultimate effects were to be felt in other regions of the mind than those in which scientific verification mattered. What had been risked and what had not been regained was the covenant conception itself. Spokesmen for the national philosophy could never again authoritatively contend that what the people suffered was caused by their sins and that repentance alone [...] could relieve them. The clergy themselves had introduced another

[45] Increase Mather, *A Relation of the Troubles Which Have Happened in New-England by Reason of the Indians there, from the Year 1614 to the Year 1675, etc.* (Boston: Foster, 1677) 6, 23.

[46] Roy Porter, *Flesh in the Age of Reason* (New York: Norton, 2003) 229.

method, and so brought a fatal confusion into the very center of their mystique.[47]

After the conflict over inoculation had subsided, a number of justified questions regarding the proper way of reconciling the belief in god-sent illness and the fruits of human-made science remained in the minds of most New Englanders: Was not any natural cure an intervention in God's divine plan and will? Were medical advances to be regarded as signs of human vanity and thus as blasphemous interferences in His providence? For Mather, such questions were but rhetorical ones. His rationale for practicing medicine in the first place was grounded in the Christian service ideal and in his firm conviction that the *vera causa* of disease could only be rooted out by (re)turning to God while the symptoms could be eased with the help of remedies that He had placed in nature for precisely this reason.[48]

## The Way to Health: *The Angel of Bethesda*

In 1724 Mather's life-long interest in science and his religious conviction to use medicine as a service for his parishioners culminated in a book that contains explanations of, and remedies for, the main illnesses that plagued humanity at the time. As he states in his diary, the idea for writing such a book had been conceived as early as March 1693, after the Salem witch trials and their ensuing damage to Mather's reputation:

---

[47] Miller 363.

[48] After the 1721/1722 smallpox epidemic had subsided, Douglass began to support inoculation in 1730. Nevertheless, Boston experienced six successive waves of smallpox until 1792, each accompanied by renewed debates over proper inoculation methods. After years of rejecting wholesale immunization measures, the Province of Massachusetts opened two inoculation hospitals in 1764. During the Revolutionary War, General Washington ordered the inoculation of all his troops to avoid thinning his already meager military ranks. Variolation became widely accepted with Edward Jenner's vaccination method developed in England in 1796. See, Elizabeth Anne Fenn, *Pox Americana: The Great Smallpox Epidemic of 1775-82* (New York: Hill, 2001) 1-27.

> To make myself more *useful* unto my Neighbours in their Afflictions; not only releeving the *Poor*, but also the *Sick*; to which purpose, I would collect, at Leisure a fit number of most parable [meaning easily procurable; M.P.] and effectual *Remedies* for all Diseases, and publish them unto the world; so, by my Hand, will be done things that the *Angels* love to do.[49]

It took Mather over thirty years to complete this ambitious project, not least because in 1693 he also proposed to write the church history of New England (*Magnalia Christi Americana*) and his extensive Bible comments (*Biblia Americana*). With another major publication—*The Christian Philosopher*—still to be written, Mather's *opus magnum* on medicine was not completed until 1724, four years before his death.

Mather reused a number of earlier writings on medicine for his book-length manuscript, among them passages from sermons, excerpts from letters addressed to the Royal Society, the section on physicians from "Bonifacius: An Essay Upon the Good" (1710), parts of the anatomical chapter "On Man" from *The Christian Philosopher*, some of his pamphlets written during the smallpox controversy, and the section on stammering from his diary. To his great disappointment, and after numerous prayers and fasts, *The Angel of Bethesda*—the title was adopted from the biblical account of the healing pool of Bethesda (John 5:4)—failed to find a publisher and was only released in its entirety almost 250 years after completion.[50] Mather designed his book on medicine as a household *vade mecum*, "A *Family-physician*, which every *Family* of any *Capacity* may find their Account in being supplied withal" (*Angel* 1). However, the diction, intellectual scope, and employment of Latin and Greek passages would have made *The Angel of Bethesda* in part inaccessible to the majority of common readers in New England. Aside from the proposed lay audience, Mather's intended

---

[49] Cotton Mather, *Diary of Cotton Mather, Part I: 1681-1708*, ed. C. Ford Worthington (Boston: Massachusetts Historical Society Collections, 1911) 163 (emphasis original).

[50] The original chapters on cancer, scrofula (king's evil), fever, febrifuges, and measles are missing from the manuscript, which is preserved at the American Antiquarian Society, and the published version.

do-it-yourself medical book is also addressed to learned men on both sides of the Atlantic. In doing so, it falls short of reconciling the author's desire to write a work of charity and to further his credentials as a writer on scientific and religious matters in a transatlantic intellectual community. Arguably, this lack of a clear audience is one of the reasons the book was not published during Mather's lifetime.

Despite its incoherent intended readership, the medical companion is a rich illustration of the author's will to do good. Its *raison d'être*, it seems, also lies in promoting Cotton Mather as an angel of Bethesda on earth, willing and able to share his medical knowledge with the sick and the poor. The text is not only a treatise on how to serve the public but also an illustration of a New England intellectual at the turn of the eighteenth century. Taken collectively, the frequent instances of authorial self-reflexivity and self-referentiality on doing good exemplify an introspective mode of writing that offers insights into the breadth and achievements, as well as the limits and shortcomings, of Puritan thought at the time. For instance, in *The Angel of Bethesda* the author's otherwise subdued pride in his intellectual accomplishments surfaces repeatedly. At the same time, Mather represents the increasing difficulty of bridging the gaps between the popular and the learned, between folk remedies and scientific medicine.

Mather attempts to integrate these force-fields contesting over proper ways of knowing, explaining, and controlling diseases by employing a plain structural design: every chapter (which he calls "capsulas") begins with a short etiology of the illness under discussion, often summarizing the current state of research on the nature and causes of the affliction. Next, the author reiterates the central message conveyed throughout the book, namely that worship and repentance should constitute the primary steps toward recovery. The majority of the sixty-six chapters that comprise the book close by offering a collection of medical treatments from a wide range of sources, from ancient Greek medicine and folk remedies (from Europe and the Americas) to contemporary medical discoveries.

The Boston minister takes pride in assembling a *"Council of Doctors"* on various diseases for the benefit of his audience (*Angel* 103). The book draws from the works of over 250 authors, many of whom had published their findings shortly before Mather began his work. Hence, the book represents the state of early eighteenth-century medical

science, which continued to echo Renaissance occultism (especially its
emphasis on magic, astrology, and alchemy), mixed with increasing
efforts to call into question the authority of the Galenic system.[51] The
transition from a medicine informed by humoral pathology to one
energized by new scientific methods is one of the central characteristics
of *The Angel of Bethesda*. When discussing the gout, for instance,
Mather explains: "Now, foul, sharp, Scorbutic Humours, bred in the
Stomach, associate themselves with the Circulating Blood" (*Angel* 67).
This is an insightful, albeit erroneous, assumption because it shows how
the author and the medical establishment he adhered to had only begun
to grasp how William Harvey's 1628 discovery of blood circulation
challenged Galenic humoralism. Mather's statement indicates how
Harvey's experiments, which in hindsight revolutionized the field of
medicine like few others of the time, was integrated into a system of
explaining the human body that had existed for almost seventeen
hundred years and that, naturally, would be slow to overcome.[52]

Although the erudite preacher is clearly fascinated by scientific
innovations, he takes repeated rhetorical swings at physicians, especially
when he detects atheistic tendencies in their writings. In "Bonifacius: An
Essay upon the Good" (1710), Mather already voiced his disapproval of
the growing interest in natural instead of spiritual causes and cures of
illness, and warned physicians not to surrender their religious devotions

---

[51] One of the main sources in Mather's book is Robert Boyle's *Medicinal
Experiments* (1688). Although he adopts Boyle's findings into his own medical
treatise, Boyle's philosophical assertion that God has set the world in motion but
is largely absent from it did not meet the approval of the Boston preacher and is
thus omitted from his text.

[52] The short quotation also illustrates Mather's overall compositional approach
in *The Angel of Bethesda* (similar to the one employed earlier in *The Christian
Philosopher*): the author cites from and paraphrases European medical experts,
often without giving due credit or signaling that he is even drawing on concepts
or remedies published previously. As Winton U. Solberg explains: "To
paraphrase and quote extensively form other works without attribution showed
both learning and proper appreciation of source material. While borrowing
freely, authors of the early modern period who wished to indicate their
authorities usually did so by mentioning sources in the body of their text. The
footnote was known but had not yet come into general use" (xlix).

to their scientific aptitudes. In addition, while Mather admired the work of some medical practitioners, he retained a life-long skepticism about human-made cures and thus held a condescending attitude toward a profession that he himself had rejected in order to follow a higher calling in life.[53]

In chapter 40 of *The Angel of Bethesda*, entitled "The Uncertainty of the Physicians," Mather complains about the recurrent disagreement among physicians with regard to explanations of illnesses and, more importantly, ways of curing them: "How rarely does, *A Council of Doctors*, do the Patient so much good, as a Single One *happens* to do!," he writes and explains that some doctors praise a specific remedy for a disease, while others deny it and/or suggest altogether different measures (*Angel* 186). Here, Mather's position toward medical science is inherently contradictory, because at the outset of the book he prides himself for offering the reader precisely what he is now criticizing: the discrepancies of medicinal knowledge provided by a "council of doctors" that promises higher chances of recovery than if the patient were at the mercy of only one physician. By parading various medical opinions and approaches, the Boston preacher makes his reader believe that a certain consensus exists, although the wide range of remedies he prescribes suggests the opposite.

While the author never discloses the premises upon which he reduces the discourse on healing for his reader, the text is clear in its repeated insistence that "*Tis from God, and not from the Physician, that my cure is to be Looked for*" (*Angel* 189). Having thus reiterated his religious convictions, the minister refrains from condemning scientific medicine based on its apparent shortcomings and inconsistencies, knowing that medicine can indeed serve humanity. He instead strikes a conciliatory note by admitting that some medical experts deserve recognition; however, he also warns physicians (and the public) that mere secular healing approaches must remain insufficient. For instance, it is not enough, Mather claims, to rationalize pain in scientific terms as "a Sensation produced on the *Tension of a Nerve*" (*Angel* 54) and to

[53] Mather remarks quite sarcastically that "A Famous Physician, Who shall be Nameless, *Died* of a Disease, which at that very Time, he had a Book in the Press, to teach the Cure of" (*Angel* 186).

prescribe remedies accordingly. More importantly, pain must first and foremost be accepted as a penalty for disobedience and as an opportunity to realize that sin is the essential cause of all human suffering. An insightful case in point is his treatment of toothache, an especially common and excruciating experience before modern dental medicine. Mather is convinced that God inflicts toothaches so widely among human beings because it is meant as a punishment for Adam tasting the fruit of the tree of knowledge. In addition, humanity is repeating original sin on a daily basis—both spiritually and physically— by using the teeth for "*Speaking* amiss" and for "*Eating* Irregularly, Inordinately; and Without a due Regard unto the Service and Glory of God" (*Angel* 62). The pain that follows these transgressions might be eased by certain natural remedies, but the crucial point for the patient is to realize the necessity for aligning his/her conduct of life with the laws of God; then, and only then, can s/he recover from and avoid painful and debilitating afflictions.[54]

Mather urges his reader to consider all forms of pain as a sign of a particular quality of the divine, of humanity's relation to God, or of an afflicted condition of the soul and, ultimately, as a blessing in disguise. In his chapter on headaches, he reminds his audience to consider "How *Empty* has my *Head* been of such *Thoughts*, as a Reasonable and a Religious Mind ought continually to have been replenish'd with!" (*Angel* 58). Similar to Michael Wigglesworth's rhetorical treatment of illness, every ailment offers a possibility for spiritual inquiry and hence Mather repeatedly includes paragraphs of advice—often beginning with the admonition to "Think"—on how to interpret ones painful affliction so as to root out its spiritual causes. This entails the duty of the afflicted

---

[54] Another painful human experience, although not an illness in the strict sense, is childbirth, which Mather felt obliged to address in accordance with the proclaimed goal of helping his flock. Of the thirteen pages the author spends on the topic roughly ten consist of extensive sermonizing designed to ease labor pains. Women should contemplate and understand that they must endure pain because of Eve's role in the expulsion from the Garden of Eden. The minister seeks to prepare women to endure the sorrows of child-bearing when he informs them that their pain will have a redeeming effect, especially when seen as an occasion for a new birth in Christ, of the child and of the mother (if they were fortunate enough to survive labor).

and his/her minister to interpret the meaning each illness contains before healing can begin. By doing so, the author not only cements the role of the church in healing matters. He also places illness in a larger cultural context which demands of each colonist to decipher natural occurrences (e.g., earthquakes, comets, prodigies, or deaths in the family) as divine signs and to practice introspection about the state of his/her soul regularly and intensively: "There is a *Self-examination* incumbent upon *All* Men: Upon *Sick* Men it is peculiarly incumbent. I pray, Lett our *Sickness* itself, be such an *Emetic*, as to make us *Vomit* up our *Sin*, with a penitent *Confession* of it" (*Angel* 7; cf. "Mens sana" 26; "A perfect recovery" 37). Mather's use of the pronouns "us" and "our" instead of "you/your" is especially noteworthy here because it indicates that the minister, instead of preaching to his congregation/audience, places himself within the community of the afflicted and, thereby, within humanity proper.

As seen earlier in this study, many colonists held that pain and suffering function as reminders that death is imminent and that the believer should use bodily afflictions as an occasion to prepare for the afterlife. A typical Matherean invocation to take illness as a god-sent opportunity to reaffirm the patient's alignment with divine law reads: "Upon the Occasion of SICKNESS on myself and others, I sett myself to consider PIETY, and the Effects of it, under the Notion of *An HEALED SOUL*" (*Angel* 20). The double typographical emphasis of "healed soul" indicates that spiritual health is indeed Mather's primary reason for writing on medical topics. Piety and devotion are a necessity for a healthy soul, which, in turn, is the precondition for a healthy body and for salvation. The state of physical and spiritual health can, as New England writers such as Mather stressed time and again, only be achieved by (re)turning to Christ, the ultimate healer, and the Bible, the true panacea.

Theorizing Disease: Nishmath-Chajim and Animalcules

After having reiterated his religious conceptualization of illness in the first four chapters of *The Angel of Bethesda*, Mather ponders theories of disease in which he supplements God's role with his own secular scientific interests and knowledge. His intellectual transgression from an orthodox alignment with the doctrine of theological pathogenesis begins in chapter five, entitled "Nishmath-Chajim. The Probable Seat of all Diseases, and a General Cure for Them, Further Discovered." In this chapter, Mather outlines a theory of disease that seeks to harmonize the realms of religion and science. He does so by locating the source of illness in a borderland between "the *Rational Soul*, and the *Corporeal Mass*" (*Angel* 28). He calls this borderland Nishmath-Chajim, the Hebrew term for "breath of life" (cf. Gen. 2:7).[55] After introducing this "vital principle," the author omits an immediate discussion which one might expect from a Puritan minister, namely how the Nishmath-Chajim transforms sin into illness; instead, he first considers biological aspects and envisions the "breath of life" as a fluid comprised of minute particles. In other words, Mather momentarily suspends his theological voice in favor of his scientific one before asserting that the Nishmath-Chajim is a life-directing principle inherent in all parts of the body and ultimately guided by God.

By employing the notion of Nishmath-Chajim, Mather syncretizes a number of thought traditions. The idea of a "vital principle" that links body and soul is similarly envisioned by Paracelsus as the spirit of the world or "fifth essence." This alchemical notion was further developed in Dutch physician Johannes Baptista van Helmont's theory of the Archeus (i.e., the threshold between matter and spirit), which Mather adopts to devise his own physico-theological approach to explaining diseases.[56] In doing so, he also modifies views of the body-soul dualism that Calvinism had inherited from Aristotelian scholasticism's partition of the soul into an irrational part (its sensitive and vegetative faculties) and a rational part (its spiritual faculty). Mather concentrates on how the

---

[55] Mather had for quite some time developed his theory of a body-soul interface, but withheld it from his religious and scientific peers on both sides of the Atlantic until after the publication of *The Christian Philosopher*. Mather's account of the Nishmath-Chajim was first printed and circulated in New London in 1722 and is hence the only section from the original manuscript of *The Angel of Bethesda* that was accessible to a wider audience before the book was published in 1972.

[56] Walter Pagel, Paracelsus: An Introduction to Philosophical Medicine in the Era of the Renaissance (Basel: Karger, 1958) 297; Michael P. Winship, "Cotton Mather, Astrologer," New England Quarterly 63.2 (1990): 308-314.

interface between a universal spirit or "breath of life" and the body influences health and illness. He regards the Nishmath-Chajim as the soul itself and, at the same time, its connecting link to the body. This implies that the "breath of life" survives the body after death, ascends to heaven, and returns at the Second Coming of Christ to reunite body and soul of the visible saints (*Angel* 32).

Mather advances his earlier conviction that body and soul are inter-implicated; yet, he is still grappling with how the two entities are connected and mutually influential. The precise connection of body and soul was one of the central questions philosophers had sought to answer since Antiquity and for seventeenth-century scientists and theologians it became one of the most important ideological battlegrounds that eventually drove both camps apart. René Descartes, for instance, had speculated that the meeting point between body and soul lies in the pineal gland, a view which attracted more ridicule than support, even from those sympathetic to the new rationality heralded by the French philosopher.[57] The main problem with Descartes, from a theological perspective, was that he considered the soul as merely a "ghost in the machine," present yet separated from the body.[58] Among the most salient contemporary medical critics of the Cartesian body-soul dualism was Georg Ernst Stahl of Halle, Germany, whose notion of *anima* (soul) claimed the ever-present influence of an immortal spirit, and thus God, over bodily functions; accordingly, diseases are caused by maladies of the soul, which work directly on the body. Stahl and others could not, however, sufficiently explain the exact connection and inter-implications of body and soul. In *The Christian Philosopher* Mather, in siding with the French anatomist Daniel Tauvry, sums up the dominant conviction of his time: "The Union between the SOUL and the BODY is altogether inexplicable, the *Soul* not having any *Surface* to touch the

---

[57] Despite this false assumption, Descartes' dualistic view of a unitary soul vis-à-vis a machine-like body was of course highly instrumental in shaping modern subjectivity well beyond the Enlightenment. For a more general and illustrative account of different conceptions of the relationship between body and soul in seventeenth- and eighteenth-century Europe (mainly Great Britain), see Porter, *Flesh*.

[58] Gilbert Ryle, *The Concept of Mind*, 1949 (London: Routledge, 2009) 5.

*Body*, and the *Body* not having any *Sentiment* as the *Soul*. The *Union* of the *Soul* and *Body* does consist [...] in the *Conformity* of our *Thoughts* to our *Corporeal* Actions."[59]

In *The Angel of Bethesda* Mather attempts to unravel the interconnectedness of the union between soul and body by introducing the notion of Nishmath-Chajim. Located in the stomach, the seat and source of illness, and responsible for regulating all bodily functions, Mather's Nishmath-Chajim not only connects mind and matter but, more importantly, the visible and invisible worlds as well as God and humanity. It marks the gateway through which God, the devil, angels, and other denizens of the invisible world can initiate and revoke diseases. For Mather, the Nishmath-Chajim hence constitutes the missing link in the chain of medical causes that begins with God, continues in the realms of spirits and natural causes, and ends in the human body. With this approach to illness, the Boston preacher continues and culminates his life-long project of explaining spiritual interventions in scientific terms and of reconciling religion and medicine by asserting that the latter "pointed to the contrivances of the body as the finest proofs of God."[60]

Mather's notion of the vital tie, essential for survival and health, furthermore exemplifies the author's modification of his mechanical explanation of bodily processes and functions presented in *The Christian Philosopher*. His unease with the atheist implications of the mechanistic worldview is in part remedied by incorporating postulates from the iatrochemical school, especially the teachings of van Helmont, who stressed that the body is an assemblage of chemical, rather than physical reactions. Instead of turning from an iatromechanist into an iatrochemist—the Boston minister cannot be placed in either camp entirely—Mather supplements medical materialism by injecting spiritual elements. As he stresses repeatedly, the mechanical model cannot sufficiently explain the divine order; man, the machine, could neither function intrinsically nor randomly but needed a guiding spirit, with which God had endowed every human being. Once disturbed by sinful thoughts and actions the Nishmath-Chajim produces illness symptoms

---

[59] Mather, *Christian Philosopher* 305 (emphasis original).

[60] Porter, *Flesh* 54.

that can only be treated by restoring its balance. With this conceptualization, the Boston minister synthesizes the views of Stahl (the soul works directly on the body) and van Helmont (chemical mediators between spirit and matter cause disease). Even though his theory lacks empirical evidence, it signals a turn from the philosophies of the body as the machine of life to a more dynamic notion of its vital properties in the late eighteenth century, continuing into modern biology and related sciences.

Mather's concept of the body-soul connection stresses the importance of the mind in causing and relieving certain afflictions. The Nishmath-Chajim represents the author's conviction that the body cannot be viewed as a separate entity and that, as a result, healing is procured by addressing the body *and* the mind. In keeping with his principal assumption that sin is the cause of all illness, Mather claims that human thoughts and imaginations are at least as important as external factors such as the environment or contagious pathogens. As Mather writes in chapter 46, "Jehoram Visited, or the Bloody-Flux remedied": "Nothing is of more Consequence in a *Dysentery*, than that the *Mind* be kept Calm, and Quite and Easy; and if it be possible, Chearful. But that the *Mind* be made *Holy,* and fill'd with proper Sentiments of *Piety,* This I am sure, will be no Prejudice, to any Intention of the Cure to be aimed at" (*Angel* 211). This quotation exemplifies the author's belief that human beings are able to influence their state of bodily health through mental exercises. As a consequence, he often prescribes measures aimed at improving the well being of the patient, for instance, prayer, introspection, interacting with persons the afflicted finds agreeable, and reading educative and/or morally uplifting books.

Mather demonstrates the healing potential of his psychogenetic approach to illness when he addresses melancholy, which was considered as an eligible and at times even fashionable disease in Elizabethan England but deemed as an imaginary malady by the Boston minister and others. In the Massachusetts Bay Colony, numerous diaries and spiritual autobiographies attest that melancholy was indeed a common distemper, often induced by morbid preoccupation with sin, religious doubt concerning personal salvation, and/or a sense of the persistent inadequacy of collective Puritan endeavors to establish a New Jerusalem.[61] Mather admits that people do actually suffer from melancholy—after all, the Greek authorities had defined it as an excess of black bile—but insinuates that the afflicted have brought this illness on themselves. "These *Melancholiks*," Mather writes, "do sufficiently *Afflict themselves*, and are Enough their *own Tormentors*. As if this *present Evil World*, would not *Really* afford Sad Things Enough, they create a World of *Imaginary Ones*, and by *Mediating Terror*, they make themselves as Miserable, as they could be from the most *Real Miseries*" (*Angel* 133). Despite his skepticism about, and even downright rejection of melancholy as an illness, the clergyman is aware that his profession forces him to take seriously all distempers which members of his flock experience, even if they are, in Edward Shorter's term, "somatizers," people who suffer from illness symptoms without a physical cause.[62] Instead of reproaching the melancholic for playing sick, Mather considers it his duty to also minister to those who are *convinced* to be ill, to speak with them and thereby heal their imbalance of soul and body. Mather's moral therapy, which concentrates on healing the Nishmath-Chajim through speaking with (and of) the patient, constitutes a proto-psychoanalytic form of treatment. His talking cure marks one of several instances in *The Angel of Bethesda* where the New England divine is at his best, displaying a farsighted, compassion-filled, and gentle understanding of human nature and its various calamities, regardless of their physiological or psychosomatic cause.

In early modern medical thought, melancholy was often linked with mental infirmities and Mather's reflections in *The Angel of Bethesda* focus repeatedly on possible natural and supernatural origins and remedies. Recalling the life of minister-physician William Thompson in

---

[61] Patricia Ann Watson, *The Angelical Conjunction: The Preacher-Physicians of Colonial New England* (Knoxville: U of Tennessee P, 1991) 12.

[62] Edward Shorter, *From Paralysis to Fatigue: A History of Psychosomatic Illnesses in the Modern Era* (New York: Free, 1992) 15. Mather himself suffered from melancholy several times in his life. For instance, while attending college he complained of the distemper, which was most likely caused by religious doubts, by the ridicule he had to face due to his stammering, and by the fact that his father was President of Harvard.

*Magnalia Christi Americana*, Mather explains how pious colonists' "melancholy indispositions," especially when the settlers feel tempted by the devil, disturb the humoral balance in their bodies, allowing Satan to further "insinuate himself, till he has gained a sort of possession in them, or at least an opportunity to shoot into the mind as many *fiery darts* as may cause a sad life unto them; yea, 'tis well if *self-murder* be not the sad end unto which these hurried people are thus precipitated."[63] In *The Angel of Bethesda*, Mather's description of mental illnesses includes references to contemporary naturalistic explanations: mania is considered as "inflammation of the animal spirits" (129); melancholy is depicted as "a flatulence in the Region of the Hypochondria" (132). Since for Mather the causes for "melancholic madness" lie in both the visible and the invisible worlds, his prescriptions for treating psychosomatic disorders center on natural and supernatural curative means. Prayer and repentance is, as in most other diseases treated in his medical *oeuvre*, the primary healing choice, but natural curatives should also be employed. The Boston minister suggests, for instance, to take a sparrow, split it in half, shave the head of the afflicted and place the hot, dissected sparrow unto the scalp in order to cure mental infirmities. The mechanistic understanding underlying this remedy once again indicates how Mather was trying to come to terms with the on-going shift from a supernatural to a natural approach in medicine. He recognized that natural causes were behind certain illnesses but nevertheless stressed that spiritual shortcomings raised God's wrath and hence, transgressions were responsible for bodily distempers. As one result, suggesting treatment methods from the realm of contemporary medical science *and* from religious doctrine were by no means deemed contradictory by the Boston minister but rather seen as complementary means to achieve recovery.

On a more abstract level, Mather's rhetorical treatment of psychosomatic disorders implicitly raises questions that are central to modern areas of inquiry in medicine and the medical humanities: What is a normal or average human condition and what constitutes a disease? What are the social, cultural, and political mechanisms behind pathologizing and medicalizing human behavior, thoughts, and speech?

---

[63] Mather, *Magnalia* I: 438 (emphasis original).

While Mather does not address these issues directly, his thoughts on melancholia illustrate how diseases are *made*, by patients who (claim to) suffer as well as by the bystanders who (mis)recognize an illness. Furthermore, his writings on mental afflictions bring to the fore the complex relations between spiritual and biological aspects of the human condition in addition to what a given society considers as normal or abnormal behavior.

These observations show that Mather's Nishmath-Chajim had not only medical, theological and, to a lesser degree, scientific and philosophical implications but also social and political ones. As Margaret Humphreys Warner further explains,

> Supported by his concept of the *nishmath-chajim*, Mather was able to make a strong case for the necessity of the preacher as healer. If, as he had established, many cures came from the invisible world, and if the spiritual condition of the patient and the tranquility of the soul could affect the health of the body, then spiritual consolation and counseling were plainly crucial to the healing process. Through the connecting link of the *nishmath-chajim* Mather created a rationale for the minister to reenter the sick room, even though the increasingly well educated physician was busily attempting to usher him out.[64]

Mather's psychogenetic disease theory was hence not only geared toward healing proper but also marked a continuation of his efforts to counter the declining influence of ministers in civil affairs in post-witch hunt New England. By postulating that illness was rooted in the realm of spirits and by advocating treatments that addressed first and foremost the welfare of the soul/mind, Mather sought to regain clerical authority and power over the body and the riddles of life against the vested interests of scientists and civic leaders. Regaining the interpretative authority over illness was especially vital after the intellectual boundary dispute over smallpox inoculation in 1721-1722. However, Mather's struggle against the waning hold of Puritanism in New England is paradoxically spurred by his flirtatious intellectual engagement and

---

[64] Margaret Humphreys Warner, "Vindicating the Minister's Medical Role: Cotton Mather's Concept of the Nishmath-Chajim and the Spiritualization of Medicine," *Journal of the History of Medicine* 36.3 (1981): 294.

agreement with certain aspects of Hermetic philosophy and the occult sciences.[65]

Toward the end of his life Mather had understood that sin was not the direct cause of all illnesses. Turning from internal (spiritual) to external (natural) causes of illness in chapter 7, "Conjecturalies, or Some Touches Upon a New Theory of Many Diseases," the colonial author postulates that some ailments are triggered by little animals, or germs, which enter the human body from the outside. Mather based this early version of germ theory, which in hindsight constituted his second main contribution to the field of medicine besides inoculation, on the discovery of animalcules (bacteria and protoza) by one of the founders of microbiology, Anton von Leeuwenhoek, and on Benjamin Marten's book *A New Theory of Consumptions* (1720).[66] No other American investigated and proposed a similar theory of airborne diseases until 1807, when John Crawford suggested that yellow fever was caused by transmission through mosquitoes and that animalcules were responsible for spreading the disease in the body. Almost a century earlier, Cotton Mather had posited similar conjectures based on second-hand medical findings and with the help of his own microscope. Centered on the assumption that germs are causative agents of disease, he writes: "Every Part of Matter is *Peopled*. Every *Green Leaf* swarms with *Inhabitants*. [...] The Eggs of these Insects (and why not the *living Insects* too!) may insinuate themselves by the *Air*, and with our *Ailments*, yea, thro' the Pores of our skin; and soon get into the Juices of our Bodies" (*Angel*

---

[65] For instance, he was interested in the millennial strains in Kabala and adopted the notion that the upper (or supernatural) world and the lower (or natural) world are guided by the same principles, a view that is also evident in ancient philosophy.

[66] Among Marten's main assumptions were that the life cycle of certain pathogens can cause specific disease symptoms and that some animalcules can survive as eggs before causing the outbreak of a disease. Marten's parasitological theorem, which were largely neglected at the time of publication, are now seen as important precedents of Louis Pasteur's and Robert Koch's bacteriological models published in the 1880s. Raymond N. Doetsch, "Benjamin Marten and His 'New Theory of Consumptions,'" *Microbiological Reviews* 42.3 (1978): 521-528.

43). While the rendering of contagion as invasion seems strikingly anticipatory of late nineteenth-century germ theory, the eighteenth-century discovery of a microbial world had almost no immediate impact on medical practice, nor did it spur further inquiry. The commonly held concept at the time was that animalcules were catalysts in chemical reactions (fermentation) but not actually involved in it. Early modern scientists recognized, but could not explain, the origin of teeming microbes, which seemed to appear out of nowhere, perhaps through the air as Mather and others held. Nor could they account for the precise role and function of pathogenic entities as causative agents of disease in ways that would generate new and more efficacious treatment methods.[67]

Mather's interest in new findings on animalcules allowed him to further conceptualize an insight that colonists had dreaded since the early settlement of New England: the "wilderness," still unknown, uncanny, and unconquered, was potentially contagious. Because English settlers generally believed that the forests were the realm of the devil and his helpers, especially demons and Native Americans, they were afraid that merely being in contact with the environment, eating the food it provided, breathing its air or interacting with the beings therein would have a de-civilizing effect, causing them to "go native."[68] Evidence of such "creolean degeneracy" exists in abundance in Cotton Mather's view. According to a widely held belief among American immigrants, common until the end of the nineteenth century, "the surrounding world seeped into newcomers' every pore, creating states of health that were as

---

[67] Joyce E. Chaplin, "Natural Philosophy and an Early Racial Idiom in North America: Comparing English and Indian Bodies," *The William and Mary Quarterly* 54.1 (1997): 238. The early eighteenth-century notion that disease is itself an invasive entity actually follows Paracelsus rather than Galen or traditional Christian notions of disease as judgment. Robert Blair St. George, *Conversing by Signs: Poetics of Implication in Colonial New England Culture* (U of North Carolina P, 1998) 196.

[68] John Canup, "Cotton Mather and 'Criolian' Degeneracy," *Early American Literature* 24 (1989): 20-34.

much environmental as they were personal."[69] Concerned with how climates affect the humors, manners, and actions of people, Mather provides in a letter to the Royal Society examples of national characteristics that have been retained and lost in migration:

> Now tis as observable, that tho' the first English Planters of this Countrey, had usually a *Government* & a *Discipline* in their *Families*, that had a sufficient *Severity* in it. Yet, as if the *Climate* had brought us to *Indianize*, the *Relaxation* of it is now such that it seems almost wholly laid aside; and a foolish *Indulgence* to Children is become an *Epidemical Miscarriage* of the Countrey & like to be attended with many evil Consequences.

He continues to explain that Natives are lazy and hate to work. Hence, English settlers need to be aware that the new climate "Indianizes" them. Mather uses a pun to indicate that he, too, is becoming transculturalized, whenever he refers to his own idleness in preparing an adequate number of reports from North America: "But you will do me more Justice if you censure me as a Tame *Indian*, tainted with the vice of the *Climate*, and rebuke me for my *Idleness*."[70]

According to Mather's *Weltanschauung* invaders from two "invisible" worlds (the body and the "wilderness"), lately uncovered by science and exploration, turned human and social bodies into contact zones, even battlegrounds, of natural and supernatural forces, and thereby produced (some) diseases. Mather's "germ theory" constituted a logical extension of the cosmology which first-generation settlers had brought to the shores of New England. The miasma/contagion approach to diseases—an approach already pointed out in Hippocrates' treatise *Air, Waters, Places*—sought to rationalize degenerative environmental influences as well as the conviction commonly held among theologians and the laity that diabolical *maleficium*, including illnesses, were transferred from one person to another. Mather's description of the

---

[69] Conevery Bolton Valenčius, *The Health of the Country: How American Settlers Understood Themselves and Their Land* (New York: Basic, 2002) 12.

[70] "Cotton Mather to James Jurin and John Woodward, 7 October 1724," Royal Society, London, EL/M2/46 (emphasis original).

common cough serves as an illustrative example of how people living in the early eighteenth-century Atlantic world envisioned the entrance of colonizing pathogens into the human body. Writes Mather:

> THE Pores (as we call 'em) of the Body, being duely kept open, they discharge an unknown Quantity of Excrementitous *Lympha* and *Serum*, from the Blood. When those Pores are stop'd, these Liquors are Increased and Stagnated, and become Sharp, and Salt, and full of Acrimony. Yea, and Whether there be such an Occasion for it, or no, the Depraved Blood sometimes is filled with ill-figures Particles, which cannot pass diverse of the *Glands*, where a Percolation is Expected from them. These Humours falling on the Membranes of the Lungs, or the vessels about the Windpipe, or on some of the Nerves that serve the Respiration, the Irritation causes a *Cough*; which is a Struggle of Nature to dislodge the Enemy. (*Angel* 172)

Mather is aware that the pores function as membranes of exchange between the body and its environment, yet he still includes Galenic premises in his explanation. In addition, he demonstrates his up-to-date knowledge about human anatomy, in particular the lungs and its surrounding organs, as well as his use of metaphor, which posits illness as a fight between forces that reside both inside and outside human bodies. Contrary to Susan Sontag's analysis of twentieth-century cancer narratives, in which she rejects military (and other) metaphors that position disease as an outside enemy invading the body, Mather repeatedly employs the terminology of warfare to describe internal battles that ensue on and underneath the human skin.[71] Explaining the causal links between animalcules, smallpox infection, and inoculation, he states:

> Behold, the Enemy at once gott into the very *Center* of the Citadel: And the Invaded Party must be very Strong indeed, if it can struggle with him, and after all Entirely Expel and conquer him. Whereas, the *Miasms* of the *Small-Pox*, being admitted in the Way of *Inoculation*, their Approaches are made only of the *Outworks* of the Citadel, and at a Considerable *Distance* from it. The Enemy, 'tis true, getts in so far, as to

---

[71] Susan Sontag, *Illness as Metaphor* (New York: Farrar, 1978).

make Some *Spoil*, yea, so much as to satisfy him, and to leave no *Prey* in the Body of the Patient, for him ever afterwards to sieze upon; but the *Vital Powers* are kept so clear from his Assaults, that they can manage the *Combat* bravely and, tho' not without a *Surrender* of those Humours in the *Blood*, which the Invader makes a Siezure on, they oblige him to *march out the same Way he came in*, and are sure of never being troubled with him any more. (*Angel* 112)

The excerpt exemplifies, almost ideally, Mather's use of language with regard to scientific matters. Steeped in military metaphors (enemy, citadel, invasion, spoil, prey, assault, seizure, marching), his imagination of how animalcules enter and suffuse the human body still lack the desired purity of eighteenth-century scientific language, which was deemed to describe natural occurrences without recourse to symbolic language. This passage also exemplifies Mather's penchant for metaphor and thus marks a deviation from Puritan plain style, a rhetoric, which actually correlated with the changes in scientific language away from allegory, symbol, and metaphor.[72]

Further into *The Angel of Bethesda*, Mather similarly conceives germs in terms of war metaphors when he attempts to grasp virulent and hereditary diseases, which "may ly dormant until the Vessels are grown more capable of bringing them into their Figure and Vigour for Operations. Thus may Diseases be convey'd from the Parents unto their Children, before they are born into the world" (*Angel* 44). Based on his inquiries of smallpox, Mather speculates that animalcules attack the blood and juices, that they may cause an array of different diseases and that they migrate from one living being to another, causing epidemics in

---

[72] Cf. Bernd Herzogenrath, "The Angel and the Animalculae: Cotton Mather and Inoculation," *Transatlantic Negotiations*, ed., Christa Buschendorf and Astrid Franke (Heidelberg: Winter, 2007) 13-24. Herzogenrath's argument that Mather anticipates modern scientific skepticism neglects Mather's continuous adherence to a *theology* of disease. Despite his intellectual flirtations with Deism, positing Mather as leaning toward secular medicine overlooks how his intense piety and religiosity suffused his thoughts and actions in all fields of knowledge until the end of his life.

different parts of the world.[73] He furthermore considers the idea that
such epidemics are not necessarily triggered by contact between human
beings alone; they can also be transmitted by insects and affect animals.
In addition, he claims that animalcules carried in the clothing or
belongings of travelers can cause epidemics and thus echoes a rational
and accurate explanation (in principle, at least) of disease transmission
at an early stage of globalization: "Tis generally Supposed, that *Europe*
is Endebted unto *America* for the *Lues Venera*. If so, *Europe* has paid its
Debt unto *America* by making unto it a Present of the *Small Pox*, in Lieu
of the *Great* One" (*Angel* 44). For Mather, the scientific observer,
diseases can no longer be understood as mere local relationships
between individuals or the collective to their environment. For Mather,
the clergyman, the assumption that a sexually transmitted disease
(syphilis) originated in America and traveled to Europe is culturally
appalling because it insinuates that the newly built society in the "New
World" is morally uncouth and intellectually inferior.[74] His emphasis on
animalcules is, as Warner explains, not inconsistent with his sin-based
explanation of disease but rather a scientific correlate: "The fact that
Mather included both sin and animalcules in his etiological thought was
thus not contradictory; one attacked the *nishmath-chajim* from the
nonmaterial side of its nature, the other from the material side."[75] What

---

[73] Mather indeed displays a correct understanding of the smallpox as a virulent
disease. He is one of few at the time who suggest that, in concordance with his
proto-germ theory, the spreading of smallpox is caused by an infectious agent, or
pathogen. "It begins now to be Vehemently Suspected That the *Small-Pox* may
be more of an *Animalculated Business*, than we have been generally aware of"
(*Angel* 94).

[74] While Mather generally shows compassion for those who have fallen ill, when
it comes to sexually transmitted diseases (chapter 21), he can hardly contain his
disgust. Unlike in most other chapters, in which the author ascribes to a
compassionate theology, Mather's God is entirely vindictive here. As a
consequence, he has virtually no treatment to offer for syphilis, even though in
1712 he reported a known Native cure to the Royal Society in London: "As for
any Remedies under this *Foul Disease*,--You are so Offensive to me, I'l do
nothing for you. You shall pay for your Cure" (*Angel* 120).

[75] Warner 287.

Warner is missing, though, is that the two main pillars of Cotton Mather's theory of disease—Nishmath-Chajim and animalcules—remain supplementary rather than complementary. Mather seems to have realized, yet had to disavow, that a full integration of religious and scientific approaches was increasingly impossible, especially when the preeminence of theology was postulated *a priori*. Rather than harmonizing religion and science, then, his representation of the two etiological conceptualizations revealed unbridgeable differences between spiritual and secular medical theories as well as their accompanying curative practices.

Treating Diseases: Heterodoxies of Healing

From a twenty-first-century medical standpoint it is fairly easy to debunk the simplicity, metaphoricity, and occasional naiveté of Cotton Mather's disease theories as mere armchair musings that are based on highly selective and inconclusive observations. In all fairness, though, Mather was not the only one groping in the (medical) dark; as Edward Shorter reminds us, "virtually all theorizing about the mechanics of disease before 1800 was like a castle built in the air: it had little empirical foundation and was completely false in modern scientific terms."[76] A more valid point of criticism concerns Mather's neglect to apply consistently his theories to the illnesses he is treating in his medical book. Babette Levy observes that the minister

> offers an elaborate hypothesis as an explanation of psychosomatic illness, tells the reader that many illnesses are psychosomatic, but ignores the whole question in his treatment of disease after disease, although he does admit once or twice that belief in a cure is the cure.[77]

His theories appear to be mere private intellectual exercises or, even worse perhaps, ostentatious displays of classical knowledge and quasi-scientific insights. One must keep in mind (again) that Mather regards the Nishmath-Chajim and animalcule theorems as inferior to the "daily

[76] Shorter 123.
[77] Levy 129.

bread" with which a devoted Calvinist deals with bodily ailments: reflection, prayer, repentance, and reform. It hence comes as no surprise that there are few, if any, references to his theorems when treating diseases, be it in his published works or in his private writings. For instance, after completing *The Angel of Bethesda*, Cotton Mather fell ill and recorded his own course of recovery in traditional Christian terms:

> I had three Maladies now [November 1724] to conflict withal. A *Cough* which proved a grievous Breast-beater; an *Asthma* which often almost suffocated me; and a *Fever*, which held me every Afternoon [...] Particularly, I imposed it as a Rule for me, that whenever any Fitt of my tedious and irksome Coughing should come upon me, I would strive to have some new Thoughts of the blessed JESUS raised in me. And I was gloriously supported by the Comforter who releeved my Soul, and caused me to triumph over the Fear of Death, and enabled me to sing the Songs of the Lord in a strange Land, and entertain my Visitors with such Flights to the Heavenly World, and Views of it, and News from it, as, I hope, honoured Him, and had a great Impression upon them.[78]

Introspection, prayer, repentance, and reform are, however, not the only measures that the Boston minister prescribes for himself and his readership. Mather is aware of, and fascinated by, other forms of healing God provides for the benefit of humanity. As a result, he advises a life-style that includes temperance, daily exercise, a balanced diet, and helping others.

Furthermore, despite his investment in treatments prescribed by contemporary medical science, Mather is wholly a man of the seventeenth century in his belief in angels and witches, and he applies his conviction about the existence of an invisible world to his practical conception of illness and healing. It is hence no surprise that Mather did not outright reject folk remedies and did not claim, as one might perhaps expect from a New England Puritan minister, that lay appropriations of the European occult tradition and non-Western approaches to healing

---

[78] Cotton Mather, *Diary of Cotton Mather, Part II: 1709-1724*, ed. C. Ford Worthington (Boston: Massachusetts Historical Society Collections, 1912) 775 (emphasis original).

constituted unlawful and dangerous flirtations with the devil.[79] In fact, throughout *The Angel of Bethesda*, Mather devotes considerable space and energy to evaluating and negotiating folk healing methods practiced by many of his New England contemporaries. For instance, in case of hemorrhoids Mather suggests: "Our common People have a common Medicine for the *Piles*. Take the *Inside Leather* on the *Sole of a Shoe*, which has been Long Worn, and had the Sweat of the Foot Sufficiently tingeing of it. Pulverize This; and lett the *Powder* be taken Inwardly" (*Angel* 221). The convenience and medical efficacy of the recipes and their ingredients is less important for the purpose of this study than the cultural insights they provide. Many folk remedies that Mather assembles in his book illustrate how ancient traditions traveled to the "New World" in the wake of the Great Migration and entered an eclectic repertoire of healing methods, especially among lay people. In chapters 54 to 56, the author appeals to and draws from New England everyday culture when he writes about remedies that are easy to acquire and to administer, for instance, water (hot and cold), various human and animal excrements, hot ashes, bread, or stroking tumorous parts of the body with a dead hand. We know from various records that colonial physicians who were familiar with advances in the sciences, and whose devotion to Calvinist tenets is unquestionable (e.g., Edward Taylor), at times prescribed means of healing drawn from, or similar to, occult practices. Mather himself was encouraged by a local physician to have his wife apply a remedy against breast cancer that she had dreamt about: the warm wool from a living sheep applied to the ailing breast. This prescription concurred with English folk healing practices, which

[79] In *The Wonders of the Invisible World* Mather reports "They say, that in some Towns it has been an usual thing for People to cure Hurts with Spells, or to use detestable Conjurations, with Sieves, Keys, and Pease, and Nails, and Horseshoes, and I know not what other Implements, to learn the things for which they have a forbidden, and an impious Curiosity." Cotton Mather, *The Wonders of the Invisible World* (1692; Early American Imprints, Series 1, no. 657) 66.

included the belief that illnesses could be transferred to animals and thus rid the human patient of his/her ailment.[80]

It is especially interesting to note that most folk recipes presented in *The Angel of Bethesda* are not explicitly framed in religious terms. In chapters 56 and 61 (on remedies that everyone should have at hand), Mather is claiming authorship as someone with a profound interest in quasi-scientific medical observations and advice. The narrative tone, content, and lack of sermonizing passages in these chapters are once again illustrative of the inherent tensions between the author's religious, scientific, and lay voices. These voices collide particularly when Mather realizes that the remedies he is presenting are drawn from pagan practices or have survived the Protestant purification of Catholic practices, especially with regard to miracle healing. In his treatment of the hiccough, for example, the preacher hence warns his audience: "There are *Magical Superstitions* practiced Sometimes on this Occasion, which a *Good Christian* must have an Abhorrence for" (*Angel* 225). These and other references to magic can be seen as descriptive rather than prescriptive. They cause the author to once again walk a fine line between paying tribute to popular healing practices, in which recourse to the occult was seen as a feasible practice, and the Protestant rejection of superstition. Like most colonial leaders, Mather was convinced that the elite may and should meddle in the sciences, including alchemy, for they would be fit to include God in their discoveries. Nevertheless, Mather remains highly selective and skeptical of alchemists and at several instances shows his rejection of Paracelsus (*Angel* 26, 296) and some of the practices undertaken in his name (*Angel* 145).

Mather's occasional uncertainty about the compliance of certain medical practices with Calvinist theology is cast aside when it comes to seemingly obvious acts of sorcery and magic. In chapter 62, "Fuga Daemonum, or Cures by Charmed Considered, and a Seventh-Son Examined," he condemns the use of amulets, charms, and other forms of superstition, which were still fairly common at the beginning of the eighteenth century, especially in more remote settlements of New

---

[80] Mather, *Diary* I: 44. Cf. Keith Thomas, *Religion and the Decline of Magic: Studies in Popular Beliefs in Sixteenth and Seventeenth-Century England* (1971; New York: Penguin, 1982) 183-186, esp. 184.

England. In addition, Mather strongly disagrees with how colonists, both from the clergy and the laity, adhered to the English physician Nicholas Culpeper's astrological medicine outlined in his *Pharamacopoeia Londinensis; or the London Dispensatory* (1653). Culpeper's work was well known in the colonies and almost every physician, clerical or secular, owned a copy of the *Pharamacopoeia*, in which the author follows and extends Galenism by suggesting a correlation between the planting, gathering, and administration of healing plants to planetary constellations. Despite the widespread application of Culpeper's method, and even though John Calvin had similarly advised that the suitable time for phlebotomies should depend on a knowledge of the stars, Mather criticized his *"Planet-Struck"* contemporaries for relying on what he considered as idolatrous and superstitious medical practice (*Angel* 301).[81]

In less obvious cases Mather struggles with suggesting cures that might be considered magic and, hence, constitute a heterodox healing practice. For example, although stones were a common and painful affliction in colonial New England, difficult to cure with available medical techniques, Mather devotes comparatively little narrative space to the spiritual aspects of healing in this case. As if prayer and repentance are insufficient, the clergyman recommends "[p]owder of a Burnt *Toad*, hung in a Bag, about the Neck."[82] And for *"Incontinency of*

---

[81] Mather follows both Calvin's defense of "natural astrology," which recognized a correlation between human bodies and the stars, and his hostile rejection of "judicial astrology" (i.e., the aim to foretell a person's destiny by consulting the stars) because it appeared to restrict the omnipotence of God. For Calvin's views on astrology, outlined in his *Advertissement contre l'astrologie judiciaire* (1549), see P. G. Maxwell-Stuart, ed. and trans., *The Occult in Early Modern Europe. A Documentary History* (London: Macmillian, 1999) 74-75.

[82] Martin Luther similarly praises the medicinal value of toads in "Tischreden" 34: "Experience has proved the toad to be endowed with valuable qualities. If you run a stick through three toads, and, after having dried them in the sun, apply them to any pestilent humor, they draw out all the poison, and the malady will disappear." Martin Luther, *The Table-Talk of Martin Luther*. 1566. trans. William Hazlitt (1566; Philadelphia: The Lutheran Publication Society, 1868) 736. The medical significance of toads is explained in Malcolm S. Beinfield,

*Urine*, a *Mouse*, flay'd and dried in a warm Oven, and powdered, and so drank at Night in a Glass of Red Wine, or any proper Vehicle; (repeated Eight of Ten times,) tis an Incomparable Remedy" (*Angel* 92). A skeptical Mather knows not what to make of this and other folk remedies that involve a good dose of superstition, yet he still reports them faithfully. One explanation for including such treatments drawn from a border zone between faith and superstition is that the author considers them not occult enough to deserve repudiation. In this sense, the text proves indicative of the difficulty to differentiate medical practices prescribed by the cunning folk from those of ordinary physicians and the clergy in colonial New England.[83] Mather wanted his book to appeal to a broad audience and, therefore, remedies that made sense to the common people could serve as a useful marketing tactic. Yet, the often extensive lists of folk remedies fail to offer a necessary hierarchy of valuation and thereby countervail his intention to write a useable health guide. Another interpretation, one that seeks to reconcile Mather's seemingly flawed efforts in presenting his recommendations, would stress, however, that by listing the medical knowledge of his time without any apparent hierarchy, the author is actually exposing the inferiority and inadequacy of folk (and scientific) knowledge in relation to theological remedies.

While proving the supremacy of religion in matters of illness and healing was certainly one of Mather's underlying motives for writing *The Angel of Bethesda*, the folk remedies he offers in essence contradict the Calvinist frame within which bodily afflictions are to be placed. When the author claims that headaches are due to the absence of proper religious thought and devotion, then a return to Christ would and should be sufficient to cure the affliction. Suggesting other ways of relieving pain and dis-ease is not contradictory *per se* within the minister's conceptual universe because the practical remedies only promise relief if proper religious care precedes it—a central assumption mirrored in the structure of virtually every chapter in his book. However, Mather glances over one of the central ambivalences in Christianity with regard

---

"The Early New England Doctor: An Adaptation to a Provincial Environment," *Yale Journal of Biology and Medicine* (1943): 123.

[83] Watson 33.

to medicine: on the one hand, bodily ailments are to be accepted as a divine blessings because they induce necessary reforms of one's conduct of life, spiritually and physically; on the other hand, illnesses should also be alleviated by charity and specific natural remedies, turning life into a gift from God. Mather neither addresses nor answers the questions why human beings need the practical remedies that he records so meticulously in the first place, if all one needs for recovery is Christ, as he repeatedly stresses. Similar to the knowledge about inoculation derived from African sources, then, Mather's attempt to assimilate Euro-American folk remedies within his theological approach to healing reveals some of the integrative limits of, and insoluble contradictions within, New England Puritanism.

Transnational Medicine

The remnants of unscientific medical prescriptions, coupled with religion-inspired healing practices, in *The Angel of Bethesda* were the main cause of ridicule by scholars who evaluated Mather's work after his death. Oliver Wendell Holmes articulated the most crushing critique of the minister's approach to illness and healing in the nineteenth century, stating that:

> The divine takes precedence over the physician in this extraordinary production. He begins by preaching a sermon at this unfortunate patient. Having thrown him into a cold sweat by his spiritual sudorific, he attacks him with his material remedies, which are often quite as unpalatable [...] Everything he could find mentioned in the seventy or eighty authors he cites, all that the old women of both sexes had ever told him of, gets into his text, or squeezes itself into his margin [...] He piles his prescriptions one upon another, without the least discrimination. He is run away with all sorts of fancies and superstitions [...].[84]

In the twentieth century some scholars sought to restore the minister's battered post-Salem reputation and to vindicate his medical

---

[84] Oliver Wendell Holmes, *Medical Essays: The Writings of Oliver Wendell Holmes,* vol. 9 (Boston: Cambridge UP, 1891) 359.

legacy, calling him "the first unmistakably American figure in the nation's history" and the "first significant figure in American medicine."[85] What is often neglected in these and other studies claiming Mather's Americanness is the extent to which Puritan contacts with Native peoples and African slaves influenced his thoughts and prescriptions, especially with regard to medicine. Mather's medical texts significantly reacted to, and were shaped by, knowledge and practices that originated outside the contemporary Euramerican discourse on illness and recovery. In addition, the contact with Otherness both changed and solidified dominant medical practices and conceptions of illness in colonial New England culture and in the minister's medical writings. This argument, and the approach to the history of U.S. medicine it entails, undercuts the national paradigm by highlighting transnational exchanges of healing methods. At the same time, it reveals how medicine, as a contact zone of cultural beliefs and practices, was employed by Mather and his contemporaries to draw lines of cultural distinction among prominent ethnic groups in colonial America.

The sources of *The Angel of Bethesda* reflect the inherently transnational constitution of the field of medicine at the beginning of the eighteenth century. Mather's text is also representative of a seminal New England Puritan stance on the healing arts: the continuous shifting between recognizing and suppressing medical knowledge that originated outside the borders of the nation. Whereas Mather acknowledges the value of African practices for devising a prophylactic treatment against smallpox, one finds only scattered remarks about Native contributions to American medicine in his book (quite in contrast to the letters sent to the Royal Society). Although he is generally open-minded toward new medical treatments, the author refuses to incorporate explicitly indigenous healing rituals, which he regards as superstitious at best, demonic at worst, and only states in passing that certain Indian plant remedies could be helpful. For instance, he briefly mentions *guajacum*, as a cure for headaches, rheumatism, dropsy, epilepsy, nightmares, tuberculosis, and ulcers in the lungs; sassafras as a diaphoretic treatment of rheumatism and tuberculosis; Cowslip water, the decoction from the Virginia bluebells (*Mertensia virginica*), probably of local Massachu-

---

[85] Silverman 426; Beall and Shryock 37.

setts use, as a remedy against smallpox. Equally succinct, Mather suggests Samp-diet, a corn meal porridge introduced by Algonquians, against stones; worm-seed (*Chenopodium anthelminticum*), also known as Jerusalem Oak, another plant of American origin, whose seeds can be used to produce oil that is toxic but effective in curing many diseases: "our Countrey-People make almost a *Panacea* of it. It strangely releeves *Pains* in the *Stomach*; and restores a ruined Appetite. It helps in *Bloody Fluxes*, and in many other Distempers" (*Angel* 207), Mather writes, fully convinced that these remedies are efficacious.[86]

In another chapter, he mentions again in passing that "[o]ur Indians cure Consumptions with a *Mullein*-Tea" (*Angel* 183), suggesting that this healing practice originated in Native culture. This statement exemplifies, rather, how transnational healing knowledge in colonial New England was often energized by multiple trajectories and borrowings. If Mather is referring to the common mullein (*verbascum thapsus*), then his reference to Indian healing signifies an appropriation of Western knowledge by the local Algonquians since mullein is native to Europe and not the Americas.[87] Furthermore, the words "our Indians" demonstrate how the author, and by extension colonial New England society, has appropriated the Other for the sake of the advancement of Western civilization, even if, ironically, that Other has already adopted European practices for its own advancement.[88] Mather thus re-inscribes

[86] Another unacknowledged native American plant, although not from New England, described by Mather is Peruvian bark from which cinchona (quinine) was won to cure malaria; Mather also recommends Peruvian or Jesuit's bark for various stomach ailments and the whooping cough. Since malaria was apparently not known to the Andean Natives, where the plant was discovered, they also did not and could not have known that the Peruvian bark could produce cinchona.

[87] Nicholas N. Smith, "Indian Medicine: Fact or Fiction?," *Bulletin of the Massachusetts Archaeological Society* 26.1 (1964): 15. Among New England indigenes mullein was used against baldness, diarrhea, and asthma (16).

[88] Martha Robinson, "New Worlds, New Medicines Indian Remedies and English Medicine in Early America," *Early American Studies* (2005): 110n11. John Josselyn, includes "Mullin" among the plants imported by the English settlers in *New-England's Rarities Discovered in Birds, Beasts, Fishes, Serpents, and Plants of that Country* (1672; Early English Books Online, J1093) 86.

Native knowledge as already part of the hegemonic colonial culture and as never really culturally Other to begin with. These (mis)recognitions of cultural repositories at once challenge the meaning of the word "Native" and indicate how Mather's *medical* narrative can only come into existence as a *national* narrative by making use of knowledge that seemingly lies beyond the nation.[89] In other words, to establish himself as an American medical expert he has to transcend national boundaries and find and integrate healing methods that could be employed in forging a (new) narrative of the nation. At the same time, however, Mather's knowledge about Native remedies and his refusal to credit them appropriately in *The Angel of Bethesda* evince his partial suppression of transnational exchanges of medical expertise.[90]

The suppression of indigenous healing methods is aptly shown in two chapters devoted to an *Ur*-American plant: tobacco. Aside from constituting a cash crop for farmers in North America, tobacco was considered a panacea until the early nineteenth century. *Nicotinia* was introduced to the "Old World" by Columbus, who had observed its medicinal use among Native Americans. Soon thereafter, physicians across the Americas and Europe learned that Indians applied tobacco as, among others, a pain-reliever, an antiseptic, an anti-diarrhoeic, a treatment for epilepsy, and as an emollient.[91]

---

[89] To be sure, this national narrative did not reach its first full fruition for at least two generations after Mather's death in 1728; however, one of its central characteristic, the ambivalent inclusions and exclusions of Otherness, are already detectable at the outset of the eighteenth century.

[90] Mather's suppression of Native medicinal applications is especially startling given the extensive account provided in John Josselyn's *New-England Rarities Discovered* (1672) which could hardly have escaped Mather's attention. One needs only to compare a typical recipe from *The Angel of Bethesda* with Josselyn's report to see how similar treatments of particular diseases were and to thus realize how much the Boston minister obviously knew about indigenous healing methods.

[91] David Harris, "Medicine in Colonial America," *California and Western Medicine* 51.1 (1939): 36; Grace G. Stewart, "A History of the Medicinal Use of Tobacco, 1492–1860," *Medical History* 11.3 (1967): 228-268; John Josselyn, *An Account of Two Voyages to New-England* (1674; Early English Books Online, J1091) 76. "With a strong decoction of Tobacco they [the Native Americans]

Inspired by the English controversy over the medical and social (dis)advantages of the plant during the mid-seventeenth century, Mather expresses his disapproval of using it for pleasure and/or because it is fashionable in Europe. He rants against what he considers a social evil and a sign of declining faith with jeremiad rhetoric and typical Matherean pathos: "My Friend, If this by they State [i.e., if you are smoking; M.P.] thou throwest away a *Liberty*, with which thy Maker and Saviour has dignified thee; and thou art *Entangled with a Yoke of Bondage* to an *Appetite*, which is not of *His*, but of *Thy own* Creating, and, when thou art *come to thyself*, thou wilt *groan to be delivered from this Bondage of Corruption*" (*Angel* 303). For the Boston minister, tobacco is a sin because it hurts the body, the temple of the soul, and compromises the mind by taking away energies better applied to praising the glory of God.[92] Aware that smoking constitutes a mental habit as well as a physical addiction, Mather disapproves of tobacco consumption because it signals the power of the body over the mind. For a staunch Puritan such a lack of control over bodily cravings marked an unacceptable reversal of the Christian mind/matter dichotomy.

In his criticism of tobacco, however, Mather is unable to fully disavow the contemporary knowledge about its presumed medical values. In *The Christian Philosopher* he has to admit that "it is doubtless a *Plant* of many Virtues," and despite his vociferous rejection of tobacco in *The Angel of Bethesda*, he advises using its ashes as toothpaste and against toothaches, and prescribes various applications in case of dizziness, deafness, asthma, worms, sores, colic, and, in modern parlance, obesity.[93] Toward the end of his medical book, he cannot but

---

Cure Burns and Scalds, boiling it in Water form a Quart to a Pint, then wash the Sore therewith, and strew on the powder of dryed Tobacco" (John Josselyn, *New England Rarities* 54).

[92] Levy 127. Levy furthermore argues that Mather's diatribe against tobacco is also meant as a counterattack on John Williams, then Boston's only tobacconist and one of the opponents of Mather's inoculation plans and practices. Cf. Levy 128; Silverman 353-354.

[93] Mather, *Christian Philosopher* 144. Mather adds: "If the *Aking Tooth,* be in any Degree an hollow One, melt a little *Bees Wax*, and mix with it a little *Tobacco Ashes*, And Stop the Tooth with it. It Eases marvellously" (*Angel* 65).

admit that "[i]t is probable That for them who have to do with Persons and in Places, where Infection may be feared, the *Smoking of Tobacco* may be a very Excellent Praeservative" (*Angel* 307).[94] Hence, as much as he desires to present a consistent argument against tobacco, Mather cannot deny its healing potentials; what he can and does deny is the *source* of knowledge about the plant's curative applications.[95]

While medical practices from America, Africa, and Europe seem to converge in the mind of the Puritan minister, knowledge about healing and illness offered by Algonquians and Africans are allowed only partial access to the first handbook American medicine and the evolving *trans*national character of the country it represents. Mather's narrative of how he learned about certain remedies from different regions of the world, successfully applied this knowledge against many odds, and then denied its origin(s) anticipates larger cultural trends of adaptation, appropriation, and acculturation in colonial and later U.S. society. At the turn of the eighteenth century Mather's medical texts relied in part on the estrangement and appropriation of the Other: in the case of Africans, the minister's ventriloquial attempt to let the slaves speak about inoculation through his narrative voice is indicative of how the self-representation of cultural alterity was inherently contained within the framework of New England Puritanism. Mather's representation of *medical* archives thus evidences the *cultural* archives instigated by Puritan endeavors in the "New World." This becomes again manifest with regard to Native American medicine, when Mather's text brings to the surface the paradox of simultaneously acknowledging and suppressing indigenous cultural knowledge, a paradox that was to be a

---

[94] Additionally, in his "Manuductio ad ministerium. Directions for a Candidate of the Ministry" (1726), Mather's last publication to include "Rules of Health," the Boston preacher grants the young, aspiring clergy the liberty to smoke if they deem it necessary: "And yet, after all, I am not so *Inflexibly sett*, as utterly to deny you the Use of Tobacco, if you are sure of any *Benefit* from it. Only I insist upon it, That you be [...] *Excessively Moderate* in it" (134; emphasis original).

[95] The only mention of Native Americans in *The Christian Philosopher* (1721) occurs in relation to corn; when it comes to tobacco, Mather does not even hint at, let alone acknowledge, who used the plant before the Europeans or for what purposes.

seminal feature of American identity formation for decades and centuries to come.

* * *

Cotton Mather's treatises on medicine reflect central colonial ideas of illness and healing: God sends disease to flush out sins; the sick body is a representation of a sinful soul and, conversely, a cured body signifies a healed soul in Christ. As a result, any illness must not only be treated physiologically but the care of the soul is to precede that of the body. Once recovered, the believer is to use his/her newfound strength to think and act according to God's laws. If the patient fails to do so, s/he has every reason to be concerned about a possible divine punishment with even more severe afflictions.

In modifying the doctrine of theological pathogenesis, the erudite Boston preacher provided increasing room for the contemporary advances of the emerging medical sciences unlike any other New England colonist before him (perhaps with the notable exception of John Winthrop Jr.). Mather's later medical writings, especially, illustrate his insistence on a providential explanation of disease; yet, at the same time, the author grapples with the integration of contemporary mechanical and chemical explanations of illness and of the human body into a larger religious frame. The *Zeitgeist* emphasis on natural causes rather than divine interventions forced him to amend traditional explanations of disease. If illnesses could no longer be interpreted as signs of God, then Mather's Calvinist cosmology would begin to lose its credibility and force. During the later stage of his writings on medicine—from the "Curiosa Americana" to *The Angel of Bethesda*—the minister voices both his continued fascination with, and partial resistance to, interpretations of illnesses that were becoming increasingly secular. Despite his efforts to harmonize science and religion, Mather inadvertently contributed to the gradual transition of interpretative authority from the ecclesiastical to the civil realms that would gain further momentum in North America in the course of the eighteenth century.

Mather's medical writings also raise the question of who should have access to new knowledge and who is responsible for keeping and disseminating it. Although written in the typical Matherean tone of spiritual admonition, authorial complacency, and occasional self-aggrandizement, *The Angel of Bethesda* marks an insightful representation of a New England minister's belief in the necessity of doing good works; not to ensure eternal life, nor as an end in itself, but rather as a means by which depraved human beings can potentially receive glimpses into their predestined state after death. The compassionate side of his physico-theological approach to disease is often overlooked in popular conceptions and scholarly investigations, which tend to depict Cotton Mather as a particularly self-righteous, denunciative, and repressive New England colonist. His contributions to the field of medicine deserve ample credit though: he was the first American intellectual to present and develop an early version of germ theory, to consider psychogenic causes of illness, and to introduce as well as support a ground-breaking method to prevent the outbreak of smallpox.

It has also often been overlooked how the philosophical, theological, and practical underpinnings of Mather's medicine emerged from a transnational framework that reached from the intra-European dissemination of medical knowledge since Antiquity, to Protestant ecumenism, to medical knowledge from cultures that resided both inside and outside colonial New England. The latter strains of early American medicine were systematically suppressed by the ideologies and prejudices of the time and also by a number of recent scholars who have ignored or underestimated the transnational sources and influences in U.S. history and culture. Mather's work on medicine illustrates not so much benign transculturations or hybridizations but rather the contagious nature of cultural meetings and interactions in the transnational arena of early America. Here, the term "contamination" aptly signifies the intellectual disease that one of the salient thinkers and representatives of colonial New England experienced when his theological cosmos came under attack by scientific advances and differential cultural knowledge, especially in the field of medicine. The Boston clergyman certainly deserves credit for fighting the intellectual infections inflicted by transnational forces through an elaborate and sophisticated religious counter-attack. In hindsight, however, Mather and New England Puritanism writ large were losing an intellectual and epistemological battle, in part due to the advances in secular medicine.

# Conclusion

By 1730 the Puritan influence on the socio-cultural and political course of the English colonies in North America was irreversibly waning. Despite a short revival during the Great Awakening (1734-c1750), and although New England Puritanism had developed certain values that post-Revolutionary Americans adopted and shaped in accordance with their own cultural, political, and economic needs, the religious supremacy established by early colonists was increasingly replaced by Enlightenment views. One of the reasons for the decline of the New England way was that scientists, philosophers, and other intellectuals on both sides of the Atlantic had introduced epistemic changes that contested an exclusive reliance on Scripture and divine providence. Instead of God's immediate and continuous involvement in earthly affairs, the eighteenth century witnessed a far-reaching transformation of His ascribed role in the universe. While most colonial Americans at the eve of the Revolution still considered God as responsible for the order and design of the world, they were increasingly investing energy in understanding and altering their natural surroundings.[1]

This general epistemic shift also encompassed the field of medicine, where eighteenth-century physicians advanced secular theories and practices of healing. God was still in the picture, but the body was now being recognized as susceptible to forces residing in nature rather than in the realm of the supernatural. Medical science, as one result, shed its earlier credulity, shunned occult and folklorist methods of truth seeking and curative approaches, and became more empirical and methodical.

---

[1] These developments, which can only be sketched here, are explained more fully in Brooke Hindle, *The Pursuit of Science in Revolutionary America, 1735-1789* (1956; New York: Norton, 1974). See, also, Frank Kelleter, *Amerikanische Aufklärung: Sprachen der Rationalität im Zeitalter der Revolution* (Paderborn: Schöningh, 2002).

Physicians benefited from discoveries in all fields related to medicine and applied new therapeutic methods with varying degrees of success. In New England, as well as in other colonies in America, the medical scene witnessed a significant rise in secularization, professionalization, and institutionalization. With the establishment of medicine as a scientific field, the figure of the minister-physician gave way to practitioners who had been educated through an apprentice system and/or had received a degree from a European university or one of the newly founded medical schools in New York (1767), Philadelphia (1769), or Boston/Cambridge (1783).[2] The gradual transformation from religious to secular approaches to the diseased body had far-reaching consequences for practitioners as well as for patients. Depending on the severity and course of the affliction, some colonists continued to rely on folk healing (including Native therapeutics), while a growing part of the population welcomed new treatment methods. Religion still played a significant role for many patients in interpreting their illness experiences, especially potentially lethal diseases such as smallpox, malaria or yellow fever, and some aspects of the earlier meaning-endowment of illness survived (e.g., sickness as a bodily dysfunction that forces the patient to reflect on the reasons for, and future consequences of, an illness). Yet, piety, prayer, and repentance were no longer considered as *necessary* preconditions for healing.

This marked a decisive move away from previous notions of illness and healing that were energized and supported by Puritan views. In seventeenth-century New England, the enigmatic boundaries between success and failure in the conquest of certain diseases often pointed to the discrepancy between the human ability to save lives and complete powerlessness vis-à-vis untreatable illnesses. The inefficacy of many medical practices tied in with the belief that God's will is inscrutable and often destructive, and this belief allowed colonists to explain why

---

[2] A thorough account of the transformations in eighteenth-century Western medicine cannot be provided here. For a more detailed overview of New England medicine, see Henry R. Viets, *A Brief History of Medicine in Massachusetts* (Boston: Houghton, 1930) 53-88; and the essays collected in Philip Cash, et al. ed., *Medicine in Colonial Massachusetts, 1620-1820* (Boston: Colonial Society of Massachusetts, 1980).

certain diseases were fatal while others were not. The lack of efficacious treatment methods was hence filled with a religiosity that addressed humanity's utter powerlessness. In contrast to Calvin's doctrine of predestination, some New England colonists employed medical discourse to actually establish a growing degree of agency over, and rationalization of, their condition. Knowledge of the body—independent of what it meant for one's spiritual estate and/or possible salvation— became increasingly important in the course of the seventeenth and eighteenth centuries because it allowed the individual to work toward salvation through healing and thus helped to counter the helplessness that Calvin had ascribed to the human race. At the same time, this knowledge helped pave the way for scientific discoveries in medicine and related fields.

Between 1620 and 1730 the majority of colonial New Englanders had understood illnesses as complicated yet potentially legible signs from God. Like no other human experience, illness connected body and spirit, and its manifestation in the body of the believer told something about his/her current and future spiritual estate. The sick and dysfunctional colonial body not only called for a firm belief in God's presence and providential intervention in the life of an individual but also induced a feeling of detestation, dislike, and repugnance of the human physical condition and the spiritual estate it signified. Hence, in many instances sickness played a central role in bringing to light the abhorrence of the human, and particularly Puritan, mind and body. At the same time, illness illustrated the capacity to transform the diseased state into an occasion for self-reflection and reform.

Throughout the first century of colonialism in New England illness tended to be conceptualized along a dual trajectory: it served as a means of convincing the individual of his/her sinfulness and also functioned as a pedagogical tool for punishing, testing, and reforming humankind, and especially His chosen people. This double coding was deemed necessary in order to explain why the chosen few were (still) suffering. Bodily ailments often created and intensified uncertainties about the salvific future of individual New England subjects who were seeking to confirm their membership among the elect. On the level of the collective, therefore, diseases were often considered as signs of crisis in the relationship between God and his chosen community.

New England colonists offered different interpretations of this relationship, depending on whether their Native neighbors or they, themselves, were affected by disease. The devastating epidemics among the indigenous population were generally read as indicators of both English corporeal and cultural superiority and divine favor. By contrast, colonists often regarded their own illnesses (especially epidemics) as a disruption of the covenant with God that, at the same time, bore the potential for covenant renewal. Hence, much as diseases posed a threat to the sustenance of settler communities, they also proved useful in strengthening New English cultural and religious orthodoxy because they called for a constant return to Puritan modes of prayer, introspection, repentance, and interaction with others. Furthermore, by embracing the illness-induced cycle of punishment and gratification, settlers were able to prove to themselves that God still cared and that the "errand into the wilderness" was still valid and worth pursuing.

The conceptualization and textualization of illness in seventeenth- and early eighteenth-century New England writings can only be understood against the background of colonists' firm belief in medical providentialism. The notion that God's will and sovereignty expressed itself in and on human bodies constituted a cultural substratum that reverberates in almost all of the illness narratives surveyed for this study. It is evident in the justification and advertisement of the colonial project in promotional texts by John Winthrop, Edward Winslow, and John Eliot, and is echoed in poems by Michael Wigglesworth and Edward Taylor. Medical providentialism, as illustrated in most of the patient letters sent to John Winthrop Jr., was part of elite conceptualizations of bodily ailments and trickled down to the laity, in whose responses to illness one often finds a fusion of official disease theology with healing approaches drawn from folk and occult traditions. Such a syncretism often met with the suspicion of colonial leaders and often led to the persecution, ostracization, and at times execution of colonists, especially women. For example, the gendering of medical providentialism became evident during the Antinomian crisis, when John Winthrop and others vociferously defended the idea that God's favor or disfavor of certain religious and social ideas manifested itself with striking immediacy in "monstrous births" of deviant women.

Aside from its gendering, medical providentialism was also repeatedly couched in racial terms. This is evident in the *Eliot Tracts* when the missionaries attempt to prove the cultural superiority of Western civilization by arguing that God has granted Europeans stronger bodies and a more advanced knowledge in medicine. This knowledge, so they claimed, clearly superseded that of Algonquian powwows, whose inefficacious healing methods and allegiance with the devil helped to facilitate the decimation of Native people before and after the arrival of the English. Medical providentialism as racial discourse once again played a salient role during the 1722 smallpox inoculation controversy when members of the Boston clergy, among them Cotton and Increase Mather, defended a preventive measure that they had learned from African slaves and Muslims. According to the main line of argument pursued by the ministers, knowledge of the inoculation procedure was as much a sign of divine providence as the disease itself and hence had to be applied by human beings, especially if they wanted to confirm their covenant with God.

These and other cultural representations of medical providentialism illustrate that in colonial New England, as elsewhere, diseases were never simply objective facts but always also social constructions that were informed by biases and expectations, some of which were undergirded by power interests, while others were energized by the sheer human longing for coping with and overcoming illness. Many personal reflections by early colonists (e.g., in poems, conversion narratives, and patient letters) demonstrate what writing can potentially bring to disease: it forces the patient to self-reflect and to arrest, as it were, the illness ordeal in language and writing. But, as Judith Butler has suggested, "[a]lthough the body depends on language to be known, the body also exceeds every possible linguistic effort of capture."[3] The texts surveyed in the previous chapters strive, albeit in different ways and by using an array of literary forms, to express suffering in language. In doing so, they raise the question whether the description of an illness can ever be congruent with its lived experience because, to cite Butler once more, "the body is the blindspot of speech, that which acts in

[3] Judith Butler, "How Can I Deny That These Hands and This Body Are Mine?" *Qui Parle* 11.1 (1997): 2. A similar argument about pain is provided by Elaine Scarry, *The Body in Pain: The Making and Unmaking of the World* (New York: New York UP, 1985).

excess of what is said, but which also acts in and through what is said."[4]
Such acts are found in a number of illness representations studied here:
in Anne Bradstreet's attempt to mold words into deeds, in the
performances of Puritan conversion by Native survivors of epidemics
recorded by missionaries, in letters revealing intimate details about the
laity's body sent to a faraway physician in New London, and in official
documents in which the staging of witchcraft unfolds with references to
the body, its ailments, and chances for healing.

Contemporary theories of body and illness narratives are, however,
not easily transferrable to historical settings, as the present study has
also shown. For instance, Arthur Frank's principal assumption that
illness writings are often marked by a life-disturbing realization of
human frailty, helplessness, and finiteness relates only tangentially to
the experiences with diseases studied here.[5] In the lives of most people
in modern Western societies, illness has become—largely owing to
advances in biomedicine—an exceptional event. Yet, the notion of
sickness as an exception would hardly have occurred to colonial New
Englanders. Since the limitations placed on health were omnipresent,
early modern patterns of coping with and describing bodily impairments
centered primarily on the idea that illness marked a divine intervention
in earthly affairs that needed to be expected and accepted. Rather than
an "alien reality," illness often signaled continuity, the familiar, the
everyday, and even the security—as paradoxical as it may seem from
today's perspective—that God was still present, still real, and still taking
an interest in the faithful.[6]

Such an interpretation of illness was actually marked by continuous
modifications, negotiations, and pluralizations at a time when social and
cultural configurations in America began to develop distinctive traits
that were still firmly tied to Europe and already subject to adaptation to
living conditions in the "New World." True, many colonists consistently

---

[4] Judith Butler, *Excitable Speech: A Politics of the Performative* (New York:
Routledge, 1997) 11.

[5] Arthur W. Frank, *The Wounded Storyteller: Body, Illness, and Ethics*
(Chicago: U of Chicago P, 1995) 53-59.

[6] David B. Morris *Illness and Culture in the Postmodern Age* (Berkeley: U of
California P, 1998) 22.

interpreted their illnesses in religious terms. Yet, one also finds a number of narratives that allude to natural causes, fail to express moments of soul-searching and reform, and/or seek alternatives to the bleed and pray approach that many seventeenth-century minister-physicians prescribed. Many illness narratives observed in this study contend with dominant theological teachings and are supplemented by discursive fragments borrowed from knowledge formations located outside the religious frame of New England society and culture, especially from the realm of science. Around the time of Cotton Mather and Edward Taylor's deaths in 1728 and 1729, respectively, diseases had contributed to, and made visible, cultural dissonances that pressed for the resolution of spiritual and epistemological riddles and questions in textual space. Colonial New England pathographies, among them Winthrop's patient letters, witchcraft depositions and court testimonies, Bradstreet's illness poems, and Mather's medical writings, shed light on the cultural tilt effect in pre-Enlightenment America from religious to scientific approaches to the world and the human body.

Colonial diseases and medical practices also challenged the stability of national borders and cultural realms that were impacted by germs, viruses, and remedies. At the same time, they manifested cultural boundary lines in early New England. The colonists' inscriptions of perceived cultural differences into narratives of the healthy and diseased body constitute an early American example of medicalization, the attempt to define social, cultural, or personal conditions within medico-biological discursive registers. These registers naturalized perceived health disparities, social inequities, and cultural differences, in this case between Algonquians and English settlers, as well as among colonists themselves. In early North America, the biocultural discourse also embodied and encoded Otherness in medical terms so as to render colonization justifiable and necessary to contemporary and future generations. Narratives of disease helped shape the colonists' mental construction of America as both a dystopian wasteland and a utopian health-land. They further served to validate encroachment on Algonquian land and emphasized the idea that English endeavors in North America were ordained by a higher power. The epidemics of 1616-1619 and 1633-1634 propelled English legitimizing narratives and the notion of American exceptionalism by suggesting that invisible, legal, and natural forces were on the side of the colonists even before the arrival of the *Mayflower*.[7]

This early form of American exceptionalism could only come into existence by assembling and syncretizing existing medical knowledge in ways that had been undertaken and continued to exist in similar fashion in many other societies around the world. Colonial New Englanders were not exçeptional in the sense that they tackled bodily afflictions significantly different from that of people in other countries. Rather, official and lay approaches to diseases in the "New World" owed significantly to the re- and deterritorializations of larger cultural formations within the British Atlantic world. The assertion that New England medical practices and illness narratives were intricately tied to a larger set of cultural transferences in the early modern Atlantic region opens the present study to seminal assumptions and problems raised in recent scholarship on transnationalism.

Since its emergence in the 1980s, transnational studies have highlighted the spatial dimensions of human relations and identities, and have challenged both the geographical basis of American studies and the exceptionalist myth at its core. Transnationalism also has impacted cross-disciplinary conversations, revealing the opportunities and limits of transposing certain assumptions and approaches raised by scholars of transnationalism in literary and cultural studies to other disciplines such as history, political science, and sociology. The field of American history, for example, has witnessed a decisive paradigm shift, from the essentialist historiography of the Consensus School towards a more sustained focus on the international connectedness of the United States

---

[7] The idea of American exceptionalism is difficult to assert for the period before the emergence of the U.S. nation-state. Since the cultural phenomenon is of a later era in American history, it seems to be more reasonable to speak of regional distinctiveness. However, since the notion of American exceptionalism is generally regarded as being rooted in colonial New England, it will be used in the following argument. In a similar vein, transnationalism, a term which usually applies to social formations organized along nineteenth-century concepts of the nation and the state, needs to be problematized. One can argue that colonial Americans had indeed a clear notion of transnationalism, for instance, when New England writers viewed England as their nation but America as their country.

in history.[8] This approach entails the deconstruction of a national(ist) narrative that especially energized and directed literary, cultural, and historical studies of the United States during most of the Cold War years, when the struggle with Communism needed an ideological underpinning. A reductive summary of this narrative reads as follows: the seeds of U.S. democracy and American culture had been planted by Puritan settlers in New England, whence "civilization" spread across the continent and eventually beyond its territorial boundaries. The "American Adam," was seen to be on a providential mission, the "errand into the wilderness," whose goal it was to bring English and European modes of living to a place conceived as "virgin land."[9] Criticized as central pillars of American exceptionalism, these assumptions have recently been discarded by a number of scholars in favor of comparative studies or those which aim to show the embeddedness of early American culture, politics, and economics in transnational networks of

---

[8] Since the early 1990s, the "transnational turn" in American studies has been the subject of intense debates. For outlines of this methodological paradigm shift in American history, see Ian Tyrrell, "American Exceptionalism in an Age of International History," *American Historical Review* 96.4 (1991): 1031-1055; Michael McGerr, "The Price of the 'New Transnational History,'" *American Historical Review* 96.4 (1991): 1056-1067; David Thelen, "The Nation and Beyond: Transnational Perspectives on United States History," *Journal of American History* 86.3 (1999): 965-975. For an overview of the debate in the field of American literary and cultural studies, see, among many others, Shelley Fisher Fishkin, "Crossroads of Cultures: The Transnational Turn in American Studies. Presidential Address to the American Studies Association, November 12, 2004," *American Quarterly* 57.1 (2005): 17-57; and the essays collected in Winfried Fluck, Donald E. Pease, and John Carlos Rowe, eds., *Re-Framing the Transnational Turn in American Studies* (Dartmouth: UP of New England, 2011).

[9] These terms refer to key texts that are often seen as foundational to the "liberal consensus" in post-WW II American studies. See R. W. B. Lewis, *The American Adam: Innocence, Tragedy, and Tradition in the Nineteenth Century* (Chicago: U of Chicago P, 1955); Perry Miller, *Errand Into the Wilderness* (Cambridge, MA: Belknap Press of Harvard UP, 1956); Henry Nash Smith, *Virgin Land: The American West as Symbol and Myth* (New York: Vintage, 1957).

transference, specifically in the Atlantic world (Africa, Europe, the Americas, and the Caribbean).[10]

It seems that with the thematic and canonic expansion of early American studies in recent years, stretching to encompass the regional, linguistic, and cultural varieties of pre-revolutionary writings in the Americas, New England society and literature has receded into the background.[11] While the extension of focus to other groups living and writing in colonial America (especially Spanish and French settler communities) marks a necessary corrective to the previous preeminence of nationalist and exceptionalist narratives, such a transnational approach does not alleviate scholars from the necessity of continuing investigations of early New England writings. Such a note of caution does not aim to reinvigorate or defend American exceptionalism or to trace contemporary U.S. culture and society back to an identifiable point

---

[10] For an overview of the major themes, topics, and approaches in the field of Atlantic history, which constitutes a subsidiary field of transnational studies, see Nicholas Canny, "Writing Atlantic History; or, Reconfiguring the History of Colonial British America," *Journal of American History* 86.3 (1999): 1093-1114; David Armitage, "Three Concepts of Atlantic History," *The British Atlantic World 1500-1800*, ed. David Armitage and Michael J. Braddick (New York: Palgrave, 2002) 11-27; Alison Games, "Atlantic History: Definitions, Challenges, and Opportunities," *American Historical Review* 111.4 (2006): 741-757. However, the present study follows the methodological retooling by Atlantic scholars only to a certain extent. Games' assertion that such a retooling "by necessity deemphasizes any single place" (749), either through comparative studies or by stressing a region's rooting in transatlantic and transnational connectivities, fails to grasp fully the textualization of illness by early New Englanders. Nevertheless, my study shows how certain medical practices and responses to diseases drew upon and constituted the British Atlantic as a cultural realm, for example, in the letters to and from John Winthrop Jr., in his father's reports on "monstrous births," Cotton Mather's medical writings, or the intellectual responses to Native American epidemics in various prose and poetic texts.

[11] See, for instance, Susan Castillo and Ivy Schweitzer, eds., *The Literatures of Colonial America: An Anthology* (Oxford: Blackwell, 2001); Carla Mulford, Angela Vietto, and Amy E. Winans, eds., *Early American Writings* (New York: Oxford UP, 2002).

of origin. Rather, my own focus on New England is owed to the observation that illnesses left numerous traces in the cultural archives of early Americans and that it resonates with larger processes of cultural adaptation in the Americas. Hence, "the shift towards considering the culture of colonial America more as a transnational phenomenon"[12] does not necessarily have to imply a renouncing of New England as an object of study. Rather, transnational studies methodologies and research foci can be employed as useful supplementary foils for studying colonial New England.[13]

A focus on medical practices and responses to illnesses in this rather limited regional setting provides insights for understanding various trajectories of, and resistances to, cultural transferences in the Atlantic world. Medical topics such as the flow of pathogens, the two-way exchange of healing knowledge between Europe and North America, or spiritual meaning-endowments of illness shaped and, at the same time, reflected networks of trade, ideas, and kinship that spanned across the Atlantic. Although intellectual and artistic responses to illness showed strong ties to the Protestant movement in Europe (which was itself marked by national and transnational networks), New England colonists consistently met the specificities of their disease burden with a mixture of treatment methods from Europe, Native America, and Africa. While New England medical practice was deeply embedded in transnational contexts, the conceptualization of illness bore significant, regionally specific and, in this sense, exceptional characteristics. The texts surveyed here hence illustrate how medical issues—from actual

---

[12] Paul Giles, "The Culture of Colonial America: Theology and Aesthetics," *A Companion to the Literatures of Colonial America*, ed. Susan Castillo and Ivy Schweitzer (Malden: Blackwell, 2005) 80.

[13] Such a focus has guided a number of studies on the transatlantic connections between Protestants in England and North America in recent years and has also influenced the present investigation. See, for instance, Francis J. Bremer, "Increase Mather's Friends: The Trans-Atlantic Congregational Network of the Seventeenth Century," *Proceedings of the American Antiquarian Society* 94.1 (1984): 59-96; Alison Searle, "'Though I Am a Stranger to You by Face, yet in Neere Bonds by Faith': A Transatlantic Puritan Republic of Letters," *Early American Literature* 43.2 (2008): 277-308.

practices to intellectual responses to illness—bring forth and illuminate a central dialectic between regional distinctiveness and international embeddings of colonial American culture.

As the preceding chapters have furthermore shown, illnesses not only raised spiritual questions for the individual and the collective but also threatened the cultural homogeneity which settlers sought to uphold. The omission of intercultural medical exchanges in many texts is, therefore, not so much a sign of their non-existence rather than an indication that colonial writers recognized the danger of admitting to adopting so-called heathen practices. In other cases, such as during the debate on smallpox inoculation, the global interplay of therapeutic systems became strikingly visible, indicating that the representation of American medicine had indeed shifted toward the transnational. The inoculation controversy and a number of other textualized illnesses hence merely represent the tip of an iceberg of the complexities that underlie intercultural exchanges in medical knowledge formations and healing practices in seventeenth- and eighteenth-century America.

# Bibliography

## I. Primary Literature

Baxter, Richard. *Reliquiae Baxterianae*. London 1696. Early English Books Online. B1370. Web.

Boyer, Paul, and Stephen Nissenbaum, eds. *Salem-Village Witchcraft: A Documentary Record of Local Conflict in Colonial New England*. Belmont: Wadsworth, 1972. Print.

Boylston, Zabdiel. *Some Account of What is Said of Inoculating or Transplanting the Small Pox*. Boston: Gerrish, 1721. Print.

---. *An Historical Account of the Small-Pox Inoculated in New-England*. London 1726. Boston: Gerrish, 1730. Print.

Bradford, William. *Of Plymouth Plantation, 1620-1647*. 1856. Ed. Samuel Eliot Morison. New York: Knopf, 1952. Print.

Bradstreet, Anne. *The Works of Anne Bradstreet*. Ed. Jeannine Hensley. Cambridge, MA: Belknap P of Harvard UP, 1967. Print.

Bunyan, John. *The Pilgrim's Progress*. 1678/1684. Ed. Cynthia Wall. New York: Norton, 2009. Print.

Calvin, John. *Institutes of the Christian Religion*. 1536. Trans. Henry Beveridge. Grand Rapids: Christian Classics Ethereal Library, 2002. Print.

Castillo, Susan, and Ivy Schweitzer, eds. *The Literatures of Colonial America: An Anthology*. Oxford: Blackwell, 2001. Print.

"The Charter of the Massachusetts Bay Company, 1629." *American Colonial Documents to 1776*. Ed. Merrill Jensen. London: Eyre & Spottiswoode, 1955. 72-84. Print.

Clarke, Daniel. "Letter to John Winthrop, Jr." 7 August 1675. Beinecke Rare Book and Manuscript Library, Yale University, New Haven. Print.

Cooper, William. *A Letter to a Friend in the Country, Attempting a Solution of the Scruples and Objections of Conscientious or Religious Nature, Commonly Made against the New Way of Receiving the Small-Pox*. Boston 1721. Early American Imprints. Series 1, no. 2247. Web.

Copeland, David E., ed. *Debating the Issues in Colonial Newspapers: Primary Documents on Events of the Period.* Westport: Greenwood, 2000. Print.

Cotta, John. *A Short Discouerie of the Vnobserued Dangers of Seuerall Sorts of Ignorant and Vnconsiderate Practisers of Physicke in England.* London 1612. Early English Books Online. STC 5833. Web.

---. *The Triall of Witch-Craft, Showing the True and Right Methode of the Discovery with the Confutation of Erroneous Wayes.* London 1616. Early English Books Online. STC 5836. Web.

Cotton, John. *Gods Promise to His Plantation.* London 1620. Early English Books Online. STC 5854.4. Web.

---. *The Whole Book of Psalms Faithfully Translated into English Metre (Bay Psalm Book).* Boston 1640. Early American Imprints. Series 1, no. 4. Web.

---. *The Way of Life, or, Gods Way and Course.* London 1641. Early English Books Online. C6470. Web.

---. *The Way of the Churches of Christ in New-England.* London 1645. Early English Books Online. C6471. Web.

Davenport, John. *Letters of John Davenport, Puritan Divine.* Ed. Isabel M. Calder. New Haven: Yale UP, 1937. Print.

Dermer, Thomas. "To His Worshipfull Friend M. Samuel Purchas, Preacher of the Word, at the Church a Little within Ludgate, London (1619)." *Sailors Narratives of Voyages along the New England Coast, 1524-1624.* Ed. George Winship Parker. Boston: Houghton, 1905. 247-258. Print.

Digby, Kenelme. "To John Winthrop, Jr." 26 January 1656. *Collections of the Massachusetts Historical Society.* Series 3, Vol. 10 (1849): 15-19. Print.

Douglass, William. *Inoculation of the Small Pox as Practised in Boston.* Boston 1722. Early American Imprints. Series 1, no. 2332. Web.

---. *The Abuses and Scandals of Some Late Pamphlets in Favour of Inoculation of the Small Pox.* Boston: Franklin, 1722. Print.

Dow, George Francis, ed. *Records and Files of the Quarterly Courts of Essex County.* Vol. II. 1656-1662. Salem, MA: Essex Institute, 1912. Print.

Eliot, John. *Tears of Repentance: or, a Further Narrative of the Progress of the Gospel amongst the Indians in New-England.* London 1653. Early English Books Online. E522. Web.

---. *A Further Accompt of the Progresse of the Gospel amongst the Indians in New-England.* London 1659. Early English Books Online. E510. Web.

---. "Rev. John Eliot's Records of the First Church in Roxbury, Mass." *The New-England Historical and Genealogical Register* 33 (April 1879): 236-239. Print.

Emerson, Everett, ed. *Letters from New England: The Massachusetts Bay Colony, 1629-1638.* Amherst: U of Massachusetts P, 1976. Print.

"An Extract of Several Letters from Cotton Mather, D. D. to John Woodward, M. D. and Richard Waller." *Philosophical Transactions* 29 (1714-1716): 62-71. Print.

Fiske, John. *The Notebook of the Reverend John Fiske, 1644-1675.* Ed. Robert G. Pope. *Collections of the Colonial Society of Massachusetts* 47. Boston: The Society, 1974. Print.

Gallope, Hannah. "To John Winthrop, Jr." 12 April 1660. *Collections of the Massachusetts Historical Society.* Series 5, Vol. 1 (1871): 98. Print.

Gookin, Daniel. *Historical Collections of the Indians in New England: Of Their Several Nations, Numbers, Customs, Manners, Religion and Government, Before the English Planted There.* 1674. Boston: Belknap & Hall, 1792. Print.

Gorges, Ferdinando. "A Briefe Narration of the Originall Undertakings of the Advancement of Plantations into the Parts of America (1658)." *Sir Ferdinando Gorges and his Province of Maine.* Vol. II. Ed. James Phinney Baxter. Boston: Prince Society, 1890. 1-81. Print.

Gorton, Samuel. "To John Winthrop, Jr." 21 October 1674. *Collections of the Massachusetts Historical Society.* Series 4, Vol. 7 (1865): 604-626. Print.

Grainger, Samuel. *The Imposition of Inoculation as a Duty Religiously Considered.* Boston: Nicholas Boone, 1721. Print.

Hale, John. *A Modest Enquiry into the Nature of Witchcraft.* Boston 1697. Early American Imprints. Series 1, no. 1050. Web.

Hall, David D., ed. *The Antinomian Controversy, 1636-1638: A Documentary History.* Durham: Duke UP, 1990. Print.

---, ed. *Witch-Hunting in Seventeenth-Century New England.* Boston: Northeastern UP, 1991. Print.

Hariot, Thomas. *A Briefe and True Report of the New Found Land of Virginia.* London 1588; Early English Books Online. STC 12785. Web.

Hartlib, Samuel. "To John Winthrop, Jr." 16 March 1660. *Proceedings of the Massachusetts Historical Society.* Third Series, Vol. 72 (1957-1960): 40-49. Print.

Hawthorne, Nathaniel. *The Scarlet Letter.* 1850. Ed. Ross C. Murfin. Boston: Bedford, 2006. Print.

Higginson, Francis. *A Direction for a Publick Profession in the Church Assembly.* Boston 1629. Early American Imprints. Series I, no. 100. Print.

---. *New-England's Plantation: Or, a Short and True Description of the Commodities and Discommodities of that Countrey.* London 1630. Early English Books Online. STC 1352:04. Web.

Holmes, Oliver Wendell. *Medical Essays: The Writings of Oliver Wendell Holmes.* Vol. 9. Boston: Cambridge UP, 1891. Print.

Johnson, Edward. *Wonder-Working Providence of Sions Saviour in New-England.* 1654. New York: Scholars' Facsimiles and Reprints, 1974. Print.

Josselyn, John. *New-England's Rarities Discovered in Birds, Beasts, Fishes, Serpents, and Plants of that Country.* London 1672. Early English Books Online. J1093. Web.

---. *An Account of Two Voyages to New-England.* London 1674. Early English Books Online. J1091. Web.

Kittredge, George Lyman, ed. "Letters of Samuel Lee and Samuel Sewall Relating to New England and the Indians." *Publications of the Colonial Society of Massachusetts* 14 (1912): 142-186. Print.

Lalemant, Hierosme. *The Jesuit Relations and Allied Documents: Travels and Explorations of the Jesuit Missionaries in New France, 1610-1791.* Vol. 19. Quebec. 1640. Ed. Reuben G. Thwaites. Trans. Finlow Alexander et al. Cleveland: Burrows, 1898. Print.

Lederer, John. *The Discoveries of John Lederer.* Ed. William P. Cumming. Charlottesville: U of Virginia P, 1958. Print.

Luther, Martin. *The Table-Talk of Martin Luther.* 1566. Trans. William Hazlitt. Philadelphia: The Lutheran Publication Society, 1868. Print.

Mather, Cotton. *Memorable Providences, Relating to Witchcrafts and Possessions.* Boston 1689. Early American Imprints, Series 1, no. 486. Web.

---. *The Wonders of the Invisible World: Observations as well Historical as Theological, upon the Nature, the Number, and the Operations of the*

*Devils*. Boston 1692. Early American Imprints. Series 1, no. 657. Web.

---. *Mens Sana in Corpore Sano: A Discourse upon Recovery from Sickness*. Boston 1698. Early American Imprints. Series 1, no. 829. Web.

---. *The Great Physician, Inviting them that are Sensible of their Internal Maladies, to Repair unto Him for His Heavenly Remedies*. Boston 1700. Early American Imprints. Series 1, no. 926. Web.

---. *Magnalia Christi Americana; or, The Ecclesiastical History of New England*. Boston 1702. Vol. II. Hartford: Andrus, 1853. Print.

---. *Magnalia Christi Americana; or, The Ecclesiastical History of New England*. Boston 1702. Vol. I. Hartford: Andrus, 1855. Print.

---. *Mare Pacificum: A Short Essay upon Those Noble Principles of Christianity, Which May Always Compose and Rejoyce, the Mind of the Afflicted Christian*. Boston 1705. Early American Imprints. Series 1, no. 1216. Web.

---. *Bonifacius: An Essay upon the Good*. Boston 1710. Early American Imprints. Series 1, no. 1460. Web.

---. "Letter to John Woodward, 17 November 1712." Royal Society, London. EL/M2/21. Print.

---. "Letter to John Woodward, 18 November 1712." Royal Society, London. EL/M2/22. Print.

---. "Letter to John Woodward, 22 November 1712." Royal Society, London. EL/M2/26. Print.

---. "Letter to John Woodward, 24 November 1712." Royal Society, London. EL/M2/27. Print.

---. "Letter to Richard Waller, 27 November 1712." Royal Society, London. EL/M2/31. Print.

---. *Wholesome Words: A Visit of Advice, Given unto Families that are Visited with Sickness*. Boston 1713. Early American Imprints. Series 1, no. 1630. Web.

---. *A Letter, about a Good Management under the Distemper of the Measles, at This Time Spreading in the Country*. Boston 1713. Early American Imprints. Series 1, no. 4376. Web.

---. *Insanabilia: An Essay upon Incurables*. Boston 1714. Early American Imprints. Series 1, no. 1691. Web.

---. *A Perfect Recovery: The Voice of the Glorious God, unto Persons, whom His Mercy Has Recovered from Sickness*. Boston 1714. Early American Imprints. Series 1, no. 1696. Web.

---. "Letter to John Woodward, 3 July 1716." British Library. Sloane Ms. 3340, folio 280-282. Print.

---. "Letter to John Woodward, 11 July 1716." British Library. Sloane Ms. 3340, folio 291-293. Print.

---. "Letter to John Woodward, 12 July 1716." British Library. Sloane Ms. 3340. Folio 294-296. Print.

---. "Letter to John Woodward, 13 July 1716." British Library, Sloane Ms. 3340, folio 296-297b. Print.

---. *The Christian Philosopher*. 1721. Ed. Winton U. Solberg. Urbana: U of Illinois P, 1994. Print.

---. "Letter to James Jurin. 4 June 1723." Royal Society, London. EL/M2/38. Print.

---. "Letter to James Jurin and John Woodward, 7 October 1724." Royal Society, London. EL/M2/46. Print.

---. "Letter to James Jurin, 22 September 1724." Royal Society, London. EL/M2/48. Print.

---. "Letter to James Jurin, 15 December 1724." Royal Society, London. EL/M2/57. Print.

---. *Diary of Cotton Mather, Part I: 1681-1708*. New York: Ungar, 1911. Print.

---. *Diary of Cotton Mather, Part II: 1709-1724*. New York: Ungar, 1911. Print.

---. *El-Shaddai: A Brief Essay, on All Supplied in an Alsufficient Saviour*. Boston 1725. Early American Imprints. Series 1, no. 2669. Web.

---. *Manuductio ad Ministerium: Directions for a Candidate of the Ministry*. Boston 1726. Early American Imprints. Series 1, no. 2772. Web.

---. *Selected Letters of Cotton Mather*. Ed. Kenneth Silverman. Baton Rouge: Louisiana State UP, 1971. Print.

---. *The Angel of Bethesda*. Ed. Gordon W. Jones. Barre, MA: American Antiquarian Society and Barre, 1972. Print.

Mather, Increase. *A Brief History of the Warr with the Indians in New England*. Boston 1676. Early American Imprints. Series 1, no. 220. Web.

---. *A Relation of the Troubles Which Have Happened in New-England by Reason of the Indians there, from the Year 1614 to the Year 1675, etc.* Boston: Foster, 1677. Print.

---. *An Essay for the Recording of Illustrious Providences*. Boston 1684. Early American Imprints. Series 1, no. 372. Web.

Mather, Richard. *Church-Government and Church-Covenant Discussed*. London 1643. Early English Books Online. M1269. Web.

Mayhew, Matthew. *A Brief Narrative of the Success which the Gospel hath had among the Indians*. Boston 1694. Early American Imprints. Series 1, no. 701. Web.

Minkema, Kenneth P., ed. "The East Windsor Conversion Narratives, 1700-1752." *The Connecticut Historical Society Bulletin* 51 (1986): 9-63. Print.

---. ed. "A Great Awakening Conversion: The Relation of Samuel Belcher." *William and Mary Quarterly* 44.1 (1987): 121-126. Print.

Morton, Thomas. *New English Canaan*. 1637. Ed. Charles F. Adams, Jr. Boston: Prince Society, 1883. Print.

Mulford, Carla, Angela Vietto, and Amy E. Winans, eds. *Early American Writings*. New York: Oxford UP, 2002. Print.

*New Englands First Fruits*. London 1643. Early English Books Online. E519. Web.

Palmer, Thomas. *The Admirable Secrets of Physick and Chyrurgery*. 1691. Ed. Thomas R. Forbes. New Haven: Yale UP, 1984. Print.

Paracelsus. *Paracelsus: Selected Readings*. Ed. and trans. Nicholas Goodrick-Clarke. Wellingborough: Crucible, 1990. Print.

"Patent of the Council for New England, Nov. 3/13, 1620." *Select Charters and Other Documents Illustrative of American History, 1606-1775*. Ed. William MacDonald. New York: Macmillan, 1904. 23-33. Print.

Perkins, William. *Two Treatises: I. Of the Nature and Practise of Repentance. II. Of the Combat of the Flesh and Spirit*. London 1593. Early English Books Online. STC 1426:02. Web.

---. *A Treatise Tending unto a Declaration, Whether a Man be in the Estate of Damnation, or in the Estate of Grace*. London: Porter, 1597. Print.

---. *The Workes of that Famous and Worthy Minister of Christ in the Universitie of Cambridge, M. William Perkins. The Second Volume*. London 1631. Early English Books Online. 19653. Web.

Rowlandson, Mary White. *The Soveraignty and Goodness of God*. 1682. Boston: Fleet for Phillips, 1720. Print.

Rush, Benjamin. *An Oration, Delivered February 4, 1774, before the American Philosophical Society, Held at Philadelphia: Containing, an Enquiry into the Natural History of Medicine among the Indians in*

*North-America*. Philadelphia 1774. Early American Imprints. Series 1, no. 13592. Web.

Shepard, Thomas. *The Clear Sun-Shine of the Gospel Breaking Forth upon the Indians in New-England*. London 1648. *Collections of the Massachusetts Historical Society*. Third Series, Vol. 4 (1834): 37-67. Print.

---. *The Parable of Ten Virgins*. London 1660. Early English Books Online. S3114A. Web.

---. *Thomas Shepard's Confessions*. Ed. George Selement and Bruce C. Woolley. *Publications of the Colonial Society of Massachusetts* 58. Boston: Society, 1981. Print.

---. "Thomas Shepard's Record of Relations of Religious Experience, 1648-1649." Ed. Mary Rhinelander McCarl. *William and Mary Quarterly* 48.3 (1991): 432-466. Print.

Shurtleff, Nathaniel B., ed. *Records of the Governor and Company of the Massachusetts Bay in New England*. Vol. 2. 1642-1649. Boston: White, 1853.

Smith, John. *A Description of New England: or, Observations and Discoveries in the North of America in the Year of our Lord 1614*. Boston: Veazie, 1865. Print.

Stafford, Edward. "To John Winthrop." 6 May 1643. *Proceedings of the Massachusetts Historical Society*. Series 1, Vol. 5 (1860-1862): 379-383. Print.

Starkey, George. *Natures Explication and Helmont's Vindication: Or a Short and Sure Way to a Long and Sound Life*. London 1657. Print.

---. *Pyrotechny Asserted and Illustrated: To Be the Surest and Fastest Means for Arts Triumph over Natures Infirmities*. London, 1658. Print.

Strong, Robert, ed. "Two Seventeenth-Century Conversion Narratives from Ipswich, Massachusetts Bay Colony." *New England Quarterly* 82.1 (2009): 136-169.

Taylor, Edward. "Dispensatory." n.d., Beinecke Rare Book and Manuscript Library. Yale University. Print.

---. "The Diary of Edward Taylor." *Proceedings of the Massachusetts Historical Society* 18 (1880-1881): 5-18. Print.

---. *The Poems of Edward Taylor*. Ed. Donald E. Stanford. New Haven: Yale UP, 1960. Print.

---. *Edward Taylor's Minor Poetry*. Ed. Thomas M. and Virginia L. Davis. Boston: Twayne, 1981. Print.

Thacher, Thomas. *A Brief Rule to Guide the Common-People of New-England How to Order Themselves and Their in the Small Pocks, or Measles*. 1677/78. Baltimore: Johns Hopkins P, 1937. Print.

Verrazano, Giovanni da. "The Written Record of the Voyage of 1524 of Giovanni da Verrazano as Recorded in a Letter to Francis I, King of France, July 8th, 1524." Trans. Susan Tarrow. *The Voyages of Giovanni da Verrazzano, 1524-1528*. Ed. Lawrence C. Wroth. New Haven: Yale UP, 1970. 133-143. Print.

Ward, George. "Letter to John Winthrop, Jr., 15 June 1652." Countway Medical Library, Harvard University, BMS C.56.2. Print.

Wheelwright, John. *Mercurius Americanus, Mr. Welds His Antitype, or, Massachusetts Great Apologie Examined*. London 1645. Early English Books Online. W1605. Web.

White, John. *The Planters Plea, Or The Grounds of Plantations Examined, and Usuall Objections Answered*. London 1630. Early English Books Online. 25399. Web.

Whitfield, Henry. *The Light Appearing More and More towards the Perfect Day*. London 1651. Early English Books Online. W1999. Web.

---. *Strength out of Weaknesse: or a Glorious Manifestation of the Further Progresse of the Gospel among the Indians of New-England*. London 1652. Early English Books Online. W2003. Web.

Wigglesworth, Michael. *The Diary of Michael Wigglesworth, 1653-1657: The Conscience of a Puritan*. Ed. Edmund S. Morgan. 1946. New York: Harper, 1965. Print.

---. *The Poems of Michael Wigglesworth*. Ed. Ronald A. Bosco. Lanham: UP of America, 1989. Print.

Williams, John. *Several Arguments, Proving, That Inoculating the Small Pox Is Not Contained in the Law of Physick, either Natural or Divine, and Therefore Unlawful*. Boston: Franklin, 1721. Print.

Williams, Roger. *A Key into the Language of America*. London 1643. Early English Books Online. W2766. Web.

---. *The Letters of Roger Williams*. Ed. John Russell Bartlett. Vol. 6. Providence: Publications of the Narragansett Club, 1874. Print.

Wilson, John. *The Day-Breaking, If not the Sun-Rising of the Gospell with the Indians in New-England*. London 1647. Early English Books Online. S3110. Web.

Winslow, Edward. *Good Newes from New England, or a True Relation of Things Very Remarkable at the Plantation of Plimoth in New-England.* London 1624. Early English Books Online. STC 25856. Web.

---. *The Glorious Progress of the Gospel amongst the Indians in New England.* London 1649. Early English Books Online. W3036. Web.

*Winthrop Papers.* Vol. I. 1498-1628. Ed. Worthington C. Ford. Boston: Massachusetts Historical Society, 1929. Print.

*Winthrop Papers.* Vol. II. 1623-1630. Ed. Stewart Mitchell. Boston: Massachusetts Historical Society, 1931. Print.

*Winthrop Papers.* Vol. III. 1631-1637. Ed. Allyn Bailey Forbes. Boston: Massachusetts Historical Society, 1943. Print.

*Winthrop Papers.* Vol. IV. 1638-1644. Ed. Allyn Bailey Forbes. Boston: Massachusetts Historical Society, 1944. Print.

*Winthrop Papers.* Vol. V. 1645-1648. Ed. Allyn Bailey Forbes. Boston: Massachusetts Historical Society, 1947. Print.

*Winthrop Papers.* Vol. VI. 1650-1654. Ed. Malcolm Freiberg. Boston: Massachusetts Historical Society, 1992. Print.

Winthrop, John. "A Modell of Christian Charity (1630)." *Collections of the Massachusetts Historical Society* 7 (1838): 31-48. Print.

---. *The History of New England from 1630-1649.* Ed. James Savage. Vol. 1. Boston: Little 1852. Print.

---. *The History of New England from 1630-1649.* Ed. James Savage. Vol. 2. Boston: Little 1853. Print.

---. *Winthrop's Journal: "History of New England": 1630-1649.* Ed. James Kendall Hosmer. Vol. 1. New York: Scribner's Sons, 1908. Print.

---. *Winthrop's Journal: "History of New England": 1630-1649.* Ed. James Kendall Hosmer. Vol. 2. New York: Charles Scribner's Sons, 1908. Print.

---. *The Journal of John Winthrop: 1630-1649.* Ed. Richard S. Dunn, James Savage, and Laetitia Yeandle. Cambridge, MA: Harvard UP, 1996. Print.

---. *A Short Story of the Rise, Reign, and Ruine of the Antinomians, Familists & Libertines* (1644). *The Antinomian Controversy, 1636-1638: A Documentary History.* Ed. David D. Hall. Durham: Duke UP, 1990. 199-310. Print.

Winthrop, John, Jr. "To John Winthrop, 17 January 1648/49." *Collections of the Massachusetts Historical Society.* Series 5, Vol. 8 (1882): 39. Print.

---. "To Fitz-John Winthrop, 8 February 1654/55." *Collections of the Massachusetts Historical Society*. Series 5, Vol. 8 (1882): 40-43. Print.

---. "To Samuel Hartlib, 25 August 1660." *Proceedings of the Massachusetts Historical Society*. Series 3, Vol. 72 (1957-1960): 49-58. Print.

---. "To Sir Robert Moray, 20 September 1664." *Proceedings of the Massachusetts Historical Society*. Series 1, Vol. 16 (1878): 223-224. Print.

---. "To Henry Oldenburg, 25 July 1668." *Collections of the Massachusetts Historical Society*. Series 5, Vol. 8 (1882): 121-125. Print.

---. "Medical Account Books." Manuscript. Hartford: Connecticut Historical Society. Print.

Winthrop, Wait. "To Fitz-John Winthrop, 2 October 1682." *Collections of the Massachusetts Historical Society*. Series 5, Vol. 8 (1882): 429. Print.

Wood, Owen. *An Alphabetical Book of Physicall Secrets*. London 1639. Early English Books Online. STC 25955. Web.

Wood, William. *New England's Prospect: A True, Lively, and Experimentall Description of that Part of America, Commonly Called New England*. London 1634. Early English Books Online. STC 25957. Web.

Woodward, William E., ed. *Records of Salem Witchcraft*. Vol. 2. Roxbury, 1864. Print.

## II. Secondary Literature

Adams, John C. "Alexander Richardson and the Ramist Poetics of Michael Wigglesworth." *Early American Literature* 25.3 (1990): 271-288. Print.

Adorno, Theodor W. *Aesthetic Theory*. 1970. Trans. C. Lenhardt. London: Routledge, 1984. Print.

Agamben, Giorgio. *Homo Sacer: Sovereign Power and Bare Life*. Trans. Daniel Heller-Roazen. Stanford: Stanford UP, 1998. Print.

Agrimi, Jole, and Chiara Crisciani. "Charity and Aid in Medieval Christian Civilization." *Western Medical Thought from Antiquity to the Middle Ages*. Ed. Mirko D. Grmek. Trans. Antony Shugaar. 1993. Cambridge, MA: Harvard UP, 1998. 170-196. Print.

Alexis, Gerhard T. "Wigglesworth's 'Easiest Room.'" *The New England Quarterly* 42.4 (1969): 573-583. Print.

Amundsen, Darrel W., and Gary B. Ferngren. "Medicine and Religion: Early Christianity through the Middle Ages." *Health/Medicine and the Faith Traditions*. Ed. Martin E. Marty and Kenneth L. Vaux. Philadelphia: Fortress, 1982. 93-131. Print.

Anderson, Virginia DeJohn. *New England's Generation: The Great Migration and the Formation of Society and Culture in the Seventeenth Century*. New York: Cambridge UP, 1991. Print.

Anselment, Raymond A. *The Realms of Apollo: Literature and Healing in Seventeenth-Century England*. Newark: U of Delaware P, 1995. Print.

Archer, David. *Fissures in the Rock: New England in the Seventeenth Century*. Hanover: UP of New England, 2001. Print.

Armitage, David. "Three Concepts of Atlantic History." *The British Atlantic World 1500-1800*. Ed. David Armitage and Michael J. Braddick. New York: Palgrave, 2002. 11-27. Print.

Arnold, David. "Introduction: Disease, Medicine and Empire." *Imperial Medicine and Indigenous Societies*. Ed. David Arnold. Manchester: Manchester UP, 1988. 1-27. Print.

Baker, Brenda J. "Pilgrim's Progress and Praying Indians: The Biocultural Consequences of Contact in Southern New England." *In the Wake of Contact: Biological Reponses to Conquest*. Ed. Clark S. Larsen and George R. Milner. New York: Wiley, 1994. 35-45.

Banerjee, Mita. *Ethnic Ventriloquism: Literary Minstrelsy in Nineteenth-Century American Literature*. Heidelberg: Winter, 2008. Print.

Bangs, Jeremy Dupertuis. *Pilgrim Edward Winslow: New England's First Diplomat*. Boston: New England Historic Genealogical Society, 2004. Print.

Banner, Stuart. *How the Indians Lost their Land: Law and Power on the Frontier*. Cambridge, MA: Harvard UP, 2005. Print.

Barnard, John. "Keats's Letters." *The Cambridge Companion to Keats*. Ed. Susan J. Wolfson. Cambridge: Cambridge UP, 2001. 120-134. Print.

Beall, Otho T., Jr. "Cotton Mather's Early 'Curiosa Americana' and the Boston Philosophical Society of 1683." *The William and Mary Quarterly* 18 (1961): 360-372. Print.

Beall, Otho T., Jr., and Richard H. Shryock. "Cotton Mather: First Significant Figure in American Medicine." *Proceedings of the American Antiquarian Society* 63.1 (1953): 37-274. Print.

Beard, George M. *The Psychology of the Salem Witchcraft Excitement of 1692*. New York: Putnam, 1882. Print.

Beinfield, Malcolm S. "The Early New England Doctor: An Adaptation to a Provincial Environment." *Yale Journal of Biology and Medicine* (1943): 99-132, 272-288. Print.

Bellin, Joshua David. "John Eliot's Playing Indian." *Early American Literature* 42.1 (2007): 1-30. Print.

Benjamin, Walter. "Critique of Violence." *Reflections: Essays, Aphorisms, Autobiographical Writings*. Ed. Peter Demetz. Trans. Edmund Jephcott. New York: Harcourt, 1978. 277-300. Print.

Benton, Robert M. "The John Winthrops and Developing Scientific Thought in New England." *Early American Literature* 7 (1973): 272-280. Print.

Bercovitch, Sacvan. *The Puritan Origins of the American Self*. New Haven: Yale UP, 1975. Print.

---. *The American Jeremiad*. Madison: U of Wisconsin P, 1978. Print.

Bever, Edward. "Witchcraft Fears and Psychosocial Factors in Disease." *The Journal of Interdisciplinary History* 30.4 (2000): 573-590. Print.

Bhabha, Homi K. *The Location of Culture*. London: Routledge, 1994. Print.

Black, Robert C. *The Younger John Winthrop*. New York: Columbia UP, 1966. Print.

Blackstock, Carrie Galloway. "Anne Bradstreet and Performativity: Self-Cultivation, Self-Deployment." *Early American Literature* 32.3 (1997): 222-248. Print.

Blake, John B. *Public Health in the Town of Boston, 1630-1822*. Cambridge, MA: Harvard UP, 1959. Print.

Bosco, Ronald A. Introduction. *The Poems of Michael Wigglesworth*. Ed. Ronald A. Bosco. Lanham: UP of America, 1989. ix-xvii. Print.

Bosco, Ronald A., and Jillmary Murphy. "New England Poetry." *The Oxford Handbook of Early American Literature*. Ed. Kevin J. Hayes. New York: Oxford UP, 2008. 115-141. Print.

Boureau, Alain. "The Letter-Writing Norm, a Medieval Invention." *Correspondence: Models of Letter-Writing from the Middle Ages to the Nineteenth Century*. Ed. Roger Chartier, Alain Boureau, and Cecile Dauphin. Princeton: Princeton UP, 1997. 24-51. Print.

Bowden, Henry Warner. *American Indians and Christian Missions: Studies in Cultural Conflict*. Chicago: U of Chicago P, 1985. Print.

Bragdon, Kathleen J. *Native People of Southern New England, 1500-1650*. Norman: U of Oklahoma P, 1996. Print.

Bratton, Timothy L. "The Identity of the New England Indian Epidemic of 1616-19." *Bulletin of the History of Medicine* 62 (1988): 351-383. Print.

Brauer, Jerald C. "Conversion: From Puritanism to Revivalism." *The Journal of Religion* 58.3 (1978): 227-243. Print.

Bremer, Francis J. "Increase Mather's Friends: The Trans-Atlantic Congregational Network of the Seventeenth Century." *Proceedings of the American Antiquarian Society* 94.1 (1984): 59-96. Print.

---. "The Puritan Experiment in New England, 1630-1660." *The Cambridge Companion to Puritanism*. Ed. John Coffey and Paul C. H. Lim. New York: Cambridge, 2008. 127-142. Print.

Brieger, Gert H. "Bodies and Borders: A New Cultural History of Medicine." *Perspectives in Biology and Medicine* 47.3 (2004): 402-421. Print.

Browne, Charles A. "Scientific Notes from the Books and Letters of John Winthrop, Jr., 1606-1676." *Isis* 11.2 (1928): 325-342. Print.

Brown, Kathleen M. "Native Americans and Early Modern Concepts of Race." *Empire and Others: British Encounters with Indigenous Peoples, 1600-1850*. Ed. Martin Daunton and Rick Halpern. Philadelphia: U of Pennsylvania P, 1999. 79-100. Print.

---. *Foul Bodies: Cleanliness in Early America*. New Haven: Yale UP, 2008. Print.

Brumm, Ursula. "The Art of Puritan Meditation in New England." *Studies in New England Puritanism*. Ed. Winfried Herget. Frankfurt: Lang, 1983. 139-167. Print.

---. "Transfer and Arrival in the Narratives of the First Immigrants to New England." *The Transit of Civilization from Europe to America: Essays in Honor of Hans Galinsky*. Ed. Winfried Herget and Karl Ortseifen. Tübingen: Narr, 1986. 29-36. Print.

Brunotte, Ulrike. *Puritanismus und Pioniergeist: Zur Faszination der Wildnis im frühen Neu-England*. Berlin: De Gruyter, 2000. Print.

Bumsted, J. M. "Emotion in Colonial America: Some Relations of Conversion Experience in Freetown, Massachusetts, 1749-1770." *New England Quarterly* 49.1 (1976): 97-108. Print.

Butler, Judith. *Gender Trouble: Feminism and the Subversion of Identity*. New York: Routledge, 1990. Print.

---. "How Can I Deny That These Hands and This Body Are Mine?" *Qui Parle* 11.1 (1997): 1-20. Print.

---. *Excitable Speech: A Politics of the Performative*. New York: Routledge, 1997. Print.

Calder, Isabel M. "A Biographical Sketch." *Letters of John Davenport, Puritan Divine*. Ed. Isabel M. Calder. New Haven: Yale UP, 1937. 1-12. Print.

Caldwell, Patricia. *The Puritan Conversion Narrative: The Beginnings of American Expression*. Cambridge: Cambridge UP, 1983. Print.

Canny, Nicholas. "Writing Atlantic History; or, Reconfiguring the History of Colonial British America." *Journal of American History* 86.3 (1999): 1093-1114. Print.

Canup, John. "Cotton Mather and 'Criolian Degeneracy.'" *Early American Literature* 24 (1989): 20-34. Print.

Caporeal, Linnda R. "Ergotism: The Satan Loosed in Salem?" *Science* 192 (1976): 21-26. Print.

Carlson, Laurie Win. *A Fever in Salem: A New Interpretation of the New England Witch Trials*. Chicago: Dee, 1999. Print.

Carré, Meyrick H. "The Formation of the Royal Society." *History Today* 10.8 (1960): 564-571. Print.

Cash, Philip, J. Worth Estes, and Eric H. Christianson, eds. *Medicine in Colonial Massachusetts, 1620-1820: Publications of the Colonial Society of Massachusetts*. Vol. 57. Boston: Society, 1980. Print.

Cassedy, James H. *Medicine in America: A Short History*. Baltimore: Johns Hopkins UP, 1991. Print.

Caulfield, Ernest. "Some Common Diseases of Colonial Children." *Publications of the Colonial Society of Massachusetts* 25 (1942): 4-65. Print.

Chaplin, Joyce E. "Natural Philosophy and an Early Racial Idiom in North America: Comparing English and Indian Bodies." *William and Mary Quarterly* 54.1 (1997): 229-252. Print.

---. *Subject Matter: Technology, the Body, and Science on the Anglo-American Frontier, 1500-1676*. Cambridge, MA: Harvard UP, 2003. Print.

Chartier, Roger, Alain Boureau, and Cécile Dauphin. *Correspondence: Models of Letter-Writing from the Middle Ages to the Nineteenth Century*. 1991. Trans. Christopher Woodall. Princeton: Princeton UP, 1997. Print.

Christianson, Eric H. "Medicine in New England." *Medicine in the New World: New Spain, New France, and New England*. Ed. Ronal L. Numbers. Knoxville: U of Tennessee P, 1987. 101-153. Rpt. in

*Sickness and Health in America*: *Readings in the History of Medicine and Public Health*. Ed. Judith W. Leavitt and Ronald L. Numbers. 3rd ed. Madison: U of Wisconsin P, 1997. 47-71. Print.

Clark, Michael P. Introduction. *The Eliot Tracts*. Ed. Michael P. Clark. Westport: Praeger, 2003. 1-53. Print.

Coffey, John, and Paul C. H. Lim. Introduction. *The Cambridge Companion to Puritanism*. Ed. John Coffey and Paul C. H. Lim. New York: Cambridge UP, 2008. 1-15. Print.

Cogley, Richard. *John Eliot's Mission to the Indians before King Philip's War*. Cambridge, MA: Harvard UP, 1999. Print.

Cohen, I. Bernard, ed. *Puritanism and the Rise of Modern Science: The Merton Thesis*. New Brunswick: Rutgers UP, 1990. Print.

Cohen, Charles Lloyd. *God's Caress: The Psychology of Puritan Religious Experience*. New York: Oxford UP, 1986. Print.

Colacurcio, Michael J. *Godly Letters: The Literature of the American Puritans*. Notre Dame: U of Notre Dame P, 2006. Print.

Como, David R. *Blown by the Spirit: Puritanism and the Emergence of an Antinomian Underground in Pre-Civil-War England*. Stanford: Stanford UP, 2004. Print.

Conforti, Joseph. *Saints and Strangers: New England in British North America*. Baltimore: Johns Hopkins UP, 2006. Print.

Cook, Sherburne F. "The Significance of Disease in the Extinction of the New England Indians." *Human Biology* 45 (1973): 485-508. Print.

Crane, E. F. "'I Have Suffer'd Much Today': The Defining Force of Pain in Early America." *Through a Glass Darkly: Reflections on Personal Identity in Early America*. Ed. Ronald Hoffman, Mechal Sobel, and Fredrika J. Teute. Williamsburg: Omohundro Institute of Early American History and Culture, 1997. 370-403. Print.

Cressy, David. *Coming Over: Migration and Communication Between England and New England in the Seventeenth Century*. New York: Cambridge UP, 1997. Print.

Cronon, William. *Changes in the Land: Indians, Colonists, and the Ecology of New England*. New York: Hill, 1983. Print.

Crosby, Alfred W. "Virgin Soil Epidemics as a Factor in the Aboriginal Depopulation in America." *The William and Mary Quarterly* 33.2 (1976): 289-299. Print.

---. "'God … Would Destroy Them, and Give Their Country to Another People.'" *American Heritage* 29 (1978): 38-43. Print.

---. *Ecological Imperialism: The Biological Expansion of Europe, 900-1900*. 2nd ed. Cambridge: Cambridge UP, 2004. Print.

Crowder, Richard. *No Featherbed to Heaven: A Biography of Michael Wigglesworth, 1631-1705*. East Lansing: Michigan State UP, 1962. Print.

Daly, Robert. *God's Altar: The World and the Flesh in Puritan Poetry*. Berkeley: U of California P, 1972. Print.

---. "Powers of Humility and the Presence of Readers in Anne Bradstreet and Phillis Wheatley." *Puritanism in America: The Seventeenth Through the Nineteenth Centuries*. Ed. Michael Schuldiner. Studies in Puritan American Spirituality. Vol. 4. Lewiston: Mellen, 1993. 1-24. Print.

Dary, David. *Frontier Medicine: From the Atlantic to the Pacific, 1492-1941*. New York: Knopf, 2008. Print.

Davis, Lennart J., and David B. Morris. "Biocultures Manifesto." *New Literary History* 38.3 (2007): 411-418. Print.

Daybell, James. *Women Letter-Writers in Tudor England*. Oxford: Oxford UP, 2006. Print.

Dean, John Ward. *Memoir of Rev. Michael Wigglesworth, Author of The Day of Doom*. 2nd ed. Albany: Munsell, 1871. Print.

Debus, Allen G. "The Paracelsian Compromise in Elizabethan England." *Ambix* 8 (1960): 71-97. Print.

---. *The English Paracelsians*. London: Osbourne, 1965. Print.

Decker, William Merrill. *Epistolary Practices: Letter Writing in America before Telecommunications*. Chapel Hill: U of North Carolina P, 1998. Print.

Deetjen, Christian. "Witchcraft and Medicine." *Bulletin of the Institute of the History of Medicine* 2 (1934): 164-175. Print.

Deleuze, Gilles, and Felix Guatarri. *Thousand Plateaus*. Trans. Brian Massumi. 1980. London: Continuum, 2004. Print.

Demos, John. "Underlying Themes in the Witchcraft of Seventeenth-Century New England." *The American Historical Review* 75.5 (1970): 1311-1326. Print.

---. *Entertaining Satan: Witchcraft and the Culture of Early New England*. New York: Oxford UP, 1982. Print.

---. *The Enemy Within: 2,000 Years of Witch-Hunting in the Western World*. New York: Viking, 2008. Print.

Dennis, Matthew. "Death and Memory in Early America." *History Compass* 4.1 (2006): 384-401. Print.

Derrida, Jacques. *Of Grammatology*. Trans. Gayatri C. Spivak. Baltimore: Johns Hopkins UP, 1976. Print.

Deutsch, Albert. "The Sick Poor in Colonial Times." *American Historical Review* 46.3 (1941): 560-579. Print.

Diamond, Jared. *Guns, Germs, and Steel: The Fates of Human Societies*. New York: Norton, 1997. Print.

Dinges, Martin, and Vincent Barras, eds. *Krankheit in Briefen im deutschen und französischen Sprachraum. 17.-21. Jahrhundert*. Stuttgart: Steiner, 2007. Print.

Ditmore, Michael G. "Preparation and Confession: Reconsidering Edmund S. Morgan's *Visible Saints*." *New England Quarterly* 67.2 (1994): 298-319. Print.

Doetsch, Raymond N. "Benjamin Marten and His 'New Theory of Consumptions.'" *Microbiological Reviews* 42.3 (1978): 521-528. Print.

Donegan, Kathleen. "'As Dying, Yet Behold We Live': Catastrophe and Interiority in Bradford's *Of Plymouth Plantation*." *Early American Literature* 37.1 (2002): 9-37. Print.

Doriani, Beth M. "'Then Have I … Said With David': Anne Bradstreet's Andover Manuscript Poems and the Influence of the Psalm Tradition." *Early American Literature* 24.1 (1989): 52-69. Print.

Drake, Samuel G. *Annals of Witchcraft in New England*. Boston: Woodward, 1869. Print.

Duden, Barbara. *The Woman beneath the Skin: A Doctor's Patients in Eighteenth-Century Germany*. Trans. Thomas Dunlap. Cambridge, MA: Harvard UP, 1991. Print.

Duffy, John. "Smallpox and the Indians in the American Colonies." *Bulletin of the History of Medicine* 25 (1951): 324-341. Print.

---. *The Healers: A History of American Medicine*. Urbana: U of Illinois P, 1976. Print.

---. *The Sanitarians: A History of American Public Health*. Urbana: U of Illinois P, 1990. Print.

Dunn, Richard. *Puritan and Yankees: The Winthrop Dynasty of New England, 1630-1717*. Princeton: Princeton UP, 1962. Print.

Eberwein, Jane Donahue. "The 'Unrefined Ore' of Anne Bradstreet's Quaternions." *Early American Literature* 9.1 (1974): 19-26. Print.

Egan, Jim. *Authorizing Experience: Refigurations of the Body Politic in Seventeenth-Century New England Writing*. Princeton: Princeton UP, 1999. Print.

Eisinger, Chester E. "The Puritan Justification for Taking the Land." *Essex Institute Historical Collections* 84 (1948): 131-143. Print.

Eldridge, Larry. "'Crazy Brained': Mental Illness in Colonial America." *Bulletin of the History of Medicine* 70.3 (1996): 361-386. Print.

Elliot, Emory. *The Cambridge Introduction to Early American Literature*. Cambridge: Cambridge UP, 2002. Print.

Elmer, Peter. "Medicine, Witchcraft and the Politics of Healing in Late Seventeenth-Century England." *Medicine and Religion in Enlightenment Europe*. Ed. Ole Peter Grell and Andrew Cunningham. Burlington: Ashgate, 2007. 223-242. Print.

Engler, Bernd, Jörg O. Fichte, and Oliver Scheiding, eds. *Millennial Thought in America: Historical and Intellectual Contexts, 1630-1860*. Trier: WVT, 2002. Print.

Estes, J. Worth. *Dictionary of Protopharmacology: Therapeutic Practices, 1700-1850*. Canton, MA: Science History, 1990. Print.

Fattore, Joan Del. "John Webster's *Metallographia*: A Source for Alchemical Imagery in the Preparatory Meditations." *Early American Literature* 18.3 (1983): 233-241. Print.

Fenn, Elizabeth A. *Pox Americana: The Great Smallpox Epidemic of 1775-82*. New York: Hill, 2001. Print.

Fenton, William N. "Contacts between Iroquois Herbalism and Colonial Medicine." *Annual Report of the Smithsonian Institution for 1941*. Washington, DC, 1942. 503-526. Print.

Ferngren, Gary B., and Darrel W. Amundsen. "Healing and Medicine: Healing and Medicine in Christianity." *Encyclopedia of Religion*. Vol. 6. Ed. Lindsay Jones. 2nd ed. Detroit: Macmillan Reference, 2005. 3843-3848. Print.

Ferszt, Elizabeth. "Rejecting a New English Aesthetic: The Early Poems of Anne Bradstreet." Diss. Wayne State University, 2006. Print.

Field, Jonathan Beecher. "The Antinomian Controversy Did Not Take Place." *Early American Studies* 6.2 (2008): 448-463. Print.

Finch, Martha L. *Dissenting Bodies: Corporealities in Early New England*. New York: Columbia UP, 2010. Print.

Fisher Fishkin, Shelley. "Crossroads of Cultures: The Transnational Turn in American Studies: Presidential Address to the American Studies

Association, November 12, 2004." *American Quarterly* 57.1 (2005): 17-57. Print.

Fissell, Mary E. "Making Meaning from the Margins: The New Cultural History of Medicine." *Locating Medical History: The Stories and their Meanings.* Ed. John Warner and Frank Huisman. Baltimore: Johns Hopkins P, 2004. 364-389. Print.

Fluck, Winfried, Donald E. Pease, and John Carlos Rowe, eds. *Re-Framing the Transnational Turn in American Studies.* Dartmouth: UP of New England, 2011. Print.

Forbes, Thomas Rogers. *The Midwife and the Witch.* New Haven: Yale UP, 1966. Print.

Foucault, Michel. *The Birth of the Clinic: An Archaeology of Medical Perception.* Trans. A. M. Sheridan Smith. 1963. London: Travistock, 1973. Print.

---. *History of Madness.* 1972. Ed. Jean Khalfa. Trans. Jonathan Murphy and Jean Khalfa. London: Routledge, 2006. Print.

---. *Discipline and Punish: The Birth of the Prison.* 1975. Trans. Alan Sheridan. New York: Vintage, 1995. Print.

---. *The History of Sexuality Vol. 1: An Introduction.* 1976. Trans. Robert Hurley. New York: Random, 1978. Print.

Fox, Sanford J. *Science and Justice: The Massachusetts Witchcraft Trials.* Baltimore: Johns Hopkins P, 1968. Print.

Frank, Arthur W. *The Wounded Storyteller: Body, Illness, and Ethics.* Chicago: U of Chicago P, 1995. Print.

French, Roger, and Andrew Wear, eds. *The Medical Revolution of the Seventeenth Century.* Cambridge: Cambridge UP, 1989. Print.

Games, Alison. "Atlantic History: Definitions, Challenges, and Opportunities." *American Historical Review* 111.4 (2006): 741-757. Print.

Gevitz, Norman. "Samuel Fuller of Plymouth Plantation: A 'Skillful Physician' or 'Quacksalver.'" *Journal of the History of Medicine* 47 (1992): 29-48. Print.

---. "'The Devil Hath Laughed at the Physicians': Witchcraft and Medical Practice in Seventeenth-Century New England." *Journal of the History of Medicine* 55.1 (2000): 5-36. Print.

Giles, Paul. "The Culture of Colonial America: Theology and Aesthetics." *A Companion to the Literatures of Colonial America.* Ed. Susan Castillo and Ivy Schweitzer. Malden: Blackwell, 2005. 78-93. Print.

Gilman, Sander L. *Disease and Representation: Images of Illness from Madness to AIDS*. Ithaca: Cornell UP, 1988. Print.

Godbeer, Richard. *The Devil's Dominion: Magic and Religion in Early New England*. Cambridge: Cambridge UP, 1992. Print.

---. *Escaping Salem: The Other Witch Hunt of 1692*. New York: Oxford UP, 2005. Print.

Goldberg, Jonathan. *Writing Matter: From the Hands of the English Renaissance*. Stanford: Stanford UP, 1990. Print.

Gonzalez-Crussi, Francisco. *A Short History of Medicine*. New York: Modern Library, 2008. Print.

Goodheart, Lawrence B. "The Distinction between Witchcraft and Madness in Colonial Connecticut." *History of Psychiatry* 13.52 (2002): 433-444. Print.

Grandjean, Katherine A. "Reckoning: The Communications Frontier in Early New England." Diss. Harvard U, 2008. Print.

Grant, William L. *Voyages of Samuel de Champlain 1604-1618*. New York: Scribner's Sons, 1907. Print.

Greenberg, Herbert. "The Authenticity of the Library of John Winthrop the Younger." *American Literature* 8 (1937): 449-452. Print.

Greenblatt, Stephen. *Renaissance Self-Fashioning: From More to Shakespeare*. Chicago: U of Chicago P, 1980. Print.

---. *Shakespearean Negotiations: The Circulation of Social Energy in Renaissance England*. Berkeley: U of California P, 1988. Print.

Grell, Ole Peter, and Andrew Cunningham, eds. *Medicine and Religion in Enlightenment Europe*. Burlington: Ashgate, 2007. Print.

Grmek, Mirko D. Introduction. *Western Medical Thought from Antiquity to the Middle Ages*. Ed. Mirko D. Grmek. Trans. Antony Shugaar. 1993. Cambridge, MA: Harvard UP, 1998. 1-21. Print.

---. "The Concept of Disease." *Western Medical Thought from Antiquity to the Middle Ages*. Ed. Mirko D. Grmek. Trans. Antony Shugaar. 1993. Cambridge, MA: Harvard UP, 1998. 241-258. Print.

Grob, Gerald N. *The Deadly Truth: A History of Disease in America*. Cambridge, MA: Harvard UP, 2002. Print.

Gordon-Grube, Karen. "The Alchemical 'Golden Tree' and Associated Imagery in the Poems of Edward Taylor." Free U Berlin, 1990. Print.

---. "Evidence of Medicinal Cannibalism in Puritan New England: 'Mummy' and Related Remedies in Edward Taylor's 'Dispensatory.'" *Early American Literature* 28 (1993): 185-221.

Guerra, Francisco. *American Medical Bibliography, 1639-1783*. New York: Harper, 1962. Print.

Hall, David D. *Worlds of Wonder, Days of Judgment: Popular Religious Belief in Early New England*. New York: Knopf, 1989. Print.

---. "New England, 1660-1730." *The Cambridge Companion to Puritanism*. Ed John Coffey and Paul C. H. Lim. New York: Cambridge, 2008. 143-158. Print.

Hammond, Jeffrey A. *Sinful Self, Saintly Self: The Puritan Experience of Poetry*. Athens: U of Georgia P, 1993. Print.

Hampshire, Stuart, ed. *The Age of Reason: The 17th Century Philosophers*. New York: New American Library, 1956. Print.

Hansen, Chadwick. *Witchcraft at Salem*. New York: Brazillier, 1969. Print.

Harley, David. "Spiritual Physic, Providence and English Medicine, 1560-1640." *Medicine and the Reformation*. Ed. Ole Peter Grell and Andrew Cunningham. London: Routledge, 1993. 101-117. Print.

Harpham, Geoffrey Galt. "Conversion and the Language of Autobiography." *Studies in Autobiography*. Ed. James Olney. New York: Oxford UP, 1988. 42-50. Print.

Harrington, Thomas F. "Dr. Samuel Fuller, of the Mayflower (1620), the Pioneer Physician." *The Johns Hopkins Hospital Bulletin* 14 (1903): 263-270. Print.

Harris, David. "Medicine in Colonial America." *California and Western Medicine* 51.1 (1939): 35-38. Print.

Harvey, Tamara. "'Now Sisters ... Impart Your Usefulnesse, And Force': Anne Bradstreet's Feminist Functionalism in *The Tenth Muse* (1650)." *Early American Literature* 35.1 (2000): 5-28. Print. Print.

Hemphill, C. Dallet. *Bowing to Necessities: A History of Manners in America, 1620-1860*. New York: Oxford UP, 1999. Print.

Herzogenrath, Bernd. "The Angel and the Animalculae: Cotton Mather and Inoculation." *Transatlantic Negotiations*. Ed. Christa Buschendorf and Astrid Franke. Heidelberg: Winter, 2007. 13-24. Print.

Hindle, Brooke. *The Pursuit of Science in Revolutionary America, 1735-1789*. 1956. New York: Norton, 1974. Print.

Hindmarsh, D. Bruce. *The Evangelical Conversion Narrative: Spiritual Autobiography in Early Modern England*. New York: Oxford UP, 2005. Print.

Hughes, Walter. "'Meat Out of the Eater': Panic and Desire in American Puritan Poetry." *Engendering Men: The Question of Male Feminist Criticism*. Ed. Joseph Allen Boone and Michael Cadden. New York: Routledge, 1990. 102-121. Print.

Hultkrantz, Ake. *Shamanic Healing and Ritual Drama: Health and Medicine in Native North American Religious Traditions*. New York: Crossroad, 1992. Print.

Hydén, Lars-Christer. "Illness and Narrative." *Sociology of Health and Illness* 19.1 (1997): 48-69. Print.

Jantz, Harold. "America's First Cosmopolitan." *Proceedings of the Massachusetts Historical Society*. Third Series, Vol. 84 (1972): 3-25. Print.

Jennings, Francis. *The Invasion of America: Indians, Colonialism, and the Cant of Conquest*. Chapel Hill: U of North Carolina P, 1975. Print.

Jeske, Jeffrey. "Edward Taylor and the Traditions of Puritan Nature Philosophy." *Essays on the Poetry of Edward Taylor in Honor of Thomas M. and Virginia L. Davis*. Ed. Michael Schuldiner. Newark: U of Delaware P, 1997. 27-67. Print.

Johnson, Parker H. "Humiliation Followed by Deliverance: Metaphor and Plot in Cotton Mather's *Magnalia*." *Early American Literature* 15 (1980/1981): 237-246. Print.

Johnson, Thomas H. "Taylor's Library." *The Poetical Works of Edward Taylor*. Ed. Thomas H. Johnson. Princeton: Princeton UP, 1966. 201-220. Print.

Jones, David S. "Virgin Soils Revisited." *William and Mary Quarterly* 60.4 (2003): 703-742. Print.

---. *Rationalizing Epidemics: Meanings and Uses of American Indian Mortality since 1600*. Cambridge, MA: Harvard UP, 2004. Print.

Karlsen, Carol F. *The Devil in the Shape of a Woman: Witchcraft in Colonial New England*. New York: Vintage, 1987. Print.

Kavasch, Barrie. "Native Foods of New England." *Enduring Traditions: The Native Peoples of New England*. Ed. Laurie Weinstein. Westport: Bergin & Garvey. 5-30. Print.

Kelleter, Frank *Amerikanische Aufklärung: Sprachen der Rationalität im Zeitalter der Revolution*. Paderborn: Schöningh, 2002. Print.

Keeble, N. H. "Puritanism and Literature." *The Cambridge Companion to Puritanism.* Ed. John Coffey and Paul C. H. Lim. New York: Cambridge UP, 2008. 309-324. Print.

Kittredge, George Lyman. "Cotton Mather's Scientific Communications to the Royal Society." *Proceedings of the American Antiquarian Society* 26 (1916): 18-57.

Kelly, Louis G. "London Apothecaries as Early Christians: Renewing the Covenant." *Healing in Religion and Society, From Hippocrates to the Puritans.* Ed. J. Kevin Coyle and Steven C. Muir. Lewiston: Mellen, 1999. 159-186.

Koehler, Lyle. "The Case of the American Jezebels: Anne Hutchinson and Female Agitation during the Years of Antinomian Turmoil, 1636-1640." *William and Mary Quarterly* 31.1 (1974): 55-78. Print.

Koo, Kathryn S. "Strangers in the House of God: Cotton Mather, Onesimus, and an Experiment in Christian Slaveholding." *Proceedings of the American Antiquarian Society* 117.1 (2007): 143-176. Print.

Kupperman, Karen Ordahl. *Settling with the Indians: The Meeting of English and Indian Cultures in America, 1580-1640.* Totowa: Rowman and Littlefield, 1980. Print.

---. "The Puzzle of the American Climate in the Early Colonial Period." *American Historical Review* 87 (1982): 1262-1289. Print.

---. "Fear of Hot Climates in the Anglo-American Colonial Experience." *The William and Mary Quarterly* 41.2 (1984): 213-240. Print.

Langdon, Carolyn. "A Complaint against Katherine Harrison, 1669." *Bulletin of the Connecticut Historical Society* 34 (1969): 18-25. Print.

Laurence, David. "William Bradford's American Sublime." *PMLA* 102.1 (1987): 55-65. Print.

Lee, Charles R. "Public Poor Relief and the Massachusetts Community, 1620-1715." *New England Quarterly* 55.4 (1982): 564-585. Print.

Leibman, Laura Arnold. Introduction. *Experience Mayhew's* Indian Converts. Ed. Laura Arnold Leibman. Amherst: U of Massachusetts P, 2008. 1-76. Print.

Leighton, Ann. *Early American Gardens: "For Meate or Medicine."* 1970. Amherst: U of Massachusetts P, 1986. Print.

Lepore, Jill. *The Name of War: King Philip's War and the Origins of American Identity.* New York: Vintage, 1998. Print.

Levin, David. "Giants in the Earth: Science and the Occult in Cotton Mather's Letters to the Royal Society." *The William and Mary Quarterly* 45 (1988): 751-770. Print.

Levy, Babette M. *Cotton Mather*. Boston: Twayne, 1979. Print.

Lewis, R. W. B. *The American Adam: Innocence, Tragedy, and Tradition in the Nineteenth Century*. Chicago: U of Chicago P, 1955. Print.

Lindman, Janet Moore, and Michele Lise Tarter, eds. *A Centre of Wonders: The Body in Early America*. Ithaca: Cornell UP, 2001. Print.

Lockridge, Kenneth. *Literacy in Colonial New England: An Enquiry into the Social Context of Literacy in the Early Modern West*. New York: Norton, 1974. Print.

Louis-Courvoisier, Micheline, and Séverine Pilloud. "Consulting by Letter in the Eighteenth Century: Mediating the Patient's View?" *Cultural Approaches to the History of Medicine: Mediating Medicine in Early Modern and Modern Europe*. Ed. Cornelie Usborne and Willem De Blécourt. New York: Palgrave, 2004. 71-88. Print.

Lovejoy, David S. "Satanizing the American Indian." *New England Quarterly* 67.4 (1994): 603-621. Print.

Lutes, Jean Marie. "Negotiating Theology and Gynecology: Anne Bradstreet's Representations of the Female Body." *Signs: Journal of Women in Culture and Society* 22.2 (1997): 309-340. Print.

Lyons, Henry. *The Royal Society, 1660-1940: A History of its Administration under its Charters*. Cambridge: The UP, 1944. Print.

MacDonald, Michael. Introduction. *Witchcraft and Hysteria in Elizabethan London: Edward Jorden and the Mary Glover Case*. Ed. Michael MacDonald. London: Routledge, 1991. vii-lxiv. Print.

Mackenthun, Gesa. *Metaphors of Dispossession: American Beginnings and the Translation of Empire, 1492-1637*. Norman: U of Oklahoma P, 1997. Print.

Macphail, Alasdair. "John Winthrop, Jr." *American Colonial Writers, 1606-1734. Dictionary of Literary Biography*. Vol. 24. Ed. Emory Elliot. Detroit: Gale, 1984. 363-369. Print.

Magner, Lois N. *A History of Medicine*. 2nd ed. Boca Raton: Taylor, 2005. Print.

Magnusson, Lynne. *Shakespeare and Social Dialogue: Dramatic Language and Elizabethan Letters*. Cambridge: Cambridge UP, 1999. Print.

Main, Gloria L. *Peoples of Spacious Land: Families and Cultures in Colonial New England*. Cambridge, MA: Harvard UP, 2001. Print.

Malinowski, Sharon, and Anna Sheets, eds. *The Gale Encyclopedia of Native American Tribes. Vol. 1: Northeast, Southeast, Caribbean*. Detroit: Gale, 1998. Print.

Mann, Charles C. *1491: New Revelations of the Americas Before Columbus*. New York: Vintage, 2005. Print.

Margerum, Eileen. "Anne Bradstreet's Public Poetry and the Tradition of Humility." *Early American Literature* 17.2 (1982): 152-160. Print.

Mayo, Lawrence Shaw. *The Winthrop Family in America*. Boston: Massachusetts Historical Society, 1948. Print.

Maxwell-Stuart, P. G. Ed. and Trans. *The Occult in Early Modern Europe: A Documentary History*. London: Macmillian, 1999. Print.

McBride, Kevin A. "Bundles, Bears, and Bibles: Interpreting Seventeenth-Century Native 'Texts.'" *Early Native Literacies in New England: A Documentary and Critical Anthology*. Ed. Kristina Bross and Hilary E. Wyss. Amherst: U of Massachusetts P, 2008. 132-141. Print.

McCray Beier, Lucinda. *Sufferers and Healers: The Experience of Illness in Seventeenth-Century England*. London: Routledge, 1987. Print.

McGerr, Michael. "The Price of the 'New Transnational History.'" *American Historical Review* 96.4 (1991): 1056-1067. Print.

McMahon, Helen. "Anne Bradstreet, Jean Bertault, and Dr. Crooke." *Early American Literature* 3.2 (1968): 118-123. Print.

Mellen, Paul F. "Coroners' Inquests in Colonial Massachusetts." *Journal of the History of Medicine and Allied Sciences* 40 (1985): 462-472. Print.

Miller, David G. *The Word Made Flesh Made Word*. London: Associated UP, 1995. Print.

Miller, Perry. *The New England Mind: The Seventeenth Century*. New York: Macmillan, 1939. Print.

---. *The New England Mind: From Colony to Province*. Cambridge, MA: Harvard UP, 1953. Print.

---. *Errand Into the Wilderness*. Cambridge, MA: Belknap P of Harvard UP, 1956. Print.

Minardi, Margot. "The Boston Inoculation Controversy of 1721-1722: An Incident in the History of Race." *William and Mary Quarterly* 61.1 (2004): 47-76. Print.

Mood, Fulmer. "John Winthrop, Jr., on Indian Corn." *New England Quarterly* 10.1 (1937): 121-133. Print.

Moore, Martin. *Memoirs of Life and Character of Rev. John Eliot*. Boston: Bedlington, 1822. Print.

Morgan, Edmund S. *The Puritan Family: Religion and Domestic Relations in Seventeenth-Century New England*. 1944. New York: Harper, 1966. Print.

---. *Visible Saints: The History of a Puritan Idea*. New York: NYUP, 1963. Print.

---. *The Puritan Dilemma: The Story of John Winthrop*. 3rd ed. New York: Pearson Longman, 2007. Print.

Morris, Amy M. E. "Plainness and Paradox: Colonial Tensions in the Early New England Religious Lyric." *A Companion to the Literatures of Colonial America*. Ed. Susan Castillo and Ivy Schweitzer. Malden: Blackwell, 2005. 501-516. Print.

Morris, David B. *Illness and Culture in the Postmodern Age*. Berkeley: U of California P, 1998. Print.

Morrison, Dane. *A Praying People: Massachusetts Acculturation and the Failure of the Puritan Mission, 1600-1690*. New York: Lang, 1995. Print.

Muir, Steven C. "Faith, Healing, and Deliverance in Mark's Gospel." *Healing in Religion and Society, From Hippocrates to the Puritans*. Ed. J. Kevin Coyle and Steven C. Muir. Lewiston: Mellen, 1999. 85-104. Print.

Muldrew, Craig. *The Economy of Obligation: The Culture of Credit and Social Relations in Early Modern England*. New York: Palgrave, 1998. Print.

Murdock, Kenneth B. *Literature and Theology in Colonial New England*. Cambridge, MA: Harvard UP, 1949. Print.

Murphey, Murray J. "The Psychodynamics of Puritan Conversion." *American Quarterly* 31.1 (1979): 135-147. Print.

Mutschler, Ben. "Illness in the 'Social Credit' and 'Money' Economies of Eighteenth-Century New England." *Medicine and the Market in England and Its Colonies, c. 1450-c. 1850*. Ed. Mark S. R. Jenner and Patrick Wallis. New York: Palgrave, 2007. 175-195. Print.

Myles, Anne G. "From Monster to Martyr: Re-Presenting Mary Dyer." *Early American Literature* 36.1 (2001): 1-30. Print.

Nagy, Doreen Evenden. *Popular Medicine in Seventeenth-Century England*. Bowling Green: Bowling Green State University Popular P, 1988. Print.

Nash Smith, Henry. *Virgin Land: The American West as Symbol and Myth.* New York: Vintage, 1957. Print.

Newman, William R. *Gehennical Fire: The Lives of George Starkey, an American Alchemist in the Scientific Revolution.* Cambridge, MA: Harvard UP, 1994. Print.

Norton, Mary Beth. *Founding Mothers and Fathers: Gendered Power and the Forming of American Society.* New York: Knopf, 1996. Print.

---. "'The Ablest Midwife That Wee Knowe in the Land': Mistress Alice Tilly and the Women of Boston and Dorchester, 1649-1650." *William and Mary Quarterly* 55.1 (1998): 105-134. Print.

---. *In the Devil's Snare: The Salem Witchcraft Crisis of 1692.* New York: Knopf, 2002. Print.

Nutton, Vivian. "The Rise of Medicine." *The Cambridge Illustrated History of Medicine.* Ed. Roy Porter. Cambridge: Cambridge UP, 1996. 52-81. Print.

Orevicz, Cheryl Z. "Edward Taylor and the Alchemy of Grace." *Seventeenth-Century News* 34 (1976): 33-34. Print.

O'Brien, Jean M. *Dispossession by Degrees: Indian Land and Identity in Natick, Massachusetts, 1650-1790.* Cambridge: Cambridge UP, 1997. Print.

---. *We Shall Remain. Episode One: After the Mayflower.* PBS. April 2010. Print. Transcript.

Pagel, Walter. *Paracelsus: An Introduction to Philosophical Medicine in the Era of the Renaissance.* Basel: Karger, 1958. Print.

Pardo-Tomás, José, and Alvar Martínez-Vidal. "Stories of Disease Written by Patients and Lay Mediators in the Spanish Republic of Letters, 1680-1720." *Journal of Medieval and Early Modern Studies* 38 (2008): 467-491. Print.

Parker, David L. "Petrus Ramus and the Puritans: The 'Logic' of Preparationist Conversion Doctrine." *Early American Literature* 8.2 (1973): 140-162. Print.

Parrish, Susan Scott. "Scientific Discourse." *The Oxford Handbook of Early American Literature.* Ed. Kevin J. Hayes. Oxford: Oxford UP, 2008. 279-299. Print.

Pearl, Valerie, and Morris Pearl. "Governor John Winthrop on the Birth of the Antinomians' 'Monster': The Earliest Reports to Reach England and the Making of a Myth." *Proceedings of the Massachusetts Historical Society* 102 (1990): 21-37. Print.

Pestana, Carla Gardina. *Quakers and Baptists in Colonial Massachusetts.* Cambridge: Cambridge UP, 1991. Print.

Pettit, Norman. *The Heart Prepared: Grace and Conversion in Puritan Spirit Life.* New Haven: Yale UP, 1966. Print.

Philbrick, Nathaniel. *Mayflower: A Story of Courage, Community, and War.* New York: Penguin, 2006. Print.

Poole, William F. "Witchcraft at Boston." *The Memorial History of Boston, including Suffolk County Massachusetts, 1630-1880.* Vol. II. Ed. Justin Winsor. Boston: Osgood, 1881. 131-172. Print.

Pope, Allan H. "Petrus Ramus and Michael Wigglesworth: The Logic of Poetic Structure." *Puritan Poets and Poetics: Seventeenth-Century American Poetry in Theory and Practice.* Ed. Peter White. University Park: Pennsylvania State UP, 1985. 210-226. Print.

Porter, Roy. "The Patient's View: Doing Medical History from Below." *Theory and Society* 14 (1985): 175-198. Print.

---. "The Patient in England, c. 1660-c. 1800." *Medicine in Society: Historical Essays.* Ed. Andrew Wear. Cambridge: Cambridge UP, 1992. 91-118. Print.

---. "Mental Illness." *The Cambridge Illustrated History of Medicine.* Ed. Roy Porter. Cambridge: Cambridge UP, 1996. 278-303. Print.

---. "What is Disease?" *The Cambridge Illustrated History of Medicine.* Ed. Roy Porter. Cambridge: Cambridge UP, 1996. 82-117. Print.

---. *Flesh in the Age of Reason.* New York: Norton, 2003. Print.

Porterfield, Amanda. "Women's Attraction to Puritanism." *Church History* 60.2 (1991): 196-209. Print.

---. *Female Piety in Puritan New England.* New York: Oxford UP, 1992.

Poynter, F. N. L. "Nicholas Culpeper and the Paracelsians." *Science, Medicine and Society in the Renaissance: Essays to Honor Walter Pagel.* Vol. 1. Ed. Allen G. Debus. London: Heinemann, 1972. 201-220. Print.

Pratt, Mary Louise. "Arts of the Contact Zone." *Profession 91* (1991): 33-40. Print.

Priewe, Marc. "Making Sense of Morbidity in Early American Autobiography." *The Morbidity of Culture: Melancholy, Trauma, Illness and Dying in Literature and Film.* Ed. Stephanie Siewert and Antonia Mehnert. Frankfurt: Lang, 2012. 69-82. Print.

---. "'Too Many My Diseases to Cite': Anne Bradstreet's Illness Poetry." *The Writing Cure: Literature and Medicine in Context.* Ed. Alexandra Lembert and Jarmila Mildorf. Münster: LIT, 2013. 115-134. Print.

Prioreschi, Plinio. *A History of Medicine. Primitive and Ancient Medicine.* Vol. 1. Lewiston: Mellen, 1991. Print.

Rainwater, Catherine. "This Brazen Serpent is a Doctors Shop": Edward Taylor's Medical Vision." *American Literature and Science.* Ed. Robert J. Scholnick. Lexington: U of Kentucky P, 1992. 18-38. Print.

Rapoza, Andrew V. "The Trials of Phillip Reade, Seventeenth-Century Itinerant Physician." *Medicine and Healing: Annual Proceedings of the Dublin Seminar for New England Folklife.* Boston: Boston UP, 1992. 82-94. Print.

Reiss, Oscar. *Medicine in Colonial America.* Lanham: UP of America, 2000. Print.

Requa, Kenneth. "Anne Bradstreet's Poetic Voices." *Early American Literature* 9.1 (1974): 3-18. Print.

Rich, Adrienne. "Anne Bradstreet and Her Poetry." *The Works of Anne Bradstreet.* Ed. Jeannine Hensley. Cambridge, MA: Belknap P of Harvard UP, 1967. ix-xxi. Print.

Richardson, Robert D., Jr., "The Puritan Poetry of Anne Bradstreet." *Texas Studies in Language and Literature* 9 (1967): 317-331. Rpt. in *The American Puritan Imagination: Essays in Revaluation.* Ed. Sacvan Bercovitch. London: Cambridge UP, 1974. 105-122. Print.

Rimmon-Kenan, Shlomith. "The Story of 'I': Illness and Narrative Identity." *Narrative* 10.1 (2002): 9-27. Print.

Rivett, Sarah. "Tokenography: Narration and the Science of Dying in Puritan Deathbed Testimonies." *Early American Literature* 42.3 (2007): 471-494. Print.

Roach, Joseph R. *Cities of the Dead: Circum-Atlantic Performance.* New York: Columbia UP, 1996. Print.

Robinson, Martha. "New Worlds, New Medicines: Indian Remedies and English Medicine in Early America." *Early American Studies* 3.1 (2005): 94-110. Print.

---. "'They Decrease in Numbers Daily': English and Colonial Perceptions of Indian Disease in Early America." Diss. U of Southern California, 2005. Print.

Rogers, Horatio. *Mary Dyer of Rhode Island.* Providence: Preston & Rounds, 1896. Print.

Rosenmeier, Rosamond. *Anne Bradstreet Revisited.* Boston: Twayne, 1991. Print.

Round, Phillip H. "Neither Here Nor There: Transatlantic Epistolarity in Early America." *A Companion to the Literatures of Colonial America*. Ed. Susan Castillo and Ivy Schweitzer. Malden: Blackwell, 2005. 426-445. Print.

Rousseau, G. S. "Literature and Medicine: Towards a Simultaneity of Theory and Practice." *Literature and Medicine* 5.2 (1986): 152-181. Print.

Russell, Bertrand. *Religion and Science*. 1935. New York: Oxford UP, 1968. Print.

Russell, Howard S. *Indian New England Before the Mayflower*. Hanover: UP of New England, 1980. Print.

Ryle, Gilbert. *The Concept of Mind*. 1949. London: Routledge, 2009. Print.

Salisbury, Neal. "Red Puritans: The 'Praying Indians' of Massachusetts Bay and John Eliot." *William and Mary Quarterly* 31.1 (1974): 27-54. Print.

---. *Manitou and Providence: Indians, Europeans, and the Making of New England, 1500-1643*. New York: Oxford UP, 1982. Print.

Scarry, Elaine. *The Body in Pain: The Making and Unmaking of the World*. New York: New York UP, 1985. Print.

Scheick, William J. "Edward Taylor's Herbalism in Preparatory Meditations." *American Poetry* 1.3 (1983): 64-71. Print.

Schneider, Gary. *The Culture of Epistolarity: Vernacular Letters and Letter Writing in Early Modern England, 1500-1700*. Newark: U of Delaware P, 2005. Print.

Scholten, Catherine. *Childbearing in American Society, 1650-1850*. New York: NYUP, 1985. Print.

Shorter, Edward. *From Paralysis to Fatigue: A History of Psychosomatic Illnesses in the Modern Era*. New York: Free, 1992. Print.

Schutte, Anne Jacobson. "'Such Monstrous Births': A Neglected Aspect of the Antinomian Controversy." *Renaissance Quarterly* 38.1 (1985): 85-106. Print.

Schweitzer, Harold. "To Give Suffering a Language." *Literature and Medicine* 14.2 (1995): 210-221. Print.

Schweitzer, Ivy. "Anne Bradstreet Wrestles With the Renaissance." *Early American Literature* 23.3 (1988): 291-312. Print.

Searle, Alison. "'Though I Am a Stranger to You by Face, yet in Neere Bonds by Faith': A Transatlantic Puritan Republic of Letters." *Early American Literature* 43.2 (2008): 277-308. Print.

Seeman, Erik R. "Lay Conversion Narratives: Investigating Ministerial Intervention." *New England Quarterly* 71.4 (1998): 629-634. Print.

Selement, George. "The Meeting of Elite and Popular Minds at Cambridge, New England, 1638-1645." *William and Mary Quarterly* 41.1 (1984): 32-48. Print.

Sena, John F. "Melancholic Madness and the Puritans." *The Harvard Theological Review* 66. 3 (1973): 293-309. Print.

Shea, Daniel B., Jr. *Spiritual Autobiography in Early America.* Princeton: Princeton UP, 1968. Print.

Shorter, Edward. "Primary Care." *The Cambridge Illustrated History of Medicine.* Ed. Roy Porter. Cambridge: Cambridge UP, 1996. 118-153. Print.

Shryock, Richard Harrison. *Medicine and Society in America, 1660-1860.* New York: New York UP, 1960. Print.

Sidney, Sir Philip. *Defence of Poesie.* 1581. Trans. Richard Bear. University of Oregon, 1992. <http://poetry.eserver.org/defense-of-poesie.txt> 3 March 2011.

Silva, Cristobal. "Miraculous Plagues: Epidemiology on New England's Colonial Landscape." *Early American Literature* 43.2 (2008): 249-275. Print.

---. *Miraculous Plagues: An Epidemiology of Early New England Narrative.* New York: Oxford UP, 2011. Print.

Silverman, Kenneth. *The Life and Times of Cotton Mather.* New York: Harper, 1984. Print.

Simmons, Williams S. *Spirit of the New England Tribes: Indian History and Folklore, 1620-1984.* Hanover: UP of New England, 1986. Print.

Sluder, Lawrence Lan. "God in the Background: Edward Taylor as Naturalist." *Early American Literature* 7.3 (1973): 265-271. Print.

Smith, Cheryl C. "Out of Her Place: Anne Hutchinson and the Dislocation of Power in New World Politics." *Journal of American Culture* 29.4 (2006): 437-453. Print.

Smith, Lisa Wynne. "'An Account of an Unaccountable Distemper': The Experience of Pain in Early Eighteenth-Century England and France." *Eighteenth-Century Studies* 41.4 (2008): 459-480. Print.

Smith, Nicholas N. "Indian Medicine: Fact or Fiction?" *Bulletin of the Massachusetts Archaeological Society* 26.1 (1964): 13-17. Print.

Smolinski, Reiner, and Kathleen B. Freels. "'Chymical Wedding': Rosicrucian Alchemy and Eucharistic Conversion Process in Edward

Taylor's Preparatory Meditations and in Early Seventeenth-Century German Tracts." *Transatlantic Encounters: Studies in European-American Relations: Presented to Winfried Herget.* Ed. Udo J. Hebel and Karl Ortseifen. Trier: WVT, 1995. 40-61. Print.

Smolinski, Reiner. "Authority and Interpretation: Cotton Mather's Response to the European Spinozists." *Shaping the Stuart World, 1603-1714: The Atlantic Connection.* Ed. Arthur Williamson and Allan MacInnes. Leyden: Brill, 2006. 175-203. Print.

Snow, Dean R., and Kim M. Lanphear. "European Contact and Indian Depopulation in the Northeast: The Timing of the First Epidemics." *Ethnohistory* 35.1 (1988): 15-33. Print.

Solberg, Winton U. Introduction. *Cotton Mather: The Christian Philosopher.* 1721. Ed. Winton U. Solberg. Urbana: U of Illinois P, 1994. xix-cxxxiv. Print.

Sontag, Susan. *Illness as Metaphor.* New York: Farrar, 1978. Print.

Spanos, Nicholas P., and Jack Gottlieb. "Ergotism and the Salem Village Witch Trials." *Science* 194 (1976): 1390-1394. Print.

Spiess, Arthur E., and Bruce D. Spiess. "New England Pandemic of 1616-1622: Cause and Archaeological Implication." *Man in the Northeast* 34 (1987): 71-83. Print.

St. George, Robert Blair. *Conversing by Signs: Poetics of Implication in Colonial New England Culture.* Chapel Hill: U of North Carolina P, 1998. Print.

Stanford, Ann. "Anne Bradstreet: Dogmatist and Rebel." *New England Quarterly* 39.3 (1966): 373-389. Print.

---. *Anne Bradstreet: The Worldly Puritan.* New York: Franklin, 1974. Print.

Stearns, Raymond Phineas. "Colonial Fellows of the Royal Society of London, 1661-1788." *Notes and Records of the Royal Society of London* 8.2 (1951): 178-246. Print.

Steiner, Walter R. "Governor John Winthrop, Jr., of Connecticut, as a Physician." *Bulletin of the Johns Hopkins Hospital* 14 (1903): 294-302. Print.

Steinke, Hubert, and Martin Stuber. "Medical Correspondence in Early Modern Europe: An Introduction." *Gesnerus* 61 (2004): 139-160. Print.

Stephen, H. L. *State Trials: Political and Social.* Vol. 1. London: Duckworth, 1899. Print.

Stewart, Alan. *Shakespeare's Letters.* Oxford: Oxford UP, 2008. Print.

Stewart, Grace G. "A History of the Medicinal Use of Tobacco, 1492-1860." *Medical History* 11.3 (1967): 228-268. Print.

Stoever, William K. B. *"A Faire and Easie Way to Heaven:" Covenant Theology and Antinomianism in Early Massachusetts*. Middletown: Wesleyan UP, 1978. Print.

Swaim, Kathleen M. "'Come and Hear': Women's Puritan Evidences." *American Women's Autobiography: Fea(s)ts of Memory*. Ed. Margo Culley. Madison: U of Wisconsin P, 1992. 32-56. Print.

Tannenbaum, Rebecca J. "'What Is Best to Be Done for These Fevers': Elizabeth Davenport's Medical Practice in New Haven Colony." *New England Quarterly* 70.2 (1997): 265-284. Print.

---. *The Healer's Calling: Women and Medicine in Early New England*. Ithaca: Cornell UP, 2002.

---. "The Housewife as Healer: Medicine as Women's Work in Colonial New England." *Women's Work in New England, 1620-1920*: *Annual Proceedings of the Dublin Seminar for New England Folklife*. Vol. 25. Boston: Boston UP, 2003. 160-169. Print.

Taylor, John M. *The Witchcraft Delusion in Colonial Connecticut*. New York: Grafton, 1908. Print.

Thacher, James. *American Medical Biography: Or Memoirs of Eminent Physicians Who Have Flourished in America*. Boston: Richardson & Lord, 1828. Print.

Thelen, David. "The Nation and Beyond: Transnational Perspectives on United States History." *Journal of American History* 86.3 (1999): 965-975. Print.

Thomas, Keith. *Religion and the Decline of Magic: Studies in Popular Beliefs in Sixteenth and Seventeenth-Century England*. 1971. New York: Penguin, 1982. Print.

Thompson, Roger. *Mobility and Migration: East Anglian Founders of New England, 1629-1640*. Amherst: U of Massachusetts P, 1994. Print.

Todorov, Tzvetan. *The Conquest of America: The Question of the Other*. Trans. Richard Howard. New York: Harper, 1984. Print.

Toulouse, Theresa. "'My Own Credit': Strategies of (E)valuation in Mary Rowlandson's Captivity Narrative." *American Literature* 64.4 (1992): 655-676. Print.

Tourney, Garfield. "The Physician and Witchcraft in Restoration England." *Medical History* 16.2 (1972): 143-155. Print.

Traister, Bryce. "Anne Hutchinson's 'Monstrous Birth' and the Feminization of Antinomianism." *Canadian Review of American Studies* 27.2 (1997): 133-158. Print.

Treichler, Paula A. *How to Have Theory in an Epidemic: Cultural Chronicles of AIDS.* Durham: Duke UP, 1999. Print.

Turnbull, George H. "George Stirk, Philosopher by Fire." *Publications of the Colonial Society of Massachusetts* 38 (1949): 219-251. Print.

Tyrrell, Ian. "American Exceptionalism in an Age of International History." *American Historical Review* 96.4 (1991): 1031-1055. Print.

Ulrich, Laurel Thatcher. *Good Wives: Image and Reality in the Lives of Women in Northern New England, 1650-1750.* New York: Knopf, 1982. Print.

---. *A Midwife's Tale: The Life of Martha Ballard, Based on her Diary, 1785-1812.* New York: Vintage, 1991. Print.

---. "John Winthrop's City of Women." *The Massachusetts Historical Review* 3 (2001): 19-48. Print.

Valenčius, Conevery Bolton. *The Health of the Country: How American Settlers Understood Themselves and Their Land.* New York: Basic, 2002. Print.

Vaughan, Alden T., ed. *New England Encounters: Indians and Euroamericans, ca. 1600-1850.* Boston: Northeastern UP, 1999. Print.

Vickers, Brian, ed. *Occult and Scientific Mentalities in the Renaissance.* Cambridge: Cambridge UP, 1984. Print.

Viets, Henry R. *A Brief History of Medicine in Massachusetts.* Boston: Houghton, 1930. Print.

Vogel, Virgil J. *American Indian Medicine.* 1970. Norman: U of Oklahoma P, 1990. Print.

Walsham, Alexandra. *Providence in Early Modern England.* Oxford: Oxford UP, 1999. Print.

Warner, Margaret Humphreys. "Vindicating the Minister's Medical Role: Cotton Mather's Concept of the Nishmath-Chajim and the Spiritualization of Medicine." *Journal of the History of Medicine* 36.3 (1981): 278-295. Print.

Waters, Thomas Franklin. *Ipswich in the Massachusetts Bay Colony.* Ipswich: Ipswich Historical Society, 1905. Print.

Watson, Patricia Ann. *The Angelical Conjunction: The Preacher-Physicians of Colonial New England.* Knoxville: U of Tennessee P, 1991. Print.

---. "The 'Hidden Ones': Women and Healing in Colonial New England." *Medicine and Healing: Annual Proceeding of the Dublin Seminar for New England Folk Life*. Vol. 25. Boston: Boston UP, 1991. 25-33. Print.

Wear, Andrew. "Puritan Perceptions of Illness in Seventeenth Century England." *Patients and Practitioners: Lay Perceptions of Medicine in Pre-Industrial Society*. Ed. Roy Porter. Cambridge: Cambridge UP, 1985. 55-99. Print.

---. "Religious Beliefs and Medicine in Early Modern England." *The Task of Healing: Medicine, Religion and Gender in England and the Netherlands, 1450-1800*. Ed. Hillary Marland and Margaret Pelling. Rotterdam: Erasmus, 1996. 145-169. Print.

---. *Health and Healing in Early Modern England*. Aldershot: Ashgate, 1998.

---. *Knowledge and Practice in English Medicine, 1550-1680*. Cambridge: Cambridge UP, 2000. Print.

---. "Place, Health, and Disease: The Airs, Waters, Places Tradition in Early Modern England and North America." *Journal of Medieval & Early Modern Studies* 38.3 (2008): 443-465. Print.

Weatherall, Miles. "Drug Treatment and the Rise of Pharmacology." *The Cambridge Illustrated History of Medicine*. Ed. Roy Porter. Cambridge: Cambridge UP, 1996. 246-277. Print.

Weber, Max. *The Protestant Ethic and the Spirit of Capitalism*. 1920. Trans. Talcott Parsons. New York: Scribner's Sons, 1958. Print.

Webster, Charles. "English Medical Reformers of the Puritan Revolution: A Background to the 'Society of Chymical Physitians.'" *Ambix* 14.1 (1967): 16-41. Print.

---. *From Paracelsus to Newton: Magic and the Making of Modern Science*. Cambridge: Cambridge UP, 1982. Print.

---. *The Great Instauration: Science, Medicine and Reform, 1626-1660*. 1975. Frankfurt: Lang, 2002. Print.

Webster, Tom. "Writing to Redundancy: Approaches to Spiritual Journeys and Early Modern Spirituality." *The Historical Journal* 39 (1996): 33-56. Print.

Weisman, Richard. *Witchcraft, Magic, and Religion in 17th-Century Massachusetts*. Amherst: U of Massachusetts P, 1984. Print.

Wess, Robert C. "Religious Tension in the Poetry of Anne Bradstreet." *Christianity and Literature* 25.2 (1976): 30-36. Print.

Wharton, Donald P. "Anne Bradstreet and the *Arabella*." *Critical Essays on Anne Bradstreet*. Ed. Pattie Cowell and Ann Stanford. Boston: Hall, 1983. 262-269. Print.

White, Peter, ed., *Puritan Poets and Poetics: Seventeenth-Century American Poetry in Theory and Practice*. University Park: Pennsylvania State UP, 1985. Print.

Whyman, Susan E. *Sociability and Power in Late-Stuart England: The Cultural Worlds of the Verneys, 1660-1720*. Oxford: Oxford UP, 1999. Print.

Wilbur, Keith. *The New England Indians*. Chester: Globe Pequot, 1978. Print.

Wilkinson, Ronald S. "The Problem of the Identity of Eirenaeus Philalethes." *Ambix* 12.1 (1964): 24-43. Print.

---. "*Hermes Christianus*: John Winthrop, Jr., and Chemical Medicine in Seventeenth Century New England." *Science, Medicine and Society in the Renaissance*. Vol. 1. Ed. Allen G. Debus. London: Heinemann, 1972. 221-241. Print.

---. *The Younger John Winthrop and Seventeenth-Century Science*. Farringdon: Classey, 1975. Print.

Wiltshire, John. "Biography, Pathography, and the Recovery of Meaning." *The Cambridge Quarterly* 29.4 (2000): 409-422. Print.

Winebrenner, Kimberly Cole. "Bradstreet's Emblematic Marriage." *Puritanism in America: The Seventeenth through the Nineteenth Centuries*. Ed. Michael Schuldiner Studies in Puritan American Spirituality. Vol. 4. Lewiston: Mellen, 1993. 45-70. Print.

Winship, Michael P. "Cotton Mather, Astrologer." *New England Quarterly* 63.2 (1990): 308-314. Print.

---. *Seers of God: Puritan Providentialism in the Restoration and Early Enlightenment*. Baltimore: Johns Hopkins UP, 2000. Print.

---. *The Times and Trials of Anne Hutchinson: Puritans.*

*Divided*. Lawrence: UP of Kansas, 2005. Print.

Winslow, Ola Elizabeth. *A Destroying Angel: The Conquest of Smallpox in Colonial Boston*. Boston: Houghton, 1974. Print.

Wisecup, Kelly. "Communicating Disease: Medical Knowledge and Literary Forms in Colonial British America." Diss. U of Maryland, 2009. Print.

Woodward, Walter William. *Prospero's America: John Winthrop, Jr., Alchemy, and the Creation of New England Culture, 1606-1676*. Chapel Hill: U of North Carolina P, 2010. Print.

# Index